Straight A's
in
Fluids &
Electrolytes

Straight A's
in
Fluids & Electrolytes

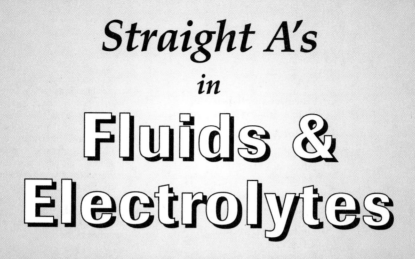

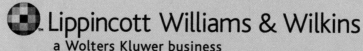 Lippincott Williams & Wilkins
a Wolters Kluwer business

Philadelphia · Baltimore · New York · London
Buenos Aires · Hong Kong · Sydney · Tokyo

STAFF

Executive Publisher
Judith A. Schilling McCann, RN, MSN

Senior Acquisitions Editor
Elizabeth Nieginski

Editorial Director
David Moreau

Clinical Director
Joan M. Robinson, RN, MSN

Senior Art Director
Arlene Putterman

Art Director
Mary Ludwicki

Senior Managing Editor
Tracy S. Diehl

Clinical Manager
Collette Bishop Hendler, RN, BS, CCRN

Editorial Project Manager
Gabrielle Mosquera

Clinical Project Managers
Mary Perrong, RN, CRNP, MSN, APRN, BC;
Kate Stout, RN, MSN, CCRN

Editors
Laura Bruck, Karen C. Comerford

Clinical Editor
Jana L. Sciarra, RN, CRNP, MSN

Copy Editors
Kimberly Bilotta (supervisor),
Scotti Cohn, Amy Furman,
Pamela Wingrod

Designer
Linda Jovinelly Franklin

Digital Composition Services
Diane Paluba (manager),
Joyce Rossi Biletz, Donna S. Morris

Associate Manufacturing Manager
Beth J. Welsh

Editorial Assistants
Megan L. Aldinger, Karen J. Kirk,
Linda K. Ruhf

Design Assistant
Georg W. Purvis IV

Indexer
Barbara Hodgson

**Library of Congress
Cataloging-in-Publication Data**

Straight A's in fluids and electrolytes.
    p. ; cm.
  Includes bibliographical references and index.
  1. Water-electrolyte imbalances—Outlines, syllabi, etc.
2. Water-electrolyte imbalances—Examinations, questions, etc. 3. Body fluid disorders—Outlines, syllabi, etc.
4. Body fluid disorders—Examinations, questions, etc.
5. Nurses—Licenses—United States—Examinations—
Study guides.   I. Lippincott Williams & Wilkins.
  [DNLM: 1. Body Fluids—physiology—Examination Questions. 2. Body Fluids—physiology—Nurses' Instruction. 3. Fluid Therapy—Examination Questions.
4. Fluid Therapy—Nurses' Instruction. 5. Water-Electrolyte Balance—physiology—Examination Questions.
6. Water-Electrolyte Balance—physiology—Nurses' Instruction. 7. Water-Electrolyte Imbalance—therapy—Examination Questions. 8. Water-Electrolyte Imbalance—therapy—Nurses' Instruction.
  QU 18.2 S896 2007]
  RC630.S765 2007
  616.3'992—dc22
ISBN13 978-1-58255-659-8
ISBN10 1-58255-659-8 (alk. paper)   2006024932

Contents

Advisory board

Contributors and consultants

Peggy Bozarth, RN, MSN
Professor
Hopkinsville (Ky.) Community & Technical College

Cheryl L. Brady, RN, MSN
Faculty
Youngstown (Ohio) State University

Marsha L. Conroy, RN, MSN, APN
Nurse Educator
Cuyahoga Community College
Cleveland

Wendy Tagan Conroy, RN, MSN, FNP
Consultant
Middletown, Conn.

Kim Cooper, RN, MSN
Nursing Department Program Chair
Ivy Tech Community College
Terre Haute, Ind.

Ronnette Chereese Langhorne, RN, MS
Assistant Professor
Thomas Nelson Community College
Hampton, Va.

Virginia D. Lester, RN, MSN, CNS (Inactive status)
Assistant Professor of Nursing
Angelo State University
San Angelo, Tex.

Catherine Shields, RN, BSN
Instructor of Practical Nursing
Ocean County Vocational Technical School
Lakehurst, N.J.

Allison J. Terry, RN, MSN, PhD
Nurse Consultant
Alabama Board of Nursing
Montgomery

Patricia Van Tine, RN, MA
Nursing Instructor
Mt. San Jacinto College
Menifee, Calif.

How to use this book

Straight A's is a multivolume study guide series developed especially for nursing students. Each volume provides essential course material in a unique two-column design. The easy-to-read interior outline format offers a succinct review of key facts as presented in leading textbooks on the subject. The bulleted exterior columns provide only the most crucial information, allowing for quick, efficient review right before an important quiz or test.

Special features appear in every chapter to make information accessible and easy to remember. **Learning objectives** encourage the student to evaluate knowledge before and after study. The **Chapter overview** highlights major concepts. **NCLEX® checks** at the end of each chapter offer additional opportunities to review material and assess knowledge gained before moving on to new information.

Other features appear throughout the book to facilitate learning. **Clinical alerts** appear in color to bring the reader's attention to important, potentially life-threatening considerations that could affect patient care. **Time-out for teaching** highlights key areas to address when teaching patients. **Go with the flow** charts promote critical thinking. Lastly, a Windows-based software program (see CD-ROM on inside back cover) poses more than 250 multiple-choice and alternate-format NCLEX-style questions in random or sequential order to assess your knowledge.

The *Straight A's* volumes are designed as learning tools, not as primary information sources. When read conscientiously as a supplement to class attendance and textbook reading, *Straight A's* can enhance understanding and help improve test scores and final grades.

Foreword

In my many years of teaching about fluid, electrolyte, and acid-base imbalances, I've found this subject to be the most difficult—yet most critical—for nursing students to fully comprehend and apply to a classroom case scenario or to an actual clinical patient.

What makes this topic so difficult? Fluid, electrolyte, and acid-base imbalances can occur anywhere at any time, in patients of all ages and in every clinical setting. They may result from illness, from a disease process, or as a complication of prescribed therapy.

What makes these imbalances critical? Their effects may range from a mild disturbance to a life-threatening condition requiring emergency intervention. As the front-line caregivers, nurses have to be alert to the early assessment cues that indicate a possible disturbance, and anticipate treatments to correct it. Early recognition and nursing intervention are vital to a patient's outcome.

Straight A's in Fluids & Electrolytes provides a mechanism for nursing students and nurses new to the profession to learn this content easily by breaking it into manageable concepts. This resource supplies many opportunities to apply these concepts using critical-thinking skills.

Through its straightforward, two-column format, *Straight A's in Fluids & Electrolytes* offers readers the option of going straight to the most critical facts or doing a more thorough review. The main text provides highlighted points that summarize such topics as types of imbalances and their causes, signs and symptoms, and diagnostics. Readers will find the book's text useful because each section summarizes key information, including nursing interventions and treatments. The outer columns feature main points every nursing student should use to brush up on key topics or study right before a quiz or exam.

The chapters cover the balances and imbalances of fluids, electrolytes, and acids-bases, and the conditions associated with these imbalances.

The *NCLEX checks* at the end of each chapter allow readers to test their knowledge of the chapter content; a rationale for the correct response provides another chance to learn. A CD-ROM with more than 250 NCLEX-style questions offers yet another opportunity to apply understanding of the material and practice test-taking skills. Repeated self-testing with these sample traditional and alternate-format NCLEX questions provides valuable preparation for the NCLEX exam and for future clinical nursing in various practice settings.

In summary, fluid, electrolyte, and acid-base imbalances may potentially impact every patient. Nurses can help patients by recognizing the early signs of potential imbalances and by knowing the rapid nursing interventions needed to manage them. A nurse's quick response in this area can make a difference in a patient's outcome. *Straight A's in Fluids & Electrolytes* is an excellent teaching tool for nursing students and practicing nurses alike. It's an invaluable resource in the effort to improve the quality of patient care!

Jennifer M. Hawley, RN, MSN
Clinical Assistant Professor
University of North Carolina School of Nursing
Chapel Hill

1

Essential concepts of fluid and electrolyte balance

LEARNING OBJECTIVES

After studying this chapter, you should be able to:

- Describe types of solutions.
- Identify the major body compartments.
- Describe how fluids and electrolytes move between body compartments.
- Discuss how to assess fluid and electrolyte balance.

CHAPTER OVERVIEW

Homeostasis—a state of internal equilibrium—is essential for optimal body function. For homeostasis to occur, fluids, electrolytes, acids, and bases must be balanced. Normally, fluids are distributed throughout the body in various compartments. These fluids consist of water and solutes (electrolytes and nonelectrolytes) that move constantly between the compartments by transport mechanisms. Determined by the hydrogen (H) ion concentration of arterial blood, pH is the common measurement that determines the body's acid-base balance.

Fluid and electrolyte balance concepts

- Fluid and electrolyte balance involves the composition and movement of body fluids.
- Body fluids are solutions composed of water and solutes.
- Solutions are classified according to their concentration, or tonicity.

Types of solutions

- Isotonic
- Hypotonic
- Hypertonic

Key facts about homeostasis

- State of internal equilibrium within the body when all body systems are in balance
- Commonly referred to as a steady state or equilibrium
- Occurs when fluid, electrolyte, and acid-base balance are all maintained within narrow limits

Homeostasis concepts

- Water and solutes distributed throughout the body's compartments
- Normal cell function maintained
- Maintained by movement and exchange of water and solutes
- Disrupted when water and solute concentrations are altered

INTRODUCTION

- **Basic concepts**
  - Knowledge of the basic concepts of fluid and electrolyte balance is necessary to provide safe, high-quality nursing care
  - Fluid and electrolyte balance involves the composition and movement of body fluids
  - Body fluids are solutions composed of water and solutes

- **Solutions**
  - Solution—liquids (solvents) containing dissolved substances (solutes)—are classified according to their concentration, or tonicity
    - Isotonic solutions: solutions that have the same solute concentration as another solution (such as body fluids)
    - Hypotonic solutions: solutions that have a lower solute concentration than another solution
    - Hypertonic solutions: solutions that have a higher solute concentration than another solution (see *Understanding solution types*)
  - Solutions ingested into the body through food, drink, or I.V. fluids as well as fluid lost from the body through vomiting, diarrhea, or excessive perspiration, can affect fluid and electrolyte balance
  - Many diseases and disorders can affect fluid and electrolyte balance

HOMEOSTASIS

- **General information**
  - State of internal equilibrium within the body when all body systems are in balance
  - Commonly referred to as a *steady state* or *equilibrium*
  - Occurs when fluid, electrolyte, and acid-base balance are all maintained within narrow limits despite a wide variation in dietary intake and metabolic rate

- **Key concepts**
  - Water and solutes distributed throughout the body's compartments
  - Normal cell function maintained by constancy of the body's compartments
  - Maintained by constant movement and continuous exchange of water and solutes
  - Disrupted when water and solute concentrations are altered within the body

Understanding solution types

Fluids are found in three types of solutions: isotonic, hypotonic, and hypertonic.

ISOTONIC SOLUTIONS
No net fluid shifts occur between isotonic solutions because the solutions are equally concentrated.

HYPOTONIC SOLUTIONS
When a less concentrated, or hypotonic, solution is placed next to a more concentrated solution, fluid shifts from the hypotonic solution into the more concentrated compartment to equalize concentrations.

HYPERTONIC SOLUTIONS
If one solution has more solutes than an adjacent solution, it has less fluid relative to the adjacent solution. Fluid will move out of the less concentrated solution into the more concentrated, or hypertonic, solution until both solutions have the same amount of solutes and fluid.

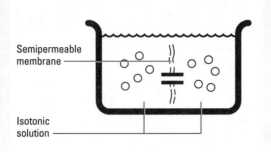

Semipermeable membrane

Isotonic solution

Semipermeable membrane

Hypotonic solution

Fluid shifts into more concentrated solution

Semipermeable membrane

Hypertonic solution

Fluid shifts into more concentrated solution

Key facts about body water
- Primary component of body fluid
- Solvent in which all solutes in the body are either dissolved or suspended
- In average-sized man, accounts for 50% to 60% of total body weight
- In women, accounts for 45% to 50% of total body weight
- In infants, represents about 80% of total body weight
- In premature infants, represents about 90% of total body weight
- In children, decreasing percentage of total weight as body water until it reaches adult percentages

WATER

● **General information**
- Is the primary component of body fluid
- Is the solvent in which all solutes in the body are either dissolved or suspended

- For an average-sized man (weight 155 lb [70.3 kg]), accounts for 50% to 60% of total body weight (approximately 40 L of body water)
- In women, accounts for 45% to 50% of total body weight
  - Have lower percentages of total body weight as body water than do men
  - Have a higher percentage of body fat (doesn't retain water well)
- In infants: represents about 80% of the total body weight; in premature infants, represents about 90% of the total body weight
- In children: percentage of total weight as body water decreases steadily until it reaches adult percentages (by about age 8)
- Obese people: lower percentage of total weight as body water (adipose tissue retains water poorly)

● **Key concepts**
  - Body water contained in two major body compartments
    - Intracellular fluid (ICF)
    - Extracellular fluid (ECF)
  - Fluid balance maintained when water intake equals water output
  - Primary source of body fluid intake: water ingestion; has two principal methods
    - Drinking fluids
    - Eating foods
  - Water in all foods
    - Accounts for almost 100% of the weight of fruit and vegetables
    - Accounts for 70% of the weight of meat
  - Approximately 350 ml of water generated daily from digestion and metabolism of carbohydrates, protein, and fat (considered intake)
  - Under certain circumstances, water introduced to the body parenterally (other than through the GI tract)—usually I.V.

SOLUTES

● **General information**
  - Are substances dissolved in a solution
  - Classified as electrolytes or nonelectrolytes
  - Nonelectrolytes: solutes without an electrical charge (glucose, proteins, lipids, oxygen, carbon dioxide, and organic acids)
  - Electrolytes: solutes that generate an electrical charge when dissolved in water (called *ions*)
  - Positively charged electrolytes: cations (sodium [Na], potassium [K], calcium [Ca], and magnesium [Mg])
  - Negatively charged electrolytes: anions (chloride, phosphorus, and bicarbonate [HCO_3^-]) (see *Differentiating anions and cations*)

● **Key concepts**
  - Concentration in body fluid: depends on body fluid compartment
  - Sodium: the major cation in the ECF

Differentiating anions and cations

Electrolytes can be either anions or cations. Anions generate a negative charge; cations produce a positive charge.

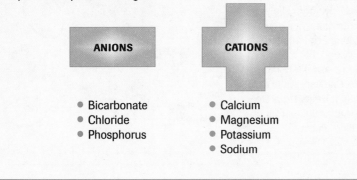

ANIONS	CATIONS
• Bicarbonate	• Calcium
• Chloride	• Magnesium
• Phosphorus	• Potassium
	• Sodium

- Potassium: the major cation in the ICF
- Electrolytes: combine in solutions based on the electrical charge they produce
- Chemical-combining power of electrolytes: measured in milliequivalent (mEq); 1 mEq of anion reacts chemically with 1 mEq of cation
- Total number of cation milliequivalent in body fluids: must always equal the total number of anion milliequivalent
- Measurement of solute concentration (the number of dissolved particles per liter) in body fluid: based on the fluid's osmotic pressure
    - Expressed as either osmolality or osmolarity
    - *Osmolality*: number of osmols (the standard unit of osmotic pressure) per kilogram of solution, expressed as milliosmols per kilogram (mOsm/kg)
    - *Osmolarity*: number of osmols per liter of solution, expressed as mOsm/L
- Osmolarity and osmolality: commonly used interchangeably
- Most calculations of body fluid solute concentrations based on osmolarity

BODY FLUID COMPARTMENTS

- **General information**
  - Body fluid: divided by semipermeable membranes into two major body compartments
      - ICF
      - ECF
  - ICF: represents fluid inside cells
      - Is the largest body compartment
      - Accounts for about two-thirds of total body fluid

Understanding fluid compartments

This illustration shows the primary fluid compartments in the body: intracellular and extracellular. Extracellular compartments are further divided into interstitial and intravascular compartments. Capillary walls and cell membranes separate intracellular fluids from extracellular fluids.

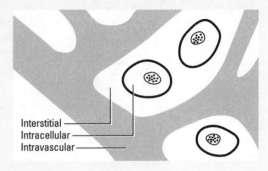

Interstitial
Intracellular
Intravascular

- ECF divided into three separate body compartments
  - Interstitial fluid (ISF)
  - Intravascular fluid (plasma)
  - Transcellular water (TSW)
- ECF: accounts for about one-third of total body fluid (see *Understanding fluid compartments*)
- ISF: occupies spaces between cells; constitutes 15% of total body fluid
- Plasma found in the intravascular space; constitutes about 4% of total body fluid (75 ml/kg of body weight)
- TSW: constitutes only 1% to 2% of total body fluid
  - Is sometimes not considered a separate compartment
  - Found in specialized compartments
    · Ocular
    · Cerebrospinal
    · Pleural
    · Synovial fluid
    · Gastric juices

Key concepts
- Body fluid not confined to one defined area or compartment; normal body membranes permeable to water—facilitates fluid movement through them
- Certain solutes more abundant in certain body compartments
  - Potassium more abundant in the ICF
  - Sodium more abundant in the ECF
- Solute movement from one body fluid compartment to another: occurs through various mechanisms
  - Active transport
  - Passive transport
- Proteins: solutes confined to the plasma that create colloid osmotic pressure in the ECF, affecting fluid and solute movement between the ECF and the ICF

Body fluid compartments concepts
- Body fluid not confined to one defined area or compartment
- Solute movement from one body fluid compartment to another occurs through various mechanisms: active transport and passive transport

BODY FLUID MOVEMENT

- **General information**
  - Maintains homeostasis
  - Affected by membrane permeability and hydrostatic and osmotic pressures
  - Water and solutes: move through active and passive transport mechanisms
    - Active transport mechanisms: involve chemical activity and the release of energy; they include the sodium-potassium pump
    - Passive transport mechanisms: don't involve chemical activity or use of energy; they include osmosis, diffusion, and capillary filtration

- **Key concepts: water movement**
  - Occurs through osmosis
    - Solvent moves through a semipermeable membrane
    - Solvent goes from an area of lower solute concentration to one of higher concentration
  - Along with distribution, depends on the concentration of solute within a compartment
    - Solute is primarily sodium
    - Referred to as the compartment's *osmolality*
  - Responds to osmolality changes because it moves freely between compartments; occurs for two reasons
    - Osmotic pressure
    - Hydrostatic pressure

- **Key concepts: solute movement**
  - Occurs through active and passive transport (see *Understanding transport mechanisms*, page 8)
  - Solute distribution dependent upon concentrations of body fluid compartments
  - Passive transport of solutes affected by the electrical potential across cell membranes
  - Works by diffusion
    - Solutes moving from an area of higher solute concentration to one of lower concentration
    - Results in an equal solute distribution
  - Filtration: requires the force of hydrostatic pressure to move water and some solutes through cell membranes via ultrafiltration (fluid produced is called *ultrafiltrate*)
  - Active transport: requires the expenditure of energy to move solutes from an area of lower solute concentration to one of higher solute concentration against a concentration gradient

Key facts about body fluid movement
- Maintains homeostasis
- Water and solutes: move through active and passive transport mechanisms
- Active transport mechanisms: involve chemical activity and release of energy; they include sodium-potassium pump
- Passive transport mechanisms: don't involve chemical activity or use of energy; they include osmosis, diffusion, and capillary filtration

Water movement
- Occurs through osmosis
- Solvent goes from area of lower solute concentration to one of higher concentration
- Occurs for two reasons: osmotic pressure and hydrostatic pressure

Solute movement
- Occurs through active and passive transport
- Works by diffusion: solutes moving from an area of higher solute concentration to one of lower concentration
- Filtration: requires force of hydrostatic pressure to move water and some solutes through cell membranes via ultrafiltration
- Active transport: requires expenditure of energy to move solutes from area of lower solute concentration to one of higher solute concentration against a concentration gradient

Cellular movement of water and solutes

- Most solutes moved by passive transport mechanisms
- Active transport, specifically sodium-potassium pump, necessary for moving sodium from the cells to the ECF
- Active transport drives potassium from the ECF into the cell
- Water moved by osmosis from the ECF to the ICF based on the osmolality of the fluid compartment

Transport mechanisms

Passive

- Diffusion: solutes move from areas of higher concentration to areas of lower concentration.
- Osmosis: fluid moves passively from areas with more fluid to areas with less fluid.
- Filtration: hydrostatic pressure builds and forces fluids and solutes through a semipermeable membrane.

Active

- Energy from the molecule adenosine triphosphate moves solutes from an area of lower concentration to an area of higher concentration.

Understanding transport mechanisms

Passive and active transport mechanisms are necessary to keep water and solutes moving throughout the body.

PASSIVE TRANSPORT MECHANISMS

In diffusion, solutes move from areas of higher concentration to areas of lower concentration until the concentration in both areas equalizes.

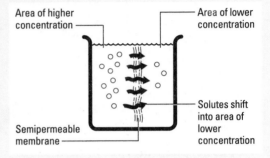

In osmosis, fluid moves passively from areas with more fluid (and fewer solutes) to areas with less fluid (and more solutes). Remember: In osmosis, fluid moves; in diffusion, solutes move.

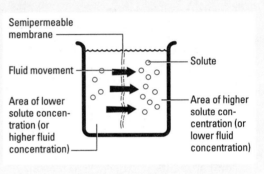

In filtration, hydrostatic pressure builds and forces fluids and solutes through a semipermeable membrane. Within the vascular system, only capillaries have walls thin enough to let solutes pass through. Capillary filtration is depicted in this illustration.

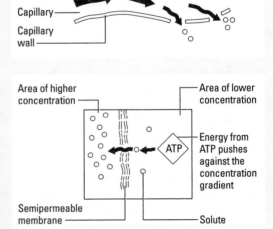

ACTIVE TRANSPORT MECHANISMS

During active transport, energy from the molecule adenosine triphosphate (ATP) moves solutes from an area of lower concentration to an area of higher concentration.

● **Key concepts: cellular movement of water and solutes**
  - Most solutes moved by passive transport mechanisms
  - Active transport, specifically the sodium-potassium pump, necessary for moving sodium from the cells to the ECF
    - Drives potassium from the ECF into the cell
    - Allows solutes to move from an area of lower solute concentration to one of higher solute concentration
  - Water moved by osmosis from the ECF to the ICF based on the osmolality of the fluid compartment
    - ICF osmolality increases: water shifts from ECF into ICF
    - ECF osmolality increases: water shifts from ICF into ECF

● **Key concepts: vascular movement of water and solutes**
  - Movement of water and solutes: occurs continuously between the vascular and ISF compartments
  - Movement of water: depends on hydrostatic and colloid osmotic pressures in the capillaries; solutes move by diffusion
  - Pressure differences in the venous and arterial ends of capillaries: influence the direction and rate of water and solute movement; process known as *Starling's law*
  - Hydrostatic pressure in the capillary's arterial end: +25 mm Hg; interstitial pressure of perivascular tissues is +11 mm Hg
    - Pressures facilitate movement of plasma water into the ICF
    - Combined forces exert pressure of +36 mm Hg
    - Pressure opposed by colloidal osmotic pressure of plasma proteins and albumins (–28 mm Hg)
    - Remaining net pressure (8 mm Hg on arterial side) moves water, solutes, and gases from vascular space to ISF
  - Hydrostatic pressure in the venous end of the capillary: normally +10 mm Hg (venous end is farther from the heart than the arterial end); interstitial pressure remains +11 mm Hg
    - Combination of positive venous pressures equals +21 mm Hg, favoring movement of water out of the capillary
    - Plasma proteins exert opposing pressure of –28 mm Hg; results in total net negative pressure of –7 mm Hg
    - Negative force draws water, metabolic cellular wastes, and carbon dioxide from the ISF into the vascular compartment; results in eventual degradation and removal of these substances by a major organ system
      · Lungs
      · Kidneys
  - Colloid osmotic pressures: help maintain plasma volumes; prevents too much fluid from leaving the capillaries
  - When fluid filters through a capillary: the protein albumin stays behind in the diminishing volume of water
    - Large molecule; normally can't pass through capillary membranes

---

Vascular movement of water and solutes

- Occurs continuously between the vascular and ISF compartments
- Movement of water: depends on hydrostatic and colloid osmotic pressures in the capillaries
- Movement of solutes: by diffusion
- Pressure differences in the venous and arterial ends of capillaries: influence the direction and rate of water and solute movement; process known as *Starling's law*

Hydrostatic pressure

- In the capillary's arterial end: facilitates movement of plasma water into the ICF and moves water, solutes, and gases from vascular space to ISF
- In the venous end of the capillary: favors movement of water out of the capillary and draws water, metabolic cellular wastes, and carbon dioxide from the ISF into the vascular compartment

Colloid osmotic pressures

- Help maintain plasma volumes
- Prevent too much fluid from leaving the capillaries

Key facts about body fluid pH

- Refers to the acidity or alkalinity of a solution, which is determined by the hydrogen ion concentration
- Hydrogen ion donor: acid
- Hydrogen ion acceptor: base
- Regulation affected by the process of large volumes of body fluids diluting metabolism products
- Arterial blood pH commonly measured to determine acid-base balance

Body fluid pH concepts

- Normal arterial blood pH: ranges from 7.35 to 7.45
- Arterial blood pH of ≤ 6.8 or ≥ 7.8: incompatible with life

Key facts about assessing fluid and electrolyte balance

- Fluid and electrolyte balance: essential for health and well-being
- Can be affected by illness, injury, surgery, and treatments
- Managing fluid and electrolyte status—one of the most difficult aspects of nursing
- Comprehensive assessment ideal
- Circumstances may require patient to be assessed quickly
- Health history: allows for exploration of the patient's chief complaint and its relationship to other symptoms

– Concentration inside capillary increases; fluid returns to capillaries through osmosis

BODY FLUID PH

- **General information**
  - Refers to the acidity or alkalinity of a solution, which is determined by the hydrogen ion concentration
    - Hydrogen ion donor: acid
    - Hydrogen ion acceptor: base
  - Regulation affected by the process of large volumes of body fluids diluting metabolism products
  - All body fluids have a pH; normal pH of different body fluids varies
  - Arterial blood pH commonly measured to determine acid-base balance
    - Regulated through the action of a buffer, the lungs, (via potassium ion exchange), and the kidneys, in that order
    - Depends on the bicarbonate-carbonic acid ratio in the plasma and ECF
- **Key concepts**
  - Normal arterial blood pH: ranges from 7.35 to 7.45
  - Despite continuous additions of metabolites from cells and food, arterial blood pH usually maintained at a fairly constant level
  - An arterial blood pH of ≤ 6.8 or ≥ 7.8: incompatible with life

ASSESSING FLUID AND ELECTROLYTE BALANCE

- **General information**
  - Is essential for health and well-being
  - Can be affected by numerous factors, such as illness, injury, surgery, and treatments
  - Even patient with minor illness at risk
  - Managing fluid and electrolyte status—one of the most difficult aspects of nursing
    - Changes that prompt disruption are usually subtle
    - Identify status changes involves keen observational skills and expertise in monitoring and assessment
- **Assessment**
  - Usually includes several steps
    - Taking a health history
    - Performing a physical examination
    - Reviewing the results of diagnostic tests
  - Comprehensive assessment ideal; circumstances may require patient to be assessed quickly

- Brief, focused assessment is best
- Obtain a more extensive history when the patient's condition improves or by interviewing family
- Reviewing patient history from referral notes and past medical records is helpful
- Health history: allows for exploration of the patient's chief complaint and its relationship to other symptoms
  - Use a systematic approach to avoid overlooking important clues
  - Be sensitive to the patient's concerns and feelings, and encourage him to respond openly
  - Be alert for nonverbal signs that seem to contradict verbal responses
- Interview: begins with questions about the patient's chief complaint
  - Focus on what brought the patient to the health care facility
  - Question the patient about signs and symptoms of fluid and electrolyte imbalance
    - Thirst, weight changes, edema
    - Altered level of consciousness (LOC)
    - Altered urine output
    - Muscle weakness
    - Paresthesia
    - Nausea and vomiting
    - Seizures
  - Have the patient characterize the problem in his own words
  - Use quantitative terms such as the number (and size) of glasses of fluids he takes in per day
- Interview: follow with information about the patient's past medical history
  - Be alert for conditions that may affect the patient's fluid and electrolyte status
    - Diabetes, ulcerative colitis, endocrine, cardiac or renal disorder
  - Note recent treatments
    - Nasogastric suction, dialysis, I.V. therapy
  - Note a history of psychiatric conditions
    - Anorexia nervosa (patient may be prone to imbalance)
    - Bulimia nervosa (patient may be prone to imbalance)
    - Depression (patient may refuse fluids and food)
- Developmental considerations impacting the patient's status; for example, fluid balance problems are more common in infants and the elderly
- Obtaining of a complete medication history
  - Prescription medications
  - Over-the-counter medications
- Investigation of the patient's lifestyle and changes affecting it

Key facts about the patient interview

- Begin with questions about the patient's chief complaint.
- Follow with information about the patient's past medical history.
- Note recent treatments.
- Note a history of psychiatric conditions.
- Consider developmental factors that may impact the patient's status.
- Obtain a complete medication history.
- Investigate the patient's lifestyle and changes affecting it.

Signs and symptoms of fluid and electrolyte disorders

- Thirst
- Weight changes
- Edema
- Altered LOC
- Altered urine output
- Muscle weakness
- Paresthesia
- Nausea and vomiting
- Seizures

Conditions that may affect the patient's fluid and electrolyte status

- Diabetes
- Ulcerative colitis
- Endocrine, cardiac, or renal disorder

Key facts about the patient's physical examination and diagnostic testing

- Physical examination: requires a systematic sequence of the inspection, palpation, auscultation, and percussion assessment techniques to elicit important findings
- Patient's general appearance: should be observed
- Patient's baseline vital signs and weight: should be obtained
- Blood chemistry tests: help evaluate and diagnose fluid and electrolyte imbalances
- Hematocrit: may vary
- Urine tests: help measure renal function and detect impairment
- Blood lactate values
- Arterial blood gas values

- Daily activities
- Exercise
- Diet
- Physical examination: requires a systematic sequence of the inspection, palpation, auscultation, and percussion assessment techniques to elicit important findings
  - Begin by observing the patient's general appearance; note body type, overall health, and muscle composition
    - Is the patient well-developed, well-nourished, alert, and energetic?
    - Does he look weak?
  - Obtain baseline vital signs and weight
    - Acute weight changes usually indicate acute fluid changes
    - Changes in vital signs, especially in pulse and blood pressure, may indicate imbalances
  - Perform a complete head-to-toe examination
- Compilation of diagnostic testing results
- Blood chemistry tests: help evaluate and diagnose fluid and electrolyte imbalances
  - Blood urea nitrogen
  - Sodium
  - Calcium
  - Magnesium
  - Creatinine
  - Chloride
  - Potassium
  - Carbon dioxide
  - Bicarbonate
  - Glucose
  - Osmolality
  - Albumin
  - Phosphate
- Hematocrit: may vary
  - Increase with dehydration
  - Decrease with water intoxication
  - Caused by plasma dilution
- Urine tests: help measure renal function and detect impairment
  - Calcium
  - Chloride
  - Osmolality
  - pH
  - Potassium
  - Sodium
  - Protein
  - Specific gravity

- Urine osmolality: can provide information about renal function and overall hydration
- Urine specific gravity: measures the concentration of urine, a valuable indication of the body's fluid status
    - The anion gap reflects serum anion-cation balance and helps distinguish among types of metabolic acidosis
    - It's also useful in monitoring renal function and total parenteral nutrition
- Blood lactate values
    - Lactic acid is a by-product of glucose's anaerobic metabolism
    - Normally, the small quantity of lactic acid that's produced daily is immediately buffered by bicarbonate, and lactate is generated
    - Excess production of lactic acid or decreased use of lactate may lead to lactic acidosis, a dangerous condition
- Arterial blood gas values measure several values
    - Partial pressures of oxygen and carbon dioxide
    - Bicarbonate concentration
    - The pH of a sample of arterial blood

NCLEX CHECKS

It's never too soon to begin your NCLEX preparation. Now that you've reviewed this chapter, carefully read each of the following questions and choose the best answer. Then compare your responses to the correct answers.

1. The largest compartment of body fluid is:
☐ **1.** ICF.
☐ **2.** ECF.
☐ **3.** ISF.
☐ **4.** intravascular space.

2. Which mechanism requires adenosine triphosphate (ATP) to function?
☐ **1.** Diffusion
☐ **2.** Osmosis
☐ **3.** Active transport
☐ **4.** Capillary filtration

3. What characterizes the process of diffusion?
☐ **1.** Solutes move from an area of higher solute concentration to an area of lower concentration.
☐ **2.** There's no movement of solutes.
☐ **3.** Solutes move from an area of lower concentration to an area of higher concentration.
☐ **4.** Hydrostatic pressure forces solutes through a semipermeable membrane.

TOP 10

Items to study for your next test on essential concepts of fluid and electrolyte balance

1. How the body maintains homeostasis
2. The classification of solutions according to concentration (isotonic, hypotonic, hypertonic)
3. The major electrolyte and nonelectrolyte solutes found in body fluid
4. Measurement of solute concentration expressed as osmolality and osmolarity
5. The two major fluid compartments (ICF, ECF) in the body
6. Key mechanisms involved in the movement of water and solutes between body fluid compartment
7. Hydrostatic pressure and colloid osmotic pressure
8. The regulation of pH in body fluids
9. Health history questions to consider for patients with fluid and electrolyte imbalance
10. Diagnostic tests used to determine fluid and electrolyte or acid-base imbalances

4. As hydrostatic pressure builds to force fluids and solutes through the capillary walls, which force acts to prevent excessive loss of intravascular fluid volume?

☐ **1.** Osmosis
☐ **2.** Colloid osmotic pressure
☐ **3.** Active transport mechanisms
☐ **4.** Diffusion

5. Because women have more body fat than men, their percentage of body water relative to their total body weight is:

☐ **1.** the same as that of men.
☐ **2.** higher than that of men.
☐ **3.** lower than that of men.
☐ **4.** the same as their percentage of body fat.

6. The nurse is infusing a hypotonic solution into her client. The nurse knows that this type of solution will affect her client's fluid status by:

☐ **1.** decreasing water content in the blood vessels.
☐ **2.** not changing water content in the blood vessels.
☐ **3.** increasing water content in the blood vessels.
☐ **4.** drawing water into the blood vessels.

7. If the osmolality of ICF increases, it can be expected that:

☐ **1.** colloid osmotic pressure will force water from ICF into ECF.
☐ **2.** there will be no water movement between compartments.
☐ **3.** water will shift from ICF into ECF.
☐ **4.** water will shift from ECF into ICF.

8. Cations are electrolytes that contain which type of charge?

☐ **1.** Negative
☐ **2.** Positive
☐ **3.** Neutral
☐ **4.** Positive or negative

9. The nurse needs to evaluate a client's acid-base balance. Which parameter should the nurse use?

☐ **1.** Hematocrit level
☐ **2.** Urine osmolality
☐ **3.** Serum calcium level
☐ **4.** Arterial blood pH

10. When taking a client's health history, the nurse should be aware of which signs and symptoms that may indicate a fluid and electrolyte imbalance? Select all that apply.

☐ **1.** Hair loss
☐ **2.** Weight change
☐ **3.** Altered LOC
☐ **4.** Paresthesia
☐ **5.** Back pain
☐ **6.** Nasal congestion

ANSWERS AND RATIONALES

1. CORRECT ANSWER: 1

ICF, representing the fluid inside the cells, is the largest compartment of body fluid.

2. CORRECT ANSWER: 3

ATP is a form of energy that's required for active transport mechanisms to function. Passive transport mechanisms—such as diffusion, osmosis, and filtration—require no energy to perform.

3. CORRECT ANSWER: 1

In diffusion, solutes passively move from an area of higher solute concentration to an area of lower concentration. Hydrostatic pressure is the key mechanism involved in filtration.

4. CORRECT ANSWER: 2

Proteins in plasma (such as albumin) draw fluids toward them creating colloid osmotic pressure, which works against hydrostatic pressure to keep adequate amounts of fluid within the blood vessel.

5. CORRECT ANSWER: 3

Because body fat, or adipose tissue, doesn't retain water well, women have a lower percentage of body water relative to their total body weight (45% to 50%) compared with that of men (50% to 60%).

6. CORRECT ANSWER: 1

Because a hypotonic solution is a less concentrated solution, fluid will be drawn from the hypotonic solution in the blood vessels to the more concentrated solution in the cells, thereby reducing water content in the blood vessels.

7. CORRECT ANSWER: 4

Because water moves by osmosis based on the osmolality (or solute concentration) of the fluid compartments, if ICF osmolality increases, then water will move from the ECF (which is less concentrated) to the ICF (which is more concentrated).

8. CORRECT ANSWER: 2

Cations are electrolytes that contain a positive charge. Examples of cations include sodium, potassium, calcium, and magnesium.

9. CORRECT ANSWER: 4

Arterial blood pH is used to assess acid-base balance. Hematocrit can indicate fluid status. Urine osmolality reflects renal function and overall hydration. Serum calcium levels reflect the level of calcium in the blood.

10. CORRECT ANSWER: 2, 3, 4

If a client complains of weight gains or losses, altered LOC, or paresthesia, a fluid or electrolyte imbalance may be suspected.

2

Fluid balance

LEARNING OBJECTIVES

After studying this chapter, you should be able to:

- State the uses of water in the body.
- Discuss the role of thirst in fluid balance.
- Describe the mechanisms of fluid regulation.
- Describe how blood pressure reflects overall fluid status.
- Identify key age-related differences in fluid balance and regulation.

CHAPTER OVERVIEW

Fluids serve various functions in the body. They're gained and lost by the body each day, but these actions must be balanced to maintain homeostasis. The kidneys, the renin-angiotensin-aldosterone system, the adrenal cortex, the thirst mechanism, and the secretion or inhibition of antidiuretic hormone (ADH) regulate fluid balance. The kidneys are the major regulatory organ.

INTRODUCTION

- **Water uses**
  - Water: most abundant component of body fluid; is required in adequate amounts for body function

Daily fluid gains and losses

Each day, the body gains and loses fluid through several different processes. This illustration shows the primary sites of fluid losses and gains as well as their average amounts. Gastric, intestinal, pancreatic, and biliary secretions are almost completely reabsorbed and aren't usually counted in daily fluid losses and gains.

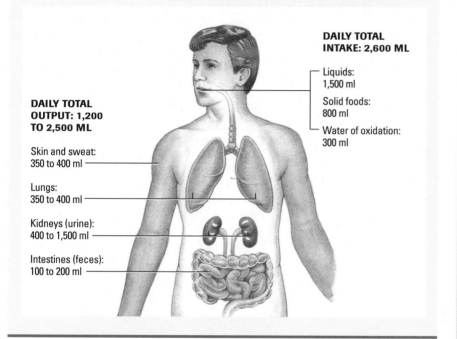

DAILY TOTAL INTAKE: 2,600 ML

Liquids:
1,500 ml

Solid foods:
800 ml

Water of oxidation:
300 ml

DAILY TOTAL OUTPUT: 1,200 TO 2,500 ML

Skin and sweat:
350 to 400 ml

Lungs:
350 to 400 ml

Kidneys (urine):
400 to 1,500 ml

Intestines (feces):
100 to 200 ml

Key facts about body water

- Most abundant component of body fluid
- Required in adequate amounts for body function
- Aids various chemical reactions
- Maintains stability of body fluids
- Aids nutrient transport to cells
- Provides a medium for waste excretion
- Acts as a lubricant and a cushion between cells
- Aids body temperature regulation

- Water: used by the body
  - Acts as a solvent for many body chemicals
  - Aids various chemical reactions
  - Maintains stability of body fluids
  - Aids nutrient transport to cells
  - Provides a medium for waste excretion
  - Acts as a lubricant between cells to permit friction-free movement
  - Aids body temperature regulation through perspiration
  - Assists in food hydrolysis
  - Conducts electric currents
  - Acts as a cushion

● **Fluid gains and losses**
  - Occur in the body each day
  - Must be balanced to maintain body fluid balance (see *Daily fluid gains and losses*)
  - Fluid intake and output monitoring: a valuable tool in determining homeostasis

Key facts about fluid gains and losses

- Must be balanced to maintain body fluid balance
- Fluid intake and output monitoring is valuable tool in determining homeostasis

Key nursing interventions for monitoring fluid balance

- Monitor fluid intake and output.
- Calculate sensible and estimate insensible losses.
- Be aware that the presence of anuria, oliguria, or polyuria signal serious problems requiring medical intervention.
- Note that daily weight is an accurate measure of fluid balance.
- Correlate daily weight with the 24-hour intake and output.
- Document use of all medications to anticipate potential fluid-related complications.
- Monitor urine specific gravity and color.
- Monitor specific diagnostic tests, serum and urine osmolality, blood urea nitrogen, serum sodium, hematocrit, and creatinine to evaluate fluid balance.

Nursing interventions

- Carefully monitor fluid intake and output
- When monitoring output, calculate sensible (measurable) losses and estimate insensible (immeasurable) losses as closely as possible
  - Insensible losses from the skin, though fairly constant, can vary depending on several factors
    - Changes in humidity levels
    - Changes in body surface area (BSA)
  - When it's difficult or impossible to measure urine output, estimate output by weighing urine-soaked diapers or incontinence pads, then subtracting the pad's or diaper's dry weight and converting the urine weight to a volume measurement
  - For a patient with watery diarrhea, estimate fluid loss by using a bedside commode, bedpan, or other collection device; fluid loss for patients with severe diarrhea may exceed 5,000 ml/day
- Obtain hourly output measurements if necessary to identify a pattern of urine output
- Monitor for anuria, oliguria, or polyuria, which would signal serious problems requiring medical intervention
- Remember that daily weight is an accurate measure of fluid balance; use a patient's weight gain (or loss) history to assess fluid, sodium, and caloric intake
  - To ensure accuracy, weigh the patient at the same time each day using the same scale; he should be wearing the same clothes and have an empty bladder
  - Correlate daily weight with the 24-hour intake and output; +500 ml equals a 1-lb (0.45-kg) weight gain and 500 ml equals a 1-lb weight loss (1-kg weight gain equals a fluid gain of 1 L)
- Document use of all medications, both over-the-counter and prescription, to anticipate potential fluid-related complications
- Monitor urine specific gravity and color
  - Overhydration: patient has normal renal function, specific gravity ≤ 1.010, and light-colored, diluted urine
  - Dehydration: patient has normal renal function, specific gravity ≥ 1.030, and dark-colored, concentrated urine
  - Remember that a falsely elevated or depressed specific gravity may occur after radiopaque dyes or diurectics are administered (respectively)
  - Be aware the specific gravity isn't reliable if the patient has renal disease associated with a concentration defect
- Monitor specific diagnostic tests such as serum and urine osmolality, blood urea nitrogen, serum sodium, hematocrit, and creatinine to evaluate fluid balance

FLUID INTAKE

● **General information**
- Necessary for metabolic use and to compensate for fluid losses
- Intake of 2,500 ml needed daily
  - Ingesting liquids (primary source): accounts for 1,500 ml/day
  - Ingesting solid foods: accounts for 800 ml/day
  - Food oxidation: accounts for 200 to 300 ml/day
- Given I.V. if water can't be ingested orally

● **Control mechanism: thirst**
- Is primarily regulated by the thirst center, located in the hypothalamus
  - Occurs as a result of even small losses of fluid
  - Is stimulated by two types of response
    • Local response (such as dry mouth)
    • Systemic response (such as the action of angiotensin II, the release of ADH, the sensation of a decrease in fluid volume, or an increase in extracellular fluid [ECF] osmolality)
  - Normal response: drinking fluid
  - Ingested fluid
    • Moves freely between fluid compartments
    • Leads to increased body fluid and decreased solute concentration
    • Balances fluid levels throughout the body
  - Also dependent on access to safe drinking water and the patient's ability to drink

FLUID REGULATION

● **General information**
- Helps maintain serum osmolarity of 280 to 295 mOsm/L; is always associated with sodium regulation
- Fluid balance regulated by kidneys, various hormones, and thirst

● **Control mechanism: kidneys**
- Play a vital role in fluid balance
- Nephrons: functional units that perform several tasks
  - Filter blood
  - Produce urine
  - Excrete excess waste
  - Constantly work to maintain fluid balance
- Nephrons: consist of two parts
  - A glomerulus (a cluster of capillaries that filters blood); surrounded by Bowman's capsule
  - A tubule (a convoluted tube that ends in a collecting duct) (see *Looking at a nephron*, page 20)

Key facts about fluid intake
● Necessary for metabolic use and to compensate for fluid losses
● Intake of 2,500 ml needed daily

Thirst and fluid intake
● Primarily regulated by the thirst center located in the hypothalamus
● Stimulated by two types of response: local and systemic
● Normal response: drinking fluid

Key facts about fluid regulation
● Helps maintain serum osmolarity
● Always associated with sodium regulation
● Fluid balance regulated by kidneys, various hormones, and thirst

The kidneys and fluid regulation
● Play a vital role in fluid balance
● Nephrons filter blood, produce urine, excrete excess waste, constantly work to maintain fluid balance
● Nephrons consist of two parts: a glomerulus and a tubule

Looking at a nephron

A nephron filters blood, produces urine, and excretes excess solutes, electrolytes, fluids, and metabolic waste products while keeping blood composition and volume constant.

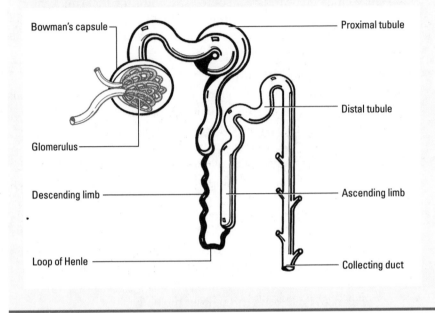

Key facts about the filtration process

- Depends on the body's needs
- If the body needs more fluid, it retains more
- If it needs less, it reabsorbs less and excretes more
- Nephrons filter about 125 ml of blood every minute, or about 180 L/day; this rate is called the *glomerular filtration rate*

ADH and fluid regulation

- ADH sometimes referred to as *vasopressin*
- Restores blood volume by reducing diuresis and increasing water retention
- Amount released dependent on body's needs

- Filtration process
  - Capillary blood pressure forces fluid through the capillary walls and into Bowman's capsule at the proximal end of the tubule
  - Along the length of the tubule, water and electrolytes are either excreted or retained
  - Depends on the body's needs
  - If the body needs more fluid, it retains more
  - If it needs less, it reabsorbs less and excretes more
  - The resulting filtrate, which eventually becomes urine, flows through the tubule into the collecting ducts and eventually into the bladder
  - Nephrons filter about 125 ml of blood every minute, or about 180 L/day; this rate is called the *glomerular filtration rate* (GFR)
- **Control mechanism: ADH**
  - Sometimes referred to as *vasopressin*
  - Produced by the hypothalamus
  - Stored and released by the posterior pituitary gland
  - Restores blood volume by reducing diuresis and increasing water retention (see *How antidiuretic hormone works*)
  - Amount released varies throughout day; dependent on body's needs

How antidiuretic hormone works

Antidiuretic hormone (ADH) regulates fluid balance through a series of steps, which are outlined here.

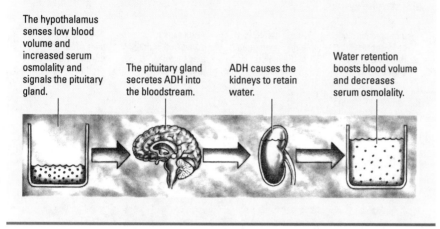

The hypothalamus senses low blood volume and increased serum osmolality and signals the pituitary gland.

The pituitary gland secretes ADH into the bloodstream.

ADH causes the kidneys to retain water.

Water retention boosts blood volume and decreases serum osmolality.

– Stimulated by increased serum osmolality or decreased blood volume
  • Increases the kidneys' reabsorption of water
  • Results in more concentrated urine
– Inhibited by decreased serum osmolality or increased blood volume
  • Decreases kidneys' reabsorption of water
  • Results in less concentrated urine

● **Control mechanism: renin-angiotensin-aldosterone system**
  • Renin: enzyme secreted by the juxtaglomerular cells near each glomerulus
    – Leads to the production of angiotensin II
      • Powerful vasoconstrictor
      • Causes peripheral vasoconstriction and stimulates aldosterone production, both of which raise blood pressure (see *Understanding aldosterone production,* page 22)
  • Amount of renin secreted depends on blood flow and level of sodium in the bloodstream
    – Blood flow to kidneys diminishes or amount of sodium reaching glomerulus drops: more renin secretes
      • Causes vasoconstriction
      • Increases blood pressure
    – Blood flow to kidneys increases or amount of sodium reaching glomerulus increases: less renin secretes
      • Causes reduction in vasoconstriction
      • Decreases blood pressure

The renin-angiotensin-aldosterone system and fluid regulation

Renin
● Leads to the production of angiotensin II, which causes peripheral vasoconstriction and stimulates aldosterone production, thereby raising blood pressure
● More renin is secreted if blood flow to kidneys diminishes or amount of sodium reaching glomerulus drops
● Increased renin secretion: causes vasoconstriction and increases blood pressure
● Less renin is secreted if blood flow to kidneys increases or amount of sodium reaching glomerulus increases
● Decreased renin secretion: causes reduction in vasoconstriction and decreases blood pressure

Aldosterone
● Regulates reabsorption of sodium and water within the nephron

Understanding aldosterone production

This illustration shows the steps involved in the production of aldosterone, which helps to regulate fluid balance through the renin-angiotensin-aldosterone system.

Juxtaglomerular cells secrete renin into the bloodstream.

Renin converts angiotensinogen in the liver to angiotensin I.

Angiotensin I is converted in the lungs into angiotensin II.

Angiotensin II stimulates the adrenal glands to produce aldosterone.

Blood flow to the glomerulus drops.

Renin travels to the liver.

Angiotensin I travels to the lungs.

Angiotensin II travels to the adrenal glands.

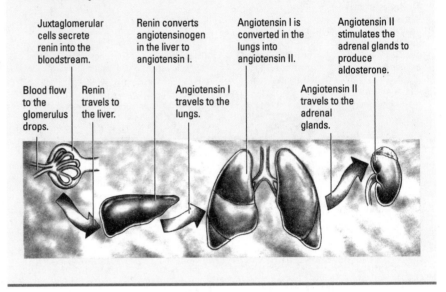

ANP and fluid regulation

- Cardiac hormone released when atrial pressure increases
- Counteracts the effects of the renin-angiotensin-aldosterone system
- Suppresses serum renin levels
- Increased release from the atria occurs in response to several conditions: chronic renal failure, heart failure, conditions that cause atrial stretching

- Aldosterone: secreted by the renal cortex, regulates reabsorption of sodium and water within the nephron (see *How aldosterone works*)

● **Control mechanism: atrial natriuretic peptide (ANP)**
- Is a cardiac hormone stored in the cells of the atria and released when atrial pressure increases
- Counteracts the effects of the renin-angiotensin-aldosterone system
  - Decreases blood pressure
  - Reduces intravascular blood volume
- Suppresses serum renin levels
  - Decreases aldosterone release from the adrenal glands
  - Increases glomerular filtration (which increases urine excretion of sodium and water)
  - Decreases ADH release from the posterior pituitary gland
  - Reduces vascular resistance by causing vasodilation
- Increased release from the atria occurs in response to several conditions
  - Chronic renal failure
  - Heart failure
  - Conditions that cause atrial stretching
    · Atrial tachycardia
    · High sodium intake
    · Use of drugs that cause vasoconstriction

How aldosterone works

Aldosterone, produced as a result of the renin-angiotensin-aldosterone system, regulates fluid volume as depicted here.

Angiotensin II stimulates the adrenal glands to release aldosterone.

Aldosterone causes the kidneys to retain sodium and water.

Sodium and water retention leads to increases in fluid volume and sodium levels.

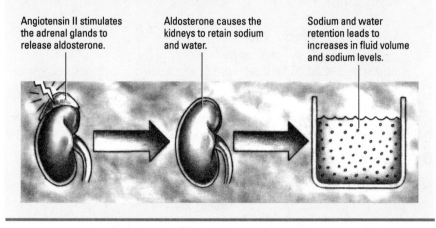

FLUID EXCRETION

- **General information**
  - Occurs through various pathways
    - Kidneys
    - Skin
    - Lungs
    - GI tract
  - Losses categorized as sensible or insensible
    - Sensible losses: through urine
    - Insensible losses: include water lost through several pathways
      - Skin
      - Respiratory system
      - GI tract
    - Immediately affect ECF; if not replaced, eventually affect intracellular fluid (ICF)
- **Control mechanisms**
  - Kidneys: major regulatory organs of fluid balance
    - Adults: lose between 1 and 2 L of fluid as urine each day
    - Urine produced influenced by ADH and aldosterone levels; averages approximately 1,500 ml/day
    - Urine excretion: should equal about 1 ml per kilogram of body weight per hour in any age-group
    - Can produce urine with a range in osmolarity (range of normal specific gravity: 1.003 to 1.030)
    - Can excrete urine with a range in osmolality
      - Range: 200 to 1,400 mOsm/L

Key facts about fluid excretion

- Losses categorized as sensible or insensible
- Sensible losses: through urine
- Insensible losses through several pathways: skin, respiratory system, GI tract
- Losses immediately affect ECF; if not replaced, eventually affect ICF

Control mechanisms for fluid excretion

- Kidneys: urine excretion should equal about 1 ml per kilogram of body weight per hour in any age-group
- Perspiration: fluid loss can reach 600 ml/day
- Lungs: may eliminate 300 to 400 ml of fluid daily
- GI: about 200 ml of fluid excreted in feces daily

- Doesn't change in amount of metabolic wastes or solutes filtered by tubules
- Perspiration: possible fluid loss of 600 ml/day
- Lungs: may eliminate 300 to 400 ml of fluid daily through several mechanisms
  - Respiration
  - Increased respiratory rate
  - Depth increase water losses
- GI: about 200 ml of fluid excreted in feces daily; may be much greater during GI illness

ASSESSING FLUID BALANCE

● General information
- Blood pressure
  - Related to the amount of blood the heart pumps and the extent of vasoconstriction present
  - Measurement: key assessment for patient's fluid status; affected by fluid volume
  - Measurement accuracy maintained via periodic comparisons of automated and direct measurement systems with manual readings
- Direct measurements
  - arterial catheter is an invasive method for measuring blood pressure
  - pulmonary artery catheters are an invasive method of measuring fluid status and left ventricular heart function
  - central venous catheters measure fluid status and right ventricular function

● Blood pressure cuff measurements
- Taken with a stethoscope and a sphygmomanometer
- One of the best tools for assessing a patient's fluid volume
- Several factors for proper measurement
  - Cuff bladder width: about 40% of the upper arm circumference
  - Patient's arm position: ensures that brachial artery is at heart level
  - Cuff position: wrapped snugly around upper arm, above the antecubital fossa
    - Adults: lower cuff border about 1″ (2.5 cm) above the antecubital fossa
    - Children: lower cuff border closer to antecubital fossa
  - Cuff bladder position: centered over medial aspect of the arm
    - Goes over the brachial artery
    - Should have a reference mark to help position correctly
  - Brachial artery palpation: stethoscope bell placed directly over the strongest pulsation point (see *Positioning a blood pressure cuff*)

Positioning a blood pressure cuff

This illustration shows how to properly position a blood pressure cuff and stethoscope bell.

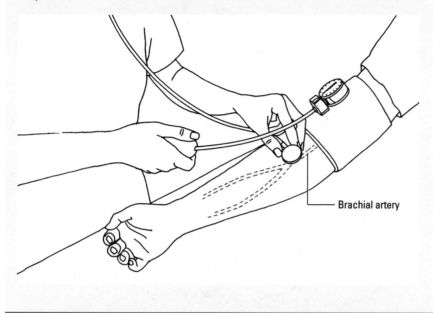

Brachial artery

- Blood pressure sometimes hard to hear; can be palpated to estimate systolic pressure (common in hypotensive patients; involves several steps)
  - Cuff placed on upper arm; brachial or radial pulse palpated
  - Cuff inflated until pulse no longer felt
  - Cuff slowly deflated, point at which pulse felt again (systolic pressure) noted
- Automated blood pressure unit: takes repeated blood pressure measurements
  - Computes, displays, and digitally records blood pressure readings
  - Cuff automatically inflates to check the blood pressure and deflates immediately afterward
  - Monitor programmable
    - Can inflate cuff as needed
    - Can set to alarm for high, low, and mean blood pressures
- Doppler device: can obtain a reading of systolic pressure in certain cases
  - Patient arm swollen
  - Patient blood pressure too low for palpable pulse (see *Taking a Doppler blood pressure,* page 26)
- Doppler device reading: involves several steps
  - Cuff inflated until pulse sound disappears

Key facts about Doppler blood pressure

- Used when you can't hear or feel a patient's blood pressure
- Probe: uses ultrasound waves directed at the blood vessel to detect blood flow

Key facts about direct measurement

- An invasive method
- Obtains hemodynamic measurements using arterial lines or venous catheters

Key facts about arterial catheters

- Used when highly accurate or frequent blood pressure measurements are required
- Can sample arterial blood
- Patient's blood pressure displayed continuously, allowing for instant notation of changes and quick response

---

Taking a Doppler blood pressure

When you can't hear or feel a patient's blood pressure, try using a Doppler ultrasound device, as shown here.

The Doppler probe uses ultrasound waves directed at the blood vessel to detect blood flow. Through the Doppler unit, you'll be able to hear the patient's blood flow with each pulse. To obtain a Doppler blood pressure:

- Place a blood pressure cuff on the arm as you usually would.
- Apply lubricant to the antecubital area where you would expect to find the brachial pulse.
- Turn the unit on and place the probe lightly on the arm over the brachial artery.
- Adjust the volume control and the placement of the probe until you hear the pulse clearly.

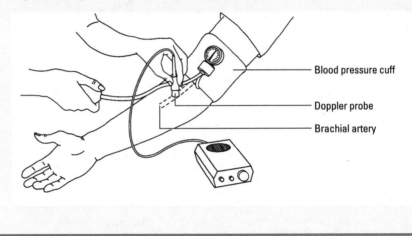

Blood pressure cuff

Doppler probe

Brachial artery

- Cuff slowly deflated; point when pulse sound returns (systolic pressure) noted (see *Correcting blood pressure measurement problems,* page 27)

● **Direct measurement**
- Is an invasive method of obtaining hemodynamic measurements using arterial or venous catheters
- Arterial catheter: continuously monitors blood pressure
  - Used when highly accurate or frequent blood pressure measurements are required
  - Can also sample arterial blood for blood gas analysis
  - Are usually inserted in the radial or the brachial artery (or the femoral artery, if needed)
  - Are connected to a transducer and then to a bedside monitor
    - Transducer: converts fluid-pressure waves from catheter into an electrical signal
    - Signal analyzed and displayed on monitor
  - Patient's blood pressure displayed continuously
    - Allows for instant notation of changes
    - Allows for quick response

Correcting blood pressure measurement problems

Use this chart to determine how to correct possible causes of a false-high or false-low blood pressure reading.

PROBLEM AND POSSIBLE CAUSE	INTERVENTIONS
False-high reading	
Cuff too small	Make sure the cuff bladder is long enough to completely encircle the extremity.
Cuff wrapped too loosely, reducing its effective width	Tighten the cuff.
Slow cuff deflation causing venous congestion in the arm or leg	Never deflate the cuff slower than 2 mm Hg/heartbeat.
Poorly timed measurement (after the patient has eaten, ambulated, appeared anxious, or flexed his arm muscles)	Postpone blood pressure measurement, or help the patient relax before taking pressures.
Multiple attempts at reading blood pressure in the same arm, causing venous congestion	Don't attempt to measure blood pressure more than twice in the same arm; wait several minutes between attempts.
False-low reading	
Incorrect position of the arm or leg	Make sure the arm or leg is level with the patient's heart.
Failure to notice auscultatory gap (sound fades out for 10 to 15 mm Hg, then returns)	Estimate systolic pressure using palpation before actually measuring it. Then check the palpable pressure against the measured pressure.
Inaudible or low-volume sounds	Before reinflating the cuff, instruct the patient to raise his arm or leg to decrease venous pressure and amplify low-volume sounds. After inflating the cuff, tell the patient to lower his arm or leg. Then deflate the cuff and listen. If you still fail to detect low-volume sounds, chart the palpable systolic pressure.

Blood pressure measurement problems

False-high reading
- Cuff too small
- Cuff wrapped too loosely, reducing its effective width
- Slow cuff deflation, causing venous congestion in the arm or leg
- Poorly timed measurement
- Multiple attempts at reading blood pressure in the same arm, causing venous congestion

False-low reading
- Incorrect position of the arm or leg
- Failure to notice auscultatory gap
- Inaudible or low-volume sounds

Key facts about pulmonary artery catheters

- Allow for measurement of PAP and PAWP, which provide information about left heart function
- Normal systolic PAP: 15 to 25 mm Hg; reflects pressure from contraction of the right atrium
- Normal diastolic PAP: 8 to 15 mm Hg; reflects lowest pressure in pulmonary vessels
- Normal PAWP: 6 to 12 mm Hg; reflects pressures coming from heart's left side
- Also measure cardiac output

- Pulmonary artery catheter: provides clearer picture of patient's fluid volume status than other techniques
  - Allows for measurement of pulmonary artery pressure (PAP) and pulmonary artery wedge pressure (PAWP), which provide information about left heart function
    - Pumping ability
    - Filling pressures
    - Vascular volume (see *Pulmonary artery catheter ports,* page 28)
  - Normal pulmonary artery systolic pressure: 15 to 25 mm Hg; reflects pressure from contraction of the right atrium

Uses for pulmonary artery catheter ports

- Pacing
- Infusing solutions
- Monitoring oxygen saturation, body temperature, cardiac output, central venous pressure, or PAWP

Key facts about cardiac output

- Refers to amount of blood pumped by the heart in 1 minute
- Normal range: 4 to 8 L/minute
- If high: patient is overloaded with fluid
- If low: patient lacks adequate blood volume

Pulmonary artery catheter ports

The ports on a pulmonary artery catheter (shown here) can be used for pacing, infusing solutions, or monitoring oxygen saturation, body temperature, cardiac output, or various intraluminal pressures, such as central venous pressure (through the proximal lumen) or pulmonary artery wedge pressure (through the distal lumen).

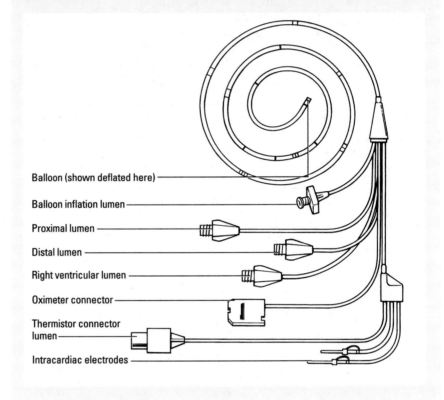

Balloon (shown deflated here)
Balloon inflation lumen
Proximal lumen
Distal lumen
Right ventricular lumen
Oximeter connector
Thermistor connector lumen
Intracardiac electrodes

- Normal diastolic PAP: 8 to 15 mm Hg; reflects lowest pressure in pulmonary vessels
- PAWP: measures pressures coming from heart's left side
  - May prove useful in gauging changes in blood volume
  - Normal PAWP range: 6 to 12 mm Hg
- Measures cardiac output
  - Refers to amount of blood pumped by the heart in 1 minute
  - Normal range: 4 to 8 L/minute
  - If high: patient is overloaded with fluid
  - If low: patient lacks adequate blood volume (assuming the heart can pump normally otherwise)
- Central venous catheter: measures central venous pressure (CVP)
  - Useful indication of fluid status

Estimating CVP

To estimate a patient's central venous pressure (CVP), use the illustration below as a guide and take these steps:

1. Place the patient at a 45- to 60-degree angle.
2. Use tangential lighting to observe the internal jugular vein.
3. Note the highest level of visible pulsation.
4. Locate the angle of Louis, or sternal notch, by palpating the point at which the clavicles join the sternum (the suprasternal notch).
5. Place two fingers on the patient's suprasternal notch and slide them down the sternum until they reach a bony protuberance—the angle of Louis. The right atrium lies about 2″ (5.1 cm) below this point.
6. Measure the distance between the angle of Louis and the highest level of visible pulsation. Normally, this distance is less than 1.2″ (3 cm).
7. Add 2 to this figure to estimate the distance between the highest level of pulsation and the right atrium. A distance greater than 4″ (10.2 cm) may indicate elevated CVP.

Key facts about central venous pressure

- Useful indication of fluid status
- Refers to pressure of the blood inside the central venous circulation
- Normal range: 0 to 7 mm Hg
- If high: patient is overloaded with fluid
- If low: patient is low on fluid
- Measured by central venous catheter

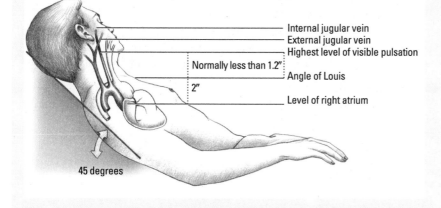

Internal jugular vein
External jugular vein
Highest level of visible pulsation
Normally less than 1.2″
Angle of Louis
2″
Level of right atrium
45 degrees

- Catheter tip typically placed in a jugular vein in neck or a subclavian vein in chest
- Refers to pressure of the blood inside the central venous circulation
- Normal range: 0 to 7 mm Hg (5 to 10 cm water)
- If high: patient is overloaded with fluid
- If low: patient is low on fluid (see *Estimating CVP*)

DEVELOPMENTAL CONSIDERATIONS

● **Pediatric patient**
  - Premature neonate's body approximately 90% water
  - Term neonate's body 70% to 80% water

Developmental considerations in fluid balance

Pediatric patient
- Premature neonate's body approximately 90% water
- Term neonate's body 70% to 80% water
- More water in infant ECF than adult ECF
- Adult body water composition attained at puberty
- Infants: ingest and excrete large volume of water daily; can't concentrate urine until about age 3 months

Older adult
- Experiences a 6% reduction in total body water
- May fail to drink enough
- Experiences decreased thirst sensation
- May need more time to return to normal if excesses or deficits occur

Pregnant patient
- Retains additional fluids (about 6 to 8 L of water) to meet maternal and fetal needs
- Late pregnancy: ADH release increases; causes water retention and increased thirst

- More water in infant ECF than adult ECF
  - As infant ages, ECF to ICF ratio decreases
    - Attributed to growth of cellular tissue
    - Also attributed to a decreased rate of growth of collagen relative to muscle growth
  - Adult body water composition attained at puberty
- Infants: ingest and excrete large volume of water daily
  - May exchange one-half of daily ECF—have higher metabolic rates, produce more waste (adult exchange: one-sixth)
  - Have greater respective BSA than adults
  - Typically lose more water from the skin than adults do; results in smaller reserve of body fluid than adults
- Infants: can't concentrate urine until about age 3 months; kidneys remain less efficient than adult's until about age 2 years

Older adult
- Experiences a 6% reduction in total body water and a decrease in ratio of ECF to ICF; result of muscle mass decline and increased fat proportion
- May fail to drink enough even when fluids are available
- May not recognize fluid deficits due to decreased thirst sensation
- Can usually maintain fluid balance under normal conditions; may need more time to return to normal if excesses or deficits occur
- Doesn't possess reserves or ability to adapt readily to rapid changes

Pregnant patient
- Retains additional fluids (about 6 to 8 L of water) to meet maternal and fetal needs
  - Increased water in ECF: accounts for 70% to 75% of patient's weight gain
  - ICF volume: increases 1.5 to 5 L; greatest accumulation occurs during second half of pregnancy
- Late pregnancy: ADH release increases; causes water retention and increased thirst

NCLEX CHECKS

It's never too soon to begin your NCLEX preparation. Now that you've reviewed this chapter, carefully read each of the following questions and choose the best answer. Then compare your responses to the correct answers.

1. The rate at which nephrons filter blood is referred to as:
   - ☐ 1. osmotic pressure.
   - ☐ 2. capillary filtration rate.
   - ☐ 3. glomerular filtration rate.
   - ☐ 4. urinary clearance time.

2. In response to the thirst sensation, fluids are ingested. This action causes:

☐ **1.** an increase in the concentration of solutes.
☐ **2.** a decrease in the concentration of solutes.
☐ **3.** no change in the concentration of solutes.
☐ **4.** an increase in serum osmolality.

3. Dry mucous membranes in the mouth stimulate the thirst center, which is located:

☐ **1.** in the thyroid gland.
☐ **2.** in the kidneys.
☐ **3.** in the stomach.
☐ **4.** in the hypothalamus.

4. How does ANP work to decrease blood pressure and reduce intravascular blood volume? Select all that apply.

☐ **1.** Decreasing aldosterone release
☐ **2.** Increasing aldosterone release
☐ **3.** Decreasing ADH release
☐ **4.** Increasing ADH release
☐ **5.** Causing vasodilation
☐ **6.** Causing vasoconstriction

5. The nurse is caring for a client with GI hemorrhage. She can expect his kidneys to respond to this condition by:

☐ **1.** secreting less renin.
☐ **2.** causing vasodilation.
☐ **3.** secreting more renin.
☐ **4.** secreting angiotensin II.

6. The nurse is testing the specific gravity of a client with hypervolemia. Which result is consistent with this condition?

☐ **1.** 1.005
☐ **2.** 1.015
☐ **3.** 1.020
☐ **4.** 1.035

7. What role does aldosterone play in fluid and electrolyte balance?

☐ **1.** Aldosterone reduces circulating blood volume.
☐ **2.** Aldosterone expands circulating blood volume.
☐ **3.** Aldosterone promotes sodium and water excretion from the kidneys.
☐ **4.** Aldosterone is responsible for converting angiotensinogen to angiotensin I in the liver.

TOP 10

Items to study for your next test on fluid balance

1. The role of water in achieving homeostasis

2. Assessment items that should be considered for total intake and output

3. The thirst center's role in maintaining fluid balance

4. Mechanisms of blood pressure regulation through chemical and vascular action

5. The role of ADH in fluid balance and shifts that occur with over- or underproduction

6. The role of aldosterone and renin in fluid balance

7. The role of ANP in relationship to aldosterone and blood pressure regulation

8. Diagnostic measurements used to evaluate fluid status (BP, PAP, PAWP, CVP)

9. Risk factors related to fluid losses based on age and maturation

10. Fluid balance changes that occur during pregnancy

8. Which of the following describes an appropriate step when obtaining blood pressure cuff measurements?
- ☐ **1.** Wrap the blood pressure cuff loosely around the client's arm.
- ☐ **2.** The cuff should have a width of about 20% of the upper arm circumference.
- ☐ **3.** Make sure the lower border of the cuff reaches the elbow joint.
- ☐ **4.** Position the client's arm so that the brachial artery is at the level of the heart.

9. PAWP readings provide information about:
- ☐ **1.** colloid osmotic pressure.
- ☐ **2.** plasma concentration.
- ☐ **3.** left heart function.
- ☐ **4.** circulating red blood cell concentration.

10. A client has a pulmonary artery catheter inserted for close monitoring after surgery. His cardiac output readings are currently 9 to 10 L/ minute. What's the most appropriate action for the nurse to take?
- ☐ **1.** Notify the practitioner and prepare to reduce the I.V. fluid rate.
- ☐ **2.** Examine the client for signs of hemorrhage.
- ☐ **3.** Notify the practitioner and prepare to increase the I.V. fluid rate.
- ☐ **4.** Assess for other signs of hypovolemia.

ANSWERS AND RATIONALES

1. CORRECT ANSWER: 3
Glomerular filtration rate (GFR) refers to the rate at which blood is filtered through the nephrons. GFR normally occurs at a rate of 125 ml/minute.

2. CORRECT ANSWER: 2
Because ingestion of fluid increases the amount of fluid in the body, the concentration of solutes will decrease. Ingestion of fluids would also decrease serum osmolality—an increase in serum osmolality indicates an increase in the concentration of solutes.

3. CORRECT ANSWER: 4
The thirst center is located in the hypothalamus.

4. CORRECT ANSWER: 1, 3, 5
By decreasing the release of aldosterone (a hormone that causes sodium and water retention) and ADH (a hormone that reduces diuresis and increases water retention), and by causing vasodilation, ANP can effectively reduce blood pressure and intravascular blood volume.

5. CORRECT ANSWER: 3
In response to a rapidly diminishing blood flow (which would occur during GI hemorrhage), the kidneys will secrete more renin to cause vasoconstriction and an increase in blood pressure.

6. CORRECT ANSWER: 1

Normal urine specific gravity ranges from 1.010 to 1.020. Conditions involving fluid excess (such as hypervolemia) cause the kidneys to excrete a more dilute urine, indicated by a specific gravity less than 1.010. Conditions involving fluid deficits (such as dehydration) cause the kidneys to excrete a more concentrated urine, indicated by a specific gravity greater than 1.030.

7. CORRECT ANSWER: 2

By causing the kidneys to retain sodium and water, aldosterone promotes blood volume expansion. The enzyme renin is responsible for the conversion of angiotensinogen to angiotensin I, which occurs in the liver.

8. CORRECT ANSWER: 4

When taking a blood pressure measurement, the brachial artery should be at heart level for most accurate results. The cuff should have a width of about 40% of the upper arm circumference. The cuff should be wrapped snugly around the client's arm, positioned about 1″ (2.5 cm) above the antecubital fossa.

9. CORRECT ANSWER: 3

PAWP provides information about left heart function and vascular volume.

10. CORRECT ANSWER: 1

Normal range for cardiac output is 4 to 8 L/minute, so the client has an increased cardiac output. A high cardiac output is indicative of fluid volume overload, so the most appropriate action would be to notify the practitioner and prepare to decrease the client's I.V. fluid rate. Examining the client for signs of hemorrhage; notifying the practitioner and preparing to increase I.V. fluid rate; and assessing for other signs of hypovolemia would be appropriate if the client had a low cardiac output.

Electrolyte balance

LEARNING OBJECTIVES

After studying this chapter, you should be able to:

● State the major electrolytes found in intracellular and extracellular fluids.

● Name at least three functions of each major electrolyte.

● Identify normal and abnormal blood level ranges for major electrolytes.

● Describe how organs, glands, and hormones function to regulate electrolyte levels.

CHAPTER OVERVIEW

Electrolytes play a vital role in maintaining life. A deficit or excess can cause life-threatening problems. The major body electrolytes include sodium (Na), potassium (K), chloride (Cl), calcium (Ca), phosphorus (P), and magnesium (Mg). These electrolytes are regulated by the renal and endocrine systems.

INTRODUCTION

● **Electrolytes**
  - Are electrically charged solutes in body fluids necessary to maintain life
  - Imbalance: abnormal excess or deficit of an electrolyte in body fluids; can cause illness
  - Balance in patients best assessed by monitoring several factors

– Normal regulation
– Functions
– Levels

● **Functions**
- Promote neuromuscular irritability
- Maintain body fluid osmolality
- Regulate acid-base balance and distribution of body fluids among body fluid compartments

● **Regulation by kidneys**
- Filtration: process of removing particles from a solution by allowing the liquid portion to pass through a membrane
- Filtration: occurs in the nephron (the anatomic and functional unit of the kidneys); is a multi-step process
    - Blood circulates through glomerulus (network of capillaries)
    - Fluids and electrolytes filtered and collected in nephron's tubules
    - Some fluids and electrolytes reabsorbed through capillaries throughout the nephron, others secreted (see *How the nephron regulates fluids and electrolytes,* page 36)
- Diuretics (drugs used to increase urine production): can affect the nephron's regulation of fluid and electrolyte balance; other drugs may do same (see *How drugs affect nephron activity,* page 37)

● **Regulation by other organs**
- Lungs and liver: part of the renin-angiotensin-aldosterone system; help regulate sodium, water balance, and blood pressure
- Adrenal glands: secrete aldosterone, which influences sodium and potassium balance in kidneys
- Heart: counteracts the renin-angiotensin-aldosterone system when it secretes atrial natriuretic peptide, causing sodium excretion
- Hypothalamus and posterior pituitary gland: produce and secrete antidiuretic hormone that causes the body to retain water, affecting solute concentration in blood
- GI tract: sodium, potassium, chloride, and water lost in sweat; however, electrolytes also absorbed from the GI tract, affecting their balance
- Parathyroid glands: usually two pairs located behind and to the side of the thyroid gland; secrete parathyroid hormone (PTH), which draws calcium into the blood from the bones, intestines, and kidneys; helps move phosphorus from the blood to the kidneys where it's excreted in urine
- Thyroid gland: secretes calcitonin, a hormone that lowers an elevated calcium level by preventing calcium release from bone and decreasing intestinal absorption and kidney reabsorption of calcium

● **Nursing interventions**
- Assess overall fluid balance by monitoring daily weight, fluid intake and output, and urine specific gravity; fluid balance is closely related to electrolyte balance

---

Key facts about electrolytes
- Electrically charged solutes in body fluids necessary to maintain life
- Abnormal excess or deficit of an electrolyte in body fluids can cause illness

Key functions of electrolytes
- Promote neuromuscular irritability
- Maintain osmolality
- Regulate acid-base balance

Role of the kidneys in electrolyte balance

Filtration
- Fluids and electrolytes filtered and collected in nephron's tubules
- Some fluids and electrolytes reabsorbed through capillaries throughout the nephron, others secreted

Diuretics
- Can affect the nephron's regulation of fluid and electrolyte balance; other drugs may do same

Role of other organs in electrolyte balance
- Lungs and liver: help regulate sodium, water balance, and blood pressure
- Adrenal glands: influence sodium and potassium balance in kidneys
- Heart: causes sodium excretion when it secretes atrial natriuretic peptide

Role of other organs in electrolyte balance
(continued)

- Hypothalamus and posterior pituitary gland: affect solute concentration in blood
- GI tract: absorbs electrolytes
- Parathyroid glands: draws calcium into the blood from the bones, intestines, and kidneys; helps move phosphorus from the blood to the kidneys, where it's excreted in urine
- Thyroid gland: lowers an elevated calcium level by preventing calcium release from bone and decreasing intestinal absorption and kidney reabsorption of calcium

Key nursing interventions for monitoring electrolyte balance

- Monitor daily weight, fluid intake and output, and urine specific gravity.
- Assess neurologic status, specifically for altered LOC.
- Evaluate motor and sensory function, especially deep tendon reflexes.
- Monitor vital signs, especially pulse and blood pressure.
- Compare ongoing ECG readings with the patient's baseline ECG to detect changes.
- Assess respiratory status for changes in rate, depth, and character.
- Monitor serum electrolyte levels for abnormalities.
- Assess nutritional status by monitoring dietary intake, weight, and serum albumin levels.
- Evaluate the patient's health history.
- Evaluate the patient's medication history.

How the nephron regulates fluids and electrolytes

In this illustration, the nephron has been stretched to show where and how fluids and electrolytes are regulated.

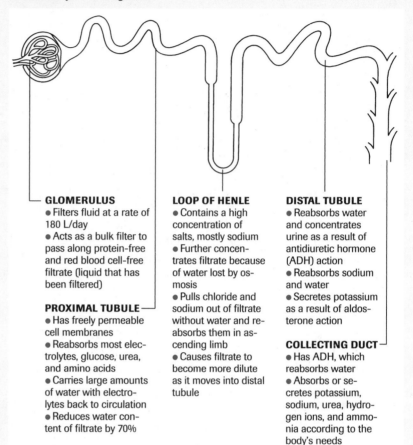

GLOMERULUS
- Filters fluid at a rate of 180 L/day
- Acts as a bulk filter to pass along protein-free and red blood cell-free filtrate (liquid that has been filtered)

PROXIMAL TUBULE
- Has freely permeable cell membranes
- Reabsorbs most electrolytes, glucose, urea, and amino acids
- Carries large amounts of water with electrolytes back to circulation
- Reduces water content of filtrate by 70%

LOOP OF HENLE
- Contains a high concentration of salts, mostly sodium
- Further concentrates filtrate because of water lost by osmosis
- Pulls chloride and sodium out of filtrate without water and reabsorbs them in ascending limb
- Causes filtrate to become more dilute as it moves into distal tubule

DISTAL TUBULE
- Reabsorbs water and concentrates urine as a result of antidiuretic hormone (ADH) action
- Reabsorbs sodium and water
- Secretes potassium as a result of aldosterone action

COLLECTING DUCT
- Has ADH, which reabsorbs water
- Absorbs or secretes potassium, sodium, urea, hydrogen ions, and ammonia according to the body's needs

- Assess neurologic status, specifically for altered level of consciousness (LOC), which may result from an electrolyte imbalance
- Evaluate motor and sensory function, especially deep tendon reflexes; neuromuscular irritability may indicate electrolyte imbalances
- Monitor vital signs, especially pulse and blood pressure; certain electrolytes, such as sodium, potassium, and magnesium, directly affect pulse and blood pressure regulation
- Compare ongoing electrocardiogram (ECG) readings with the patient's baseline ECG to detect changes that may indicate an imbalance
- Assess respiratory status for changes in rate, depth, and character
- Monitor serum electrolyte levels for abnormalities (see *Interpreting serum electrolyte test results,* page 38)

How drugs affect nephron activity

Here's a look at how certain diuretics and other drugs affect the nephron's regulation of fluid and electrolyte balance.

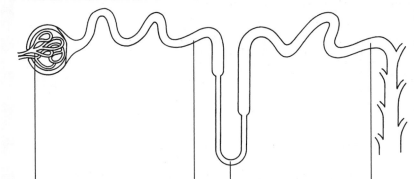

GLOMERULUS
- *Dopamine (Intropin)*. Dopamine may increase urine output. Dopaminergic receptor sites exist along the afferent arterioles (tiny vessels that bring blood to the glomerulus). In low doses (0.5 to 3 mcg/kg/minute), dopamine dilates these vessels in the glomerulus to increase blood flow to it. This in turn increases filtration in the nephron.

PROXIMAL TUBULE
- *Carbonic anhydrase inhibitors* (acetazolamide [Diamox]). These drugs reduce hydrogen ion (acid) concentration in the tubule, which causes increased excretion of bicarbonate, water, sodium, and potassium.
- *Glucose*. High blood levels of osmotic diuretic cause excess glucose to spill over into the tubules. The osmotic effect of glucose also results in increased urine output.
- *Mannitol (Osmitrol)*. Osmotic diuretic mannitol isn't reabsorbed in the tubule; it remains in high concentrations throughout its journey, increasing filtrate osmolality and hindering water, sodium, and chloride reabsorption, thereby increasing their excretion.

LOOP OF HENLE
- *Loop diuretics* (furosemide [Lasix], bumetanide [Bumex], and ethacrynic acid [Edecrin]). Loop diuretics act on the ascending loop of Henle to prevent water and sodium reabsorption. As a result, volume in the tubules is increased and blood volume is decreased. Potassium and chloride are also excreted here.

DISTAL TUBULE
- *Potassium-sparing diuretics* (spironolactone [Aldactone]). These diuretics interfere with sodium and chloride reabsorption in the tubule. Potassium is spared, and sodium, chloride, and water are excreted. Urine output increases, and the body retains potassium.
- *Thiazide diuretics* (hydrochlorothiazide [HydroDIURIL] and metolazone [Zaroxolyn]). Thiazide diuretics act high in the distal tubule to prevent sodium reabsorption, which increases the amount of tubular fluid and electrolytes farther down the nephron. Blood volume decreases, aldosterone increases sodium reabsorption and, in exchange, potassium is lost from the body.

Effect of drugs on nephron activity

Dopamine
- May increase urine output
- Dilates afferent arterioles in the glomerulus to increase blood flow and filtration in the nephron

Carbonic anhydrase inhibitors
- Reduce hydrogen ion (acid) concentration in the tubule
- Causes increased excretion of bicarbonate, water, sodium, and potassium

Glucose
- High blood levels of osmotic diuretic cause excess glucose to spill over into the tubules
- Osmotic effect results in increased urine output

Mannitol
- Increases filtrate osmolality and hinders water, sodium, and chloride reabsorption, thereby increasing their excretion

Loop diuretics
- Prevent water and sodium reabsorption
- Cause potassium and chloride excretion

Potassium-sparing diuretics
- Interfere with sodium and chloride reabsorption in the tubule
- Urine output increases, and the body retains potassium

Thiazide diuretics
- Prevent sodium reabsorption
- Blood volume decreases, aldosterone increases sodium reabsorption and, in exchange, potassium is lost from the body

- Remember that electrolytes may be obtained through food intake; be aware of fluids and foods high in certain electrolytes (see *Dietary sources of major electrolytes,* page 39)
- Assess nutritional status by monitoring dietary intake, weight, and serum albumin levels; if indicated, obtain anthropometric measurements and compare with standards

Normal serum electrolyte levels

- Calcium: 8.9 to 10.1 mg/dl
- Calcium, ionized: 4.5 to 5.1 mg/dl
- Chloride: 96 to 106 mEq/L
- Magnesium: 1.5 to 2.5 mEq/L
- Phosphates: 2.5 to 4.5 mg/dl or 1.8 to 2.6 mEq/L
- Potassium: 3.5 to 5 mEq/L
- Sodium: 135 to 145 mEq/L

Interpreting serum electrolyte test results

Use the quick-reference chart to interpret serum electrolyte test results in adult patients. This chart also includes disorders that can cause imbalances.

ELECTROLYTE	RESULTS	IMPLICATIONS	COMMON CAUSES
Calcium	8.9 to 10.1 mg/dl	Normal	
	< 8.9 mg/dl	Hypocalcemia	Acute pancreatitis
	> 10.1 mg/dl	Hypercalcemia	Hyperparathyroidism
Calcium, ionized	4.5 to 5.1 mg/dl	Normal	
	< 4.5 mg/dl	Hypocalcemia	Massive transfusion
	> 5.1 mg/dl	Hypercalcemia	Acidosis
Chloride	96 to 106 mEq/L	Normal	
	< 96 mEq/L	Hypochloremia	Prolonged vomiting
	> 106 mEq/L	Hyperchloremia	Hypernatremia
Magnesium	1.5 to 2.5 mEq/L	Normal	
	< 1.5 mEq/L	Hypomagnesemia	Malnutrition
	> 2.5 mEq/L	Hypermagnesemia	Renal failure
Phosphates	2.5 to 4.5 mg/dl or 1.8 to 2.6 mEq/L	Normal	
	< 2.5 mg/dl or 1.8 mEq/L	Hypophosphatemia	Diabetic ketoacidosis
	> 4.5 mg/dl or 2.6 mEq/L	Hyperphosphatemia	Renal insufficiency
Potassium	3.5 to 5 mEq/L	Normal	
	< 3.5 mEq/L	Hypokalemia	Diarrhea
	> 5 mEq/L	Hyperkalemia	Burns and renal failure
Sodium	135 to 145 mEq/L	Normal	
	< 135 mEq/L	Hyponatremia	Syndrome of inappropriate antidiuretic hormone
	> 145 mEq/L	Hypernatremia	Diabetes insipidus

Dietary sources of major electrolytes

This chart highlights key dietary sources of the major electrolytes in the body.

ELECTROLYTE	DIETARY SOURCES
Sodium	• Canned soups and vegetables • Cheese • Ketchup • Processed meats • Seafood • Snack foods • Table salt
Potassium	• Chocolate • Dried fruit, nuts, and seeds • Peanut butter • Fruits, such as oranges, bananas, apricots, and cantaloupe • Meats • Vegetables, especially avocados, beans, potatoes, mushrooms, tomatoes, and carrots
Magnesium	• Chocolate • Dry beans and peas • Green, leafy vegetables • Meats • Nuts • Seafood • Whole grains
Calcium	• Bonemeal • Dairy products, such as milk, cheese, and yogurt • Green, leafy vegetables • Legumes • Molasses • Nuts • Whole grains
Phosphorus	• Cheese • Dried beans • Eggs • Fish • Milk products • Nuts and seeds • Organ meats (such as brain and liver) • Poultry • Whole grains
Chloride	• Canned vegetables • Fruits • Processed meats • Raw vegetables, such as lettuce and celery • Salty foods • Table salt

Key dietary sources of major electrolytes

• Sodium: table salt
• Potassium: fruits
• Magnesium: seafood
• Calcium: dairy products
• Phosphorus: eggs
• Chloride: salty foods

- Evaluate the patient's health history for medical conditions that might alter electrolyte balance
- Evaluate the patient's medication history for prescription and over-the-counter drugs that could interfere with electrolyte balance, such as diuretics, antacids, laxatives, and salt substitutes

SODIUM

General information
- Is the major cation in the extracellular fluid (ECF), accounting for 90% of ECF cations
- Normal ECF serum concentration: 135 to 145 mEq/L
- Normal intracellular fluid (ICF) concentration: 10 mEq/L
- Excreted or absorbed via proportionate excretion or absorption of water and chloride
- Minimum daily requirement: 0.5 to 2.7 grams; adults in the United States consume an average of 6 grams/day

Functions
- Maintains appropriate ECF osmolality
- Maintains ECF volume by attracting fluid; influences body water distribution (with chloride)
- Affects the concentration, excretion, and absorption of potassium and chloride
- Combines readily with bicarbonate (HCO_3^-) and chloride to help regulate acid-base balance
- Aids impulse transmission in nerve and muscle fibers

Regulation
- Mainly balanced through kidneys via aldosterone action
- Also excreted from the body through several processes
    - Perspiration
    - Vomiting
    - Diarrhea
    - Diuretic therapy
    - Burn injuries
- Excretion can match sodium intake (kidneys adjust)
- Serum sodium level: change usually reflects a change in total body water balance
- Controlled by a feedback loop and hormones aldosterone and antidiuretic hormone (ADH)
    - Increased level in ECF: decreases aldosterone production, which increases renal sodium excretion; also raises ECF osmolality, which stimulates ADH release that increases renal water reabsorption
    - Decreased sodium level in ECF: increases aldosterone production, which decreases renal sodium excretion; also lowers ECF osmolal-

Sidebar

Key facts about sodium
- Major cation in the ECF
- Normal serum level: 135 to 145 mEq/L
- Excreted or absorbed via proportionate excretion or absorption of water and chloride

Key functions of sodium
- Maintains ECF osmolality
- Influences body water distribution (with chloride)
- Affects the concentration, excretion, and absorption of potassium and chloride
- Helps regulate acid-base balance
- Aids impulse transmission in nerve and muscle fibers

Key facts about sodium regulation
- Mainly balanced through kidneys via aldosterone action
- Also excreted through: perspiration, vomiting, diarrhea, diuretic therapy, and burn injuries
- Change in level: reflects a change in total body water balance
- Serum levels: controlled by ADH and sodium-potassium pump

GO WITH THE FLOW

Regulating sodium and water

This flowchart shows two of the body's compensatory mechanisms for restoring sodium and water balance.

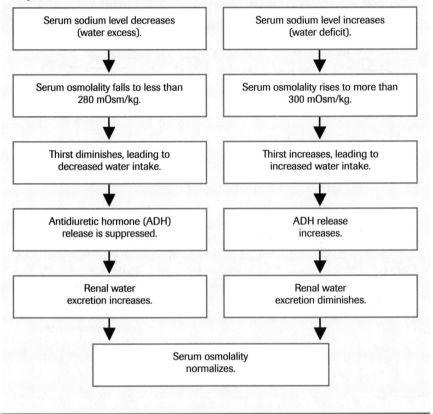

Serum sodium level decreases (water excess).	Serum sodium level increases (water deficit).
Serum osmolality falls to less than 280 mOsm/kg.	Serum osmolality rises to more than 300 mOsm/kg.
Thirst diminishes, leading to decreased water intake.	Thirst increases, leading to increased water intake.
Antidiuretic hormone (ADH) release is suppressed.	ADH release increases.
Renal water excretion increases.	Renal water excretion diminishes.

Serum osmolality normalizes.

ity, which inhibits ADH release and increases renal water excretion (see *Regulating sodium and water*)

- *Sodium-potassium pump:* active transport mechanism; also helps maintain normal sodium levels
  - Extracellular sodium levels normally extremely high compared with intracellular sodium levels; produces several results
    - Sodium ions: normally most abundant outside the cells; tend to diffuse inward
    - Potassium ions: normally most abundant inside the cells; tend to diffuse outward
  - Diffusion counteracted by pump; maintains normal sodium and potassium levels
  - Each sodium ion linked with carrier; can't get through the cell wall alone

Key facts about the sodium-potassium pump

- Active transport mechanism
- Helps maintain normal sodium levels
- Sodium ions: normally most abundant outside the cells; tend to diffuse inward
- Potassium ions: normally most abundant inside the cells; tend to diffuse outward
- Stimuli: affect membrane permeability to move sodium inward and potassium outward
- ATP: combines with magnesium and an enzyme to create energy for ion/carrier movement

Understanding the sodium-potassium pump

These illustrations show how the sodium-potassium pump carries ions when their concentrations change.

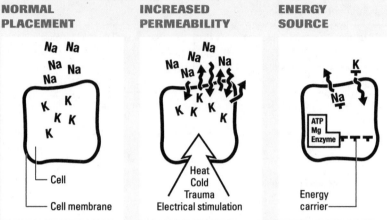

NORMAL PLACEMENT

INCREASED PERMEABILITY

ENERGY SOURCE

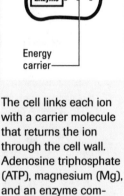

Normally, more sodium (Na) ions exist outside the cells than inside. More potassium (K) ions exist inside the cells than outside.

Certain stimuli increase the membrane's permeability. Sodium ions diffuse inward; potassium ions diffuse outward.

The cell links each ion with a carrier molecule that returns the ion through the cell wall. Adenosine triphosphate (ATP), magnesium (Mg), and an enzyme commonly found in cells create the energy that returns the ion to the cell.

– Energy required for ion/carrier movement—comes from adenosine triphosphate (ATP); made up of several components
  · Phosphorus
  · Magnesium
  · An enzyme (see *Understanding the sodium-potassium pump*)
– Serves several major functions
  · Allows the body to carry out its essential functions
  · Helps prevent cellular swelling caused by too many ions inside the cell attracting excessive amounts of water
  · Creates an electrical charge in the cell from the movement of ions; permits transmission of neuromuscular impulses

POTASSIUM

● **General information**
  • Is the major cation in the ICF
  • Normal serum level range: 3.5 to 5 mEq/L

Key facts about potassium

● Major cation in the ICF
● Normal serum level: 3.5 to 5 mEq/L
● Found in saliva, perspiration, and stomach and intestinal secretions

Potassium's role in acid–base balance

These illustrations show the movement of potassium ions (K+) in response to changes in extracellular hydrogen ion (H+) concentration. H+ concentration changes with acidosis and alkalosis.

NORMAL BALANCE

Under normal conditions, the K+ content in intracellular fluid (ICF) is much greater than in extracellular fluid (ECF). H+ concentration is low in both compartments.

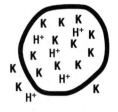

ACIDOSIS

In acidosis, H+ content in ECF increases and the ions move into the ICF. To keep the ICF electrically neutral, an equal number of K+ leave the cell, causing hyperkalemia.

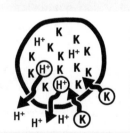

ALKALOSIS

In alkalosis, more H+ are present in ICF than in the ECF. Therefore, H+ move from the ICF into the ECF. To keep the ICF electrically neutral, K+ move from the ECF into the ICF, causing hypokalemia.

- Cellular concentration: about 140 mEq/L; usually not measured clinically
- Daily dietary requirement: about 40 mEq; the average daily intake in the United States is 60 to 100 mEq
- Found in saliva, perspiration, and stomach and intestinal secretions

● **Functions**
- Maintains cell electroneutrality and cell osmolality
- Directly affects skeletal and cardiac muscle contraction and electrical conductivity
- Aids neuromuscular transmission of nerve impulses
- Plays a major role in acid-base balance; any alteration in potassium balance will result in acid-base imbalance (see *Potassium's role in acid-base balance*)

Key facts about potassium regulation

- Daily potassium ingestion necessary; body doesn't conserve it
- About 80% of ingested potassium eliminated through kidneys
- Has a reciprocal relationship with sodium
- No effective mechanism for kidneys to combat loss; may excrete it even when the serum level is low
- Also excreted in sweat and feces
- Sodium-potassium pump also regulates levels
- Levels possibly affected by change in pH

Key facts about chloride

- Most abundant anion in the ECF
- Normal serum level: 96 to 106 mEq/L

Key functions of chloride

- Maintains serum osmolality and water balance
- Forms CSF
- Combines with major cations to create sodium chloride, HCl, potassium chloride, and calcium chloride
- Helps maintain acid-base balance
- Assists in carbon dioxide transport in the RBCs

● Regulation

- Daily potassium ingestion necessary; body doesn't conserve it
- About 80% of ingested potassium eliminated through kidneys
- About 20 to 40 mEq of potassium lost in each liter of urine
- Rise in serum potassium levels produces several effects
    - Renal tubules excrete more potassium
    - Increased potassium loss in urine
- Has a reciprocal relationship with sodium; kidneys reabsorb sodium, excrete potassium when aldosterone (hormone) secreted
- No effective mechanism for kidneys to combat loss; may excrete it even when the serum level is low
- Remaining potassium excreted in sweat and feces
    - Bowel condition influenced by absorption
    - 5 to 10 mEq lost in each liter of GI fluid
- Sodium-potassium pump also regulates
    - Moves sodium from the cell into the ECF
    - Maintains high intracellular potassium levels by pumping potassium into the cell
- Serum levels possibly affected by change in pH
    - Hydrogen (H) and potassium ions freely exchanged across plasma cell membranes
    - Acidosis: excess hydrogen moves into cells, pushes potassium into ECF for balance; may cause hyperkalemia
    - Hypokalemia possibly caused by alkalosis; increases potassium movement into cell, maintains balance

CHLORIDE

● General information

- Is the most abundant anion in the ECF
- Normal serum level: 96 to 106 mEq/L
- Normal concentration in the ICF: 4 mEq/L
- High levels in cerebrospinal fluid (CSF); also found in bile and in gastric and pancreatic juices
- Normal daily requirement for adults: 750 mg

● Functions

- Has negative charge
    - Travels with positively charged sodium
    - Maintains serum osmolality and water balance
- Forms CSF
    - Works with sodium to do so
    - Choroid plexus (mass of tiny blood vessels inside the ventricles of the brain) dependent on sodium and chloride to attract water to form CSF fluid component
- Combines with major cations to create important compounds
    - Sodium chloride

– Hydrochloric acid (HCl)

– Potassium chloride

– Calcium chloride

• Works through HCl production

– Helps maintain acid-base balance

– Assists in carbon dioxide transport in the red blood cells (RBCs)

● **Regulation**

• Depends on chloride intake and excretion and reabsorption of chloride ions in the kidneys

– Most is absorbed in the intestines; only a small portion lost in stools

– Is excreted through the kidneys, perspiration, diarrhea, and diuretic use

• Sufficient dietary chloride provided by salt (usually sodium chloride)

• Balance tied most closely to sodium balance; one electrolyte level changes, other changes comparably

• Is indirectly affected by aldosterone

– Causes renal tubules to reabsorb sodium

– Positively charged sodium ions reabsorbed, negatively charged chloride ions passively reabsorbed because of electrical attraction to sodium

• Also involves acid balance

– Reabsorbed and excreted in direct opposition to bicarbonate (negatively charged ion; alkaline)

– Levels change, body attempts to keep its positive-negative balance, makes corresponding changes in bicarbonate levels in kidneys

– Levels decrease, kidneys retain bicarbonate and bicarbonate levels increase

– Levels increase, kidneys excrete bicarbonate and bicarbonate levels decrease

CALCIUM

● **General information**

• Is a cation found in both the ECF and the ICF

• About 99% of the body's calcium found in the bones and teeth

• Only 1% found in serum and soft tissue (matters when measuring blood calcium levels)

• Two methods to measure calcium levels

– Serum calcium level

· Most commonly ordered calcium test

· Measures the total amount of calcium in the blood

· Normal range: 8.5 to 10.5 mg/dl

– Ionized calcium level

· Measures various forms of calcium in ECF

Key facts about chloride regulation

• Most is absorbed in the intestines; only a small portion lost in stools

• Excreted through the kidneys, perspiration, diarrhea, and diuretic use

• Sufficient dietary chloride provided by salt

• Balance tied most closely to sodium balance

• Indirectly affected by aldosterone

• Also involves acid balance

Key facts about calcium

• Cation found in both the ECF and the ICF

• About 99% of the body's calcium found in the bones and teeth

• Two methods to measure calcium levels: serum calcium level and ionized calcium level

• Serum calcium level is most commonly ordered calcium test; normal range, 8.5 to 10.5 mg/dl

• Most of ion's physiologic functions carried out by ionized calcium; normal adult range, 4.5 to 5.1 mg/dl

• Total serum levels possibly influenced by serum protein abnormalities, but ionized calcium levels remain unchanged

• Serum albumin levels considered when evaluating total serum calcium levels

• Has an inverse relationship with phosphorus

Calculating calcium and albumin levels

- The formula for correcting a patient's calcium level:

  total serum calcium level + 0.8
  (4 – albumin level) =
  corrected calcium level

Key functions of calcium

- Responsible for formation and structure of bones and teeth
- Helps maintain cell membrane structure, function, and membrane permeability
- Affects activation, excitation, and contraction of cardiac and skeletal muscle
- Participates in neurotransmitter release at synapses
- Helps activate specific steps in blood coagulation
- Activates serum complement

Calculating calcium and albumin levels

A noncritically ill patient's total calcium decreases by 0.8 mg/dl for every 1 g/dl that his serum albumin level drops. Use this calculation to determine what your patient's calcium level would be if his serum albumin level were normal—and to help determine if treatment is necessary.

CORRECTING A LEVEL

The normal albumin level is 4 g/dl. The formula for correcting a patient's calcium level is:

total serum calcium level + 0.8 (4 – albumin level) = corrected calcium level

CALCULATING THE ANSWER

For example, if a patient's serum calcium level is 8.2 mg/dl and his albumin level is 3 g/dl, what would his corrected calcium be?

8.2 + 0.8 (4 – 3) = 9 mg/dl

The corrected calcium level is within normal range and probably wouldn't be treated.

- · About 41% of all extracellular calcium bound to protein; 9% bound to citrate or other organic ions; remaining 50% ionized (or free) calcium, its only active form
- · Most of ion's physiologic functions carried out by ionized calcium
- · Normal adult range: 4.5 to 5.1 mg/dl
- Almost half bound to albumin (protein)
- Total serum levels possibly influenced by serum protein abnormalities, but ionized calcium levels remain unchanged
- Serum albumin levels considered when evaluating total serum calcium levels (see *Calculating calcium and albumin levels*)
- Has an inverse relationship with phosphorus
  - Increased serum calcium level: results in decreased serum phosphorus level
  - Decreased serum calcium level: results in increased serum phosphorus level
- Recommended daily dietary intake: 800 to 1,200 mg
- Normal concentration in ICF: 10 mEq/L

● **Functions**
  - Responsible, with phosphorus, for formation and structure of bones and teeth
  - Helps maintain cell membrane structure, function, and membrane permeability
  - Affects activation, excitation, and contraction of cardiac and skeletal muscle
  - Participates in neurotransmitter release at synapses

- Helps activate specific steps in blood coagulation
- Activates serum complement, a major factor in immune system function

● **Regulation**
- Absorbed in the small intestine in the presence of vitamin D
- Excreted in urine and feces
- Body levels have several regulators
    - PTH
    - Calcitonin
    - Vitamin D
    - Phosphorus
    - Serum pH
- PTH: when released from the parathyroid glands, draws calcium from bones
    - Promotes transfer (with phosphorus) into plasma
    - Increases serum calcium levels
    - Also promotes kidney reabsorption of calcium and stimulates the intestines to absorb the mineral; phosphorus excreted simultaneously
    - Released when serum calcium levels are low; is suppressed when serum calcium is high
- Calcitonin: produced in the thyroid gland; also helps regulate levels
    - Acts as PTH antagonist
    - Released by the thyroid when calcium levels are too high
    - High levels inhibit bone resorption
        · Decreases amount of calcium available from bone
        · Ultimately decreases serum calcium level
    - Decreases absorption of calcium and enhances its excretion by the kidneys
- Absorption promoted by vitamin D (in active form) through several pathways
    - Intestines
    - Calcium resorption from bone
    - Kidney reabsorption of calcium
    - All raise serum calcium level (see *Calcium in balance,* page 48)
- Ingested with foods (particularly dairy products) and synthesized when skin exposed to ultraviolet light
- Intestinal absorption inhibited by phosphorus
    - Has inverse relationship with calcium; when calcium levels low and the kidneys retain calcium, phosphorus excreted
    - Calcium levels rise: phosphorus levels drop
    - Calcium levels drop: phosphorus levels rise
- Serum pH has inverse relationship with the ionized calcium level
    - Serum pH rises and blood becomes more alkaline: more calcium binds with protein, ionized calcium level drops

Key facts about phosphorus

- Primary anion found in the ICF
- About 85% found in bone and teeth in combination with calcium
- Normal serum level range: 2.5 to 4.5 mEq/dl (1.8 to 2.6 mEq/L)

Key functions of phosphorus

- With calcium, is an essential component of bones and teeth
- Helps maintain cell membrane integrity
- Plays a major role in acid-base balance
- Plays essential roles in muscle and neurologic function and in carbohydrate, protein, and fat metabolism
- Primary ingredient in 2,3-DPG, a compound in RBCs that facilitates oxygen delivery from RBCs to the tissues
- Promotes energy transfer to cells through the formation of energy-storing substances such as ATP
- Important for WBC phagocytosis and platelet function

Calcium in balance

Extracellular calcium levels are normally kept constant by several interrelated processes that move calcium ions into and out of extracellular fluid (ECF). Calcium enters the extracellular space through resorption of calcium ions from bone, through the absorption of dietary calcium in the GI tract, and through reabsorption of calcium from the kidneys. Calcium leaves ECF as it's excreted in stools and urine and deposited in bone tissues. This illustration shows how calcium moves throughout the body.

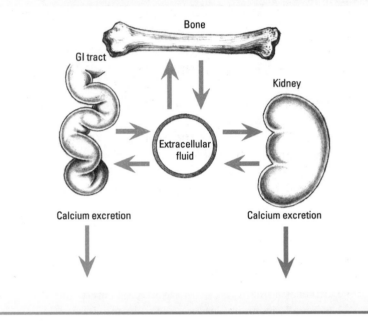

– Serum pH drops and blood becomes more acidotic: less calcium binds to protein, ionized calcium level rises

PHOSPHORUS

General information
- Is the primary anion found in the ICF
- About 85% found in bone and teeth in combination with calcium (1:2 ratio of phosphorus to calcium)
- About 14% in soft tissue
- Less than 1% in ECF
- Normal serum level range: 2.5 to 4.5 mEq/dl (1.8 to 2.6 mEq/L)
- Normal concentration inside cells: 100 mEq/L
- Recommended adult daily requirement: 800 to 1,200 mg

Functions
- With calcium, is an essential component of bones and teeth
- Helps maintain cell membrane integrity (phospholipids make up cell membranes)

- Plays a major role in acid-base balance through acting as urinary buffer; 600 to 900 mg excreted in urine daily
- Plays essential roles in muscle and neurologic function and in carbohydrate, protein, and fat metabolism
- Is a primary ingredient in 2,3-diphosphoglycerate (2-3 DPG), a compound in RBCs that facilitates oxygen delivery from RBCs to the tissues
- Promotes energy transfer to cells through the formation of energy-storing substances such as ATP
- Is important for white blood cell (WBC) phagocytosis and platelet function

● **Regulation**
  - Total body amount related to multiple factors
    – Dietary intake
    – Hormonal regulation
    – Kidney excretion
    – Transcellular shifts
  - Is readily absorbed through the GI tract; amount absorbed is proportional to amount ingested
  - Kidneys excrete about 90% as they regulate serum levels; GI tract excretes remainder
    – Dietary intake of phosphorus increases, kidneys increase excretion to maintain normal phosphorus levels
    – Low-phosphorus diet: causes the kidneys to reabsorb more phosphorus in proximal tubules to conserve it
  - Hormonal regulation controlled by parathyroid glands
    – Also affect PTH activity
    – PTH release affected by changes in calcium, not phosphorus, levels
  - Affected by PTH
    – Influences renal excretion of phosphorus
    – Increases calcium reabsorption in response to decreased calcium level in the ECF
  - Mobilization from bone influenced by PTH levels
  - Has inverse relationship with calcium

MAGNESIUM

● **General information**
  - Is a major cation in the ICF (second to potassium in abundance in ICF)
  - About 60% contained in bone; ECF contains less than 1%, ICF holds remainder
  - Approximately 25 mEq daily supplied by normal diet; of this, about 40% absorbed in the small intestine

Key facts about phosphorus regulation

- Total body amount related to multiple factors
- Readily absorbed through the GI tract
- Kidneys excrete about 90%; GI tract excretes remainder
- Hormonal regulation controlled by parathyroid glands
- Mobilization from bone influenced by PTH levels
- Has inverse relationship with calcium

Key facts about magnesium

- Major cation in the ICF
- About 60% contained in bone
- Approximately 25 mEq daily supplied by normal diet; of this, about 40% absorbed in the small intestine
- Normal serum level: 1.8 to 2.5 mEq/L

Key functions of magnesium

- Promotes enzyme reactions within the cell during carbohydrate metabolism
- Helps the body produce and use ATP for energy
- Takes part in DNA and protein synthesis
- Affects neuromuscular irritability and contractility of cardiac and skeletal muscle
- Affects peripheral vasodilation
- Facilitates transport of sodium and potassium across cell membranes
- Influences intracellular calcium level through its effect on PTH secretion

Key facts about magnesium regulation

- Regulated by GI and urinary systems through absorption, excretion, and retention
- GI tract: tries to adjust to any level change
- Balanced by kidneys

Developmental considerations in electrolyte balance

Pediatric patient
- Vary little from adults in terms of plasma electrolyte concentrations
- Potassium and chloride concentrations highest in first few months of life
- Serum calcium levels correlated with gestational age
- Magnesium and calcium levels low in the first 24 hours after birth
- Normal phosphorus levels significantly higher in children than adults in relation to respective growth needs

- Normal serum level range: 1.8 to 2.5 mEq/L
  - 33% bound to protein
  - Remainder exists as free cations
- Normal concentration in ICF: 40 mEq/L

● **Functions**
- Promotes enzyme reactions within the cell during carbohydrate metabolism
- Helps the body produce and use ATP for energy
- Takes part in deoxyribonucleic acid (DNA) and protein synthesis
- Acts on the myoneural junction, affecting neuromuscular irritability and contractility of cardiac (antiarrhythmic action) and skeletal muscle
- Affects peripheral vasodilation, resulting in changes in blood pressure and cardiac output
- Facilitates transport of sodium and potassium across cell membranes; affects sodium and potassium ion levels both inside and outside the cell
- Influences intracellular calcium level through its effect on PTH secretion

● **Regulation**
- Regulated by GI and urinary systems through absorption, excretion, and retention
  - Dietary intake
  - Output via urine and stools
- GI tract: tries to adjust to any level change
  - Serum magnesium level drops, GI tract may absorb more magnesium
  - Magnesium level rises, GI tract excretes more in stools
- Balanced by kidneys via altered reabsorption at proximal tubule and loop of Henle
  - Serum levels climb, excess secreted by kidneys in urine; effect heightened by diuretics
  - Serum levels fall, kidneys conserve efficiently (daily loss of circulating ionized magnesium can be restricted to just 1 mEq)

DEVELOPMENTAL CONSIDERATIONS

● **Pediatric patient**
- Vary little from adults in terms of plasma electrolyte concentrations
- Potassium and chloride concentrations highest in first few months of life
- Serum calcium levels correlated with gestational age; transient physiologic hyperparathyroidism experienced by neonates
- Magnesium and calcium levels low in the first 24 hours after birth
- Normal phosphorus levels significantly higher in children than adults in relation to respective growth needs

- **Older adult**
  - Water balance influenced by physiologic changes associated with aging
    - Renal function: decreases by 10% after age 65
    - Decreased aldosterone secretion: results in diminished ability to conserve sodium and excrete potassium
    - Decreased calcium absorption: results in greater need for dietary calcium and vitamin D
  - May salt food heavily to compensate for decreased acuity for salt taste
  - Can usually maintain electrolyte balance under normal conditions; may need more time to return to normal after excesses or deficits
  - Don't possess the reserves or ability to adapt readily to rapid changes in fluid balance
  - Disease processes and drug therapy: cause increased risk for electrolyte imbalances

- **Pregnant patient**
  - To meet maternal and fetal needs, retains additional sodium (about 950 mEq [3 to 6 mEq/day])
    - About 60% used by the fetus and placenta
    - Remainder distributed in maternal blood and ECF
  - Plasma sodium concentrations: decrease approximately 5 mEq/L during pregnancy
  - Total serum calcium concentrations: decrease during second or third month of pregnancy; reach lowest level during third trimester
  - Serum magnesium levels: drop from 6% to 8% during pregnancy
  - Approximately 350 mEq of potassium retained during pregnancy
    - Stored in fetus, uterus, breasts, and RBCs
    - Maternal plasma concentrations: remain at prepregnancy levels or slightly lower

Developmental considerations in electrolyte balance
(continued)

Older adult
- Water balance influenced by physiologic changes associated with aging
- May need more time to return to normal after excesses or deficits
- Disease processes and drug therapy: cause increased risk for electrolyte imbalances

Pregnant patient
- Retains additional sodium
- Plasma sodium concentrations: decrease
- Total serum calcium concentrations: decrease during second or third month of pregnancy
- Serum magnesium levels: drop
- Potassium levels: may drop slightly

NCLEX CHECKS

It's never too soon to begin your NCLEX preparation. Now that you've reviewed this chapter, carefully read each of the following questions and choose the best answer. Then compare your responses to the correct answers.

1. Although electrolytes exist inside and outside of cells, measurement of electrolyte levels occurs:
- ☐ **1.** only inside the cells.
- ☐ **2.** outside the cells in the bloodstream.
- ☐ **3.** outside the cells in the interstitial fluid.
- ☐ **4.** in the transcellular spaces.

TOP 10

Items to study for your next test on electrolyte balance

1. Role of electrolyte balance (through regulation by active and passive actions) in maintaining homeostasis
2. Normal ranges for serum levels of each electrolyte (sodium, potassium, chloride, calcium, phosphorus, magnesium)
3. Sodium-potassium pump and ATP activation
4. Organ, gland, and hormonal impact on electrolyte balance
5. Role of each major electrolyte
6. Major cation and anion in body compartments (ICF, ECF)
7. Assessment findings that reflect imbalances of each electrolyte
8. Nursing role in electrolyte maintenance, including awareness of drugs that alter electrolyte balance
9. How electrolytes are replaced, including daily needs
10. Electrolyte variations based upon age, maturation, development, and pregnancy

2. The most abundant cation in ICF is:
- ☐ **1.** potassium.
- ☐ **2.** sodium.
- ☐ **3.** phosphorus.
- ☐ **4.** calcium.

3. Sodium is one of the most important elements in the body. Which statements about sodium are true? Select all that apply.
- ☐ **1.** Sodium is the most abundant anion found in ECF.
- ☐ **2.** Sodium maintains proper ECF osmolality.
- ☐ **3.** 99% of sodium is found in the bones and teeth.
- ☐ **4.** Sodium preserves ECF volume and fluid distribution throughout the body.
- ☐ **5.** Sodium aids in nerve and muscle fiber impulse transmission.
- ☐ **6.** Sodium plays a crucial role in cell membrane integrity.

4. Which electrolyte must be ingested daily?
- ☐ **1.** Calcium
- ☐ **2.** Magnesium
- ☐ **3.** Phosphorus
- ☐ **4.** Potassium

5. A client's serum calcium level is 7 mg/dl. Which would be the most appropriate action for the nurse to take?
- ☐ **1.** Encourage the client to eat peanut butter and bananas.
- ☐ **2.** Remove all calcium from his I.V. fluids.
- ☐ **3.** Encourage him to eat yogurt and green, leafy vegetables.
- ☐ **4.** Prepare to administer phosphorus supplements because that level is probably low.

6. What effect does calcitonin have on serum calcium levels?
- ☐ **1.** No effect
- ☐ **2.** Increases serum calcium level
- ☐ **3.** Decreases serum calcium level
- ☐ **4.** Regulates calcium levels indirectly by altering phosphorus levels

7. How does the sodium-potassium pump function?
- ☐ **1.** It allows for sodium to diffuse inside cells and potassium to diffuse outside cells.
- ☐ **2.** It prevents solute movement across cell membranes.
- ☐ **3.** It's a passive transport mechanism that maintains normal sodium and potassium levels.
- ☐ **4.** It allows sodium to move out of the cell and returns potassium to inside the cell.

8. A client receiving furosemide (Lasix) should be monitored closely for which electrolyte imbalance?
- ☐ **1.** Hypermagnesemia
- ☐ **2.** Hypophosphatemia
- ☐ **3.** Hypokalemia
- ☐ **4.** Hypercalcemia

9. Which structure plays a major role in balancing calcium and phosphorus levels?
- ☐ **1.** Lungs
- ☐ **2.** Parathyroid glands
- ☐ **3.** Adrenal cortex
- ☐ **4.** Hypothalamus

10. A state of acidosis places a client at risk for which electrolyte imbalance?
- ☐ **1.** Hypokalemia
- ☐ **2.** Hyperkalemia
- ☐ **3.** Hypomagnesemia
- ☐ **4.** Hypermagnesemia

ANSWERS AND RATIONALES

1. CORRECT ANSWER: 2
Electrolyte levels are only measured outside the cells (extracellular) in the bloodstream.

2. CORRECT ANSWER: 1
Potassium is the most abundant cation in ICF. Sodium is the most abundant cation in ECF. Calcium is found in both ICF and ECF. Phosphorus is the primary anion found in ICF.

3. CORRECT ANSWER: 2, 4, 5
Sodium is the most abundant cation found in ECF. 99% of calcium is found in the bones and teeth. Phosphorus plays a crucial role in cell membrane integrity.

4. CORRECT ANSWER: 4
Because the body can't conserve potassium, it must be ingested daily. Calcium, magnesium, and phosphorus are stored in the bones and, in lesser amounts, in other areas of the body.

5. CORRECT ANSWER: 3
Normal calcium ranges from 8.9 to 10.1 mg/dl, so the client's calcium level is low. The client's albumin level would determine if supplements were needed, and that information wasn't supplied. The most appropriate action would be to encourage calcium-rich foods such as yogurt and green, leafy vegetables. Peanut butter and bananas are good sources of potassium. Removing calcium from his I.V. fluid would further decrease serum calcium

levels. His phosphorus level is most likely high (remember, calcium and phosphorus have an inverse relationship), so phosphorus supplementation isn't necessary.

6. CORRECT ANSWER: 3

Calcitonin decreases calcium levels by decreasing the amount of calcium available from the bone, decreasing the absorption of calcium, and enhancing its excretion from the kidneys.

7. CORRECT ANSWER: 4

The sodium-potassium pump, an active transport mechanism, uses energy in the form of ATP to move sodium out of cells and potassium back into cells.

8. CORRECT ANSWER: 3

Because Lasix allows for potassium excretion, the client should be monitored for hypokalemia.

9. CORRECT ANSWER: 2

The parathyroid glands secrete PTH, which is released to promote kidney reabsorption of calcium and excretion of phosphorus to maintain normal serum levels.

10. CORRECT ANSWER: 2

Hydrogen ions and potassium ions freely exchange across cell membranes to keep the ICF electrically neutral. In acidosis, excess hydrogen moves into cells and potassium moves out of the cells to maintain balance. This process increases serum potassium levels and places the client at risk for hyperkalemia.

4

Acid-base balance

LEARNING OBJECTIVES

After studying this chapter, you should be able to:

- Differentiate between acids and bases.
- Discuss the role of buffering chemicals in the body.
- Describe how the respiratory and renal systems regulate acid-base balance.
- Identify normal and abnormal arterial blood gas results.

CHAPTER OVERVIEW

Acid-base balance is maintained by controlling the hydrogen ion concentration of the extracellular fluid (ECF). Buffer systems in the body regulate the acid-base balance by taking up or adding hydrogen or hydroxyl ions. The lungs and kidneys are the major regulators of acid-base balance. The lungs compensate for metabolic disturbances; the kidneys compensate for respiratory disturbances. Acid-base balance is measured using arterial blood gas (ABG) levels and anion gap results.

Interpreting normal pH

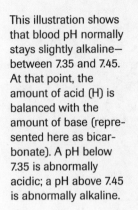

This illustration shows that blood pH normally stays slightly alkaline—between 7.35 and 7.45. At that point, the amount of acid (H) is balanced with the amount of base (represented here as bicarbonate). A pH below 7.35 is abnormally acidic; a pH above 7.45 is abnormally alkaline.

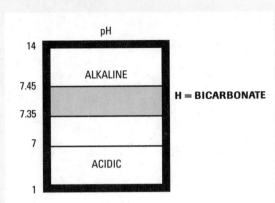

INTRODUCTION

- **Definition**
  - *Acid-base balance:* refers to homeostasis of hydrogen ion concentration in body fluids
  - Concentration of hydrogen ions in body fluid expressed as pH
  - Body fluids classified as acids or bases according to hydrogen ion concentration
    - Acid: hydrogen ion donor
      - Solution containing more acid than base has more hydrogen and a lower pH
      - Solution with a pH below 7: classified as an acid, or acidic (carbonic acid is an example)
    - Base: hydrogen ion acceptor
      - Solution containing more base than acid has less hydrogen and a higher pH
      - Solution with a pH above 7: classified as a base, or alkaline (bicarbonate [HCO_3^-] is an example)

- **Hydrogen ion concentration**
  - Acid-base balance maintained by controlling hydrogen ion concentration of body fluids, specifically ECF
  - pH numerical value inversely proportional to number of hydrogen ions in solution
    - Hydrogen ion concentration rises, pH falls
    - Hydrogen ion concentration falls, pH rises
  - Normal blood pH range: 7.35 to 7.45
  - pH below 6.8 or above 7.8 incompatible with life (see *Interpreting normal pH*)

Recognizing acidosis

Acidosis, a condition in which pH is below 7.35, occurs when acids (H) accumulate or bases, such as bicarbonate, are lost.

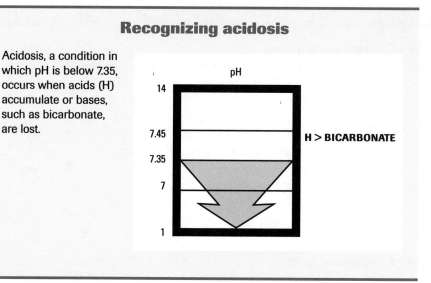

Recognizing alkalosis

Alkalosis, a condition in which pH is higher than 7.45, occurs when bases (such as bicarbonate) accumulate or acids (H) are lost.

● **Imbalances**
  • *Acidosis*: an excess of hydrogen ions
    – Results from either acid excess or base deficit
    – Marked by pH less than 7.35 (see *Recognizing acidosis*)
  • *Alkalosis*: a deficit of hydrogen ions
    – Results from either base excess or acid deficit
    – Marked by pH more than 7.45 (see *Recognizing alkalosis*)

Types of acid–base imbalances

Acidosis
● Excess of hydrogen ions
● Marked by pH less than 7.35

Alkalosis
● Deficit of hydrogen ions
● Marked by pH more than 7.45

Key facts about buffer regulation of acid-base balance

- Body pH fairly constant; hydrogen ion concentration affected by water-diluted products of metabolism
- Cells: buffer by taking up or releasing extra hydrogen ions
- Buffers: regulate hydrogen ion concentration

Key facts about buffers

Bicarbonate

- Mainly responsible for buffering blood and interstitial fluid
- Rely on a series of chemical reactions in which pairs of weak acids and bases combine with stronger acids and bases to weaken them
- Assisted by organs: kidneys and lungs

Phosphate

- Depend on a series of chemical reactions to minimize pH changes
- React with either acids or bases to form compounds that slightly alter pH
- Especially effective in renal tubules

Protein

- Most abundant buffers in the body
- Work both inside and outside of cells
- Bind with acids and bases to neutralize them

BUFFER REGULATION OF ACID-BASE BALANCE

● General information

- Body pH fairly constant; hydrogen ion concentration affected by water-diluted products of metabolism
  - Kidneys excrete only 1%
  - Lungs and other buffers handle remainder
- Cells: buffer by taking up or releasing extra hydrogen ions
  - Involves exchanging potassium for hydrogen
  - Affects potassium balance
- Buffers: regulate hydrogen ion concentration
  - Take up or release hydrogen or hydroxyl ions
  - Temporarily minimize the effect of hydrogen or HCO_3^- on blood pH until renal or respiratory system takes effect

● Bicarbonate buffers

- Make up the body's primary buffer system
- Mainly responsible for buffering blood and interstitial fluid
- Rely on a series of chemical reactions in which pairs of weak acids and bases (such as carbonic acid and bicarbonate) combine with stronger acids (such as hydrochloric acid) and bases to weaken them
- Decrease the strength of potentially damaging acids and bases, reducing the danger those chemicals pose to pH balance
- Assisted by organs
  - Kidneys: regulate bicarbonate production
  - Lungs: regulate carbonic acid production, which itself results from combining carbon dioxide (CO_2) and water

● Phosphate buffers

- Like bicarbonate buffers, depend on a series of chemical reactions to minimize pH changes
- React with either acids or bases to form compounds that slightly alter pH; can provide extremely effective buffering
- Prove especially effective in renal tubules, where phosphates exist in greater concentration

● Protein buffers

- Are the most abundant buffers in the body
- Work both inside and outside of cells
- Are made up of hemoglobin as proteins
- Behave chemically like bicarbonate buffers; bind with acids and bases to neutralize them (for example, in red blood cells, hemoglobin combines with hydrogen to act as a buffer)

RESPIRATORY SYSTEM REGULATION AND COMPENSATION

● **General information**
- System: has multiple functions
  - Serves as second line of defense against acid-base imbalance
  - As buffer, can maintain acid-base balance twice as effectively as chemical buffers (can handle twice the amount of acids and bases)
  - Responds to pH changes within minutes
    - Can only restore normal pH temporarily
    - Kidneys responsible for long-term pH adjustments

● **Regulation**
- Blood levels of CO_2 (gas that combines with water to form carbonic acid) regulated by lungs; decreased pH caused by increased levels of carbonic acid
- Chemoreceptors in brain's medulla sense pH changes; vary breathing rate and depth to compensate
  - Body responds to low pH
    - Breathes faster or deeper to eliminate more CO_2 from the lungs
    - CO_2 level in blood drops while pH increases
  - Body responds to high pH
    - Breathes slower or less deeply
    - Reduces CO_2 excretion and lowers pH
- Partial pressure of arterial CO_2 in arterial blood ($Paco_2$) used to assess effectiveness of ventilation
  - Normal $Paco_2$ level: 35 to 45 mm Hg
  - $Paco_2$ levels reflect CO_2 levels in the blood; levels increase concurrently

● **Compensation**
- Lungs: compensate for metabolic disturbances by retaining or removing CO_2, minimizing change in serum pH
- *Metabolic alkalosis:* bicarbonate excess
  - Suppresses the rate and depth of respirations
  - Causes CO_2 retention and carbonic acid buildup
- *Metabolic acidosis:* bicarbonate deficit
  - Causes increased rate and depth of respirations
  - Causes greater elimination of CO_2

RENAL SYSTEM REGULATION AND COMPENSATION

● **General information**
- System has several functions and characteristics
  - Slowest of all regulating systems
  - Takes from a few hours to several days to adjust to changes
  - Can permanently adjust blood pH

Key facts about respiratory system regulation and compensation

- Serves as second line of defense against acid-base imbalance
- Responds to pH changes within minutes
- Can only restore normal pH temporarily; kidneys responsible for long-term pH adjustments

Regulation
- Blood levels of CO_2 regulated by lungs
- Chemoreceptors in brain's medulla sense pH changes
- Body responds to low pH: breathes faster or deeper to eliminate more CO_2 from the lungs; CO_2 level in blood drops while pH increases
- Body responds to high pH: breathes slower or less deeply; reduces CO_2 excretion and lowers pH
- Normal $Paco_2$ level: 35 to 45 mm Hg

Compensation
- Metabolic alkalosis: bicarbonate excess; suppresses the rate and depth of respirations; causes CO_2 retention and carbonic acid buildup
- Metabolic acidosis: bicarbonate deficit; causes increased rate and depth of respirations; causes greater elimination of CO_2

Key facts about renal system regulation and compensation

- Slowest of all regulating systems
- Takes from a few hours to several days to adjust to changes
- Can permanently adjust blood pH
- Kidneys: can reabsorb acids and bases or excrete them into urine; can also produce bicarbonate to replenish lost supplies

Regulation: if too much acid, not enough base

- pH drops, kidneys reabsorb sodium bicarbonate
- Hydrogen, along with phosphate or ammonia, excreted by kidneys
- Bicarbonate level in blood rises; increases pH

Regulation: if more base and less acid

- pH rises: kidneys excrete bicarbonate and retain more hydrogen ions
- Blood bicarbonate levels drop, pH decreases

Compensation

- Kidneys: excrete or retain hydrogen and bicarbonate
- Respiratory acidosis: kidneys excrete hydrogen and conserve bicarbonate to restore balance
- Respiratory alkalosis: kidneys retain hydrogen and excrete bicarbonate to restore balance

Key facts about measurement of acid-base balance

- ABG measurements: the major diagnostic tool for evaluating acid-base balance
- Anion gap helps differentiate acidotic conditions

- Kidneys: can reabsorb acids and bases or excrete them into urine; can also produce bicarbonate to replenish lost supplies

● **Regulation**
  - Kidneys: regulate bicarbonate level (reflects metabolic component of acid-base balance)
    – Level reported with ABG results (normal level: 22 to 26 mEq/L)
    – Level also reported with serum electrolyte levels as total serum CO_2 content
  - Problems apparent if blood contains too much acid or not enough base
    – pH drops, kidneys reabsorb sodium bicarbonate
    – Hydrogen, along with phosphate or ammonia, excreted by kidneys
    – Urine more acidic than normal
    – Bicarbonate formed in the renal tubules by bicarbonate reabsorption and increased hydrogen excretion; eventually retained in body
    – Bicarbonate level in blood rises to a more normal level; increases pH
  - Problems also apparent if blood contains more base and less acid
    – pH rises, kidneys excrete bicarbonate and retain more hydrogen ions
    – Urine becomes more alkaline, blood bicarbonate levels drop, pH decreases

● **Compensation**
  - Kidneys: excrete or retain hydrogen and bicarbonate
    – Carbonic acid excess (respiratory acidosis): kidneys excrete hydrogen and conserve bicarbonate to restore balance
    – Carbonic acid deficit (respiratory alkalosis): kidneys retain hydrogen and excrete bicarbonate to restore balance
  - Hydrogen exchanges for potassium; raises or lowers pH

MEASUREMENT OF ACID-BASE BALANCE

● **General information**
  - Acids and bases: mainly leave body through gas exchange between cells and external environment; gas measurement reflects acid-base balance
  - Arterial blood gas measurements: the major diagnostic tool for evaluating acid-base balance; anion gap result helps differentiate various acidotic conditions
  - Related methods of measurement
    – Transcutaneous blood gas measurements
    – Pulse oximetry
    – Serum potassium levels
    – Total CO_2 and chloride levels

ABG analysis

- Help determine a patient's acid-base status, evaluate pulmonary gas exchange efficiency, assess the respiratory system, evaluate blood oxygenation, and monitor respiratory therapy
- ABG levels analyzed in blood samples obtained from one of several arteries
    - Radial
    - Brachial
    - Femoral
    - May also come from an arterial line
- Six parameters included in ABG measurements
    - pH
    - $PaCO_2$
    - Bicarbonate (HCO_3^-) concentration
    - Base excess
    - Partial pressure of oxygen in arterial blood (PaO_2)
    - Oxygen saturation (SaO_2)
- pH levels: indicate blood acidity
    - Normal range: 7.35 to 7.45
    - pH greater than 7.45: indicates alkalosis
    - pH less than 7.35: indicates acidosis
    - Normal or borderline pH: has several possible indications
        - Normal acid-base balance
        - Body attempting to compensate for slightly abnormal or chronic acid-base imbalance
- $PaCO_2$ levels: indicate the partial pressure of CO_2 in arterial blood
    - Used to evaluate the respiratory acid-base component
    - Normal range: 35 to 45 mm Hg
    - $PaCO_2$ values greater than 45 mm Hg: hypoventilation or excessive CO_2 retention (hypercapnia) and therefore acidosis
    - $PaCO_2$ values less than 35 mm Hg: hyperventilation or excessive CO_2 exhalation (hypocapnia) and therefore alkalosis (see *Quick look at ABG results,* page 62, and *Inaccurate ABG results,* page 62)
- HCO_3^- levels: reflect the arterial blood's HCO_3^- concentration
    - Used to evaluate the metabolic acid-base component
    - Normal range: 22 to 26 mEq/L
    - HCO_3^- values greater than 26 mEq/L: alkalosis
    - HCO_3^- values less than 22 mEq/L: acidosis
- Base excess: reflects level of HCO_3^- and other bases such as plasma proteins and hemoglobin
    - Used to evaluate metabolic acid-base component
    - Normal range: −2 to +2
    - Base excess values greater than +2: base excess (acid deficit) in metabolic alkalosis
    - Base excess values less than −2: base deficit (acid excess) in metabolic acidosis

(see *Quick look at ABG results,* page 62, and *Inaccurate ABG results,* page 62)

Key facts about ABG analysis

- Determine acid-base status
- Evaluate pulmonary gas exchange efficiency
- Evaluate blood oxygenation
- Monitor respiratory therapy

Six parameters included in ABG measurements

- pH
- $PaCO_2$
- HCO_3^- concentration
- Base excess
- PaO_2
- SaO_2

Key facts about levels

pH
- Indicates blood acidity
- Normal range: 7.35 to 7.45

$PaCO_2$
- Indicates partial pressure of CO_2 in arterial blood
- Normal range: 35 to 45 mm Hg

HCO_3^-
- Reflects the arterial blood's HCO_3^- concentration
- Normal range: 22 to 26 mEq/L

Base excess
- Reflects level of HCO_3^-
- Normal range: −2 to +2

PaO_2
- Reveals lungs' ability to oxygenate blood
- Normal range: 80 to 100 mm Hg

SaO_2
- Reflects oxygen-carrying capacity of hemoglobin
- Normal range: 95% to 100%

Quick look at ABG results

Here's a quick look at how to interpret arterial blood gas (ABG) results and the questions you need to ask:

- Check the pH. Is it normal (7.35 to 7.45), acidotic (below 7.35), or alkalotic (above 7.45)?
- Determine the partial pressure of arterial carbon dioxide ($Paco_2$) level. Is it normal (35 to 45 mm Hg), low, or high?
- Watch the bicarbonate (HCO_3^-) level. Is it normal (22 to 26 mEq/L), low, or high?
- Look for signs of compensation. Which value ($Paco_2$ or HCO_3^-) more closely corresponds to the change in pH?
- Determine the partial pressure of arterial oxygen (Pao_2) and oxygen saturation (Sao_2) levels. Is the Pao_2 normal (80 to 100 mm Hg), low, or high? Is the Sao_2 normal (95% to 100%), low, or high?

Inaccurate ABG results

To avoid altering arterial blood gas (ABG) results, be sure to use proper technique when drawing a sample of arterial blood. Remember:

- A delay in getting the sample to the laboratory or in drawing blood for ABG analysis within 15 to 20 minutes of a procedure (such as suctioning or administering a respiratory treatment) could alter results.
- Air bubbles in the syringe could affect the oxygen level.
- Venous blood in the syringe could alter carbon dioxide and oxygen levels and pH.

- Pao_2 levels: reflect partial pressure of oxygen in arterial blood
  – Reveals lungs' ability to oxygenate blood
  – Normal range: 80 to 100 mm Hg (varies with age)
  – Pao_2 levels not used to evaluate acid-base status
  – Pao_2 values less than 80 mm Hg: hypoxemia
- Sao_2 levels: reflect oxygen-carrying capacity of hemoglobin
  – Help evaluate respiratory function
  – Not used to evaluate acid-base status
  – Normal range: 95% to 100%

● Anion gap result

- Is the arithmetical difference between the concentration of routinely measured cations (sodium and potassium) and routinely measured anions (chloride and bicarbonate)
- Cations (positively charged ions) and anions (negatively charged ions): must be equal in the blood to maintain a proper balance of electrical charges

Key facts about anion gap result

- Difference between the concentration of cations and anions
- Cations and anions: must be equal in the blood to maintain a proper balance of electrical charges

Calculating the anion gap

This illustration depicts the normal anion gap. The gap is calculated by adding the chloride level and the bicarbonate level and then subtracting that total from the sodium level. The value normally ranges from 8 to 14 mEq/L and represents the level of unmeasured anions in extracellular fluid.

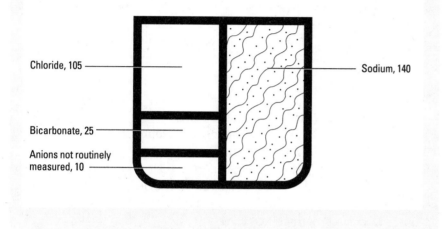

Chloride, 105

Sodium, 140

Bicarbonate, 25

Anions not routinely
measured, 10

● Anion gap identification

- 90% of circulating cations accounted for by sodium; 85% of counter-balancing anions accounted for by chloride and bicarbonate together (potassium generally omitted because it occurs in such low, stable amounts)
- Gap between the two measurements represents anions not routinely measured
    - Sulfates
    - Phosphates
    - Proteins
    - Organic acids such as lactic acid and ketone acids (see *Calculating the anion gap*)

● Anion gap interpretation

- Normal result range: 8 to 14 mEq/L
- Increase greater than 14 mEq/L: indicates increase in percentage of one or more unmeasured anions in bloodstream
- Increases: can occur with acidotic conditions characterized by higher-than-normal amounts of organic acids
    - Lactic acidosis
    - Ketoacidosis
- Anion gap: normal for certain other conditions
    - Hyperchloremic acidosis
    - Renal tubular acidosis

Key facts about anion gap identification

- 90% of cations comprised of sodium
- 85% of anions comprised of chloride and bicarbonate
- Anion gap: represents anions not routinely measured

Key facts about anion gap interpretation

- Normal result range: 8 to 14 mEq/L
- Increase greater than 14 mEq/L: indicates increase in percentage of one or more unmeasured anions in bloodstream; can occur with acidotic conditions

Developmental considerations in acid-base balance

Pediatric patient
- Neonates: have less homeostatic buffering capacity than older children and adults
- Tend toward slight metabolic acidosis (pH: 7.30 to 7.35)

Older adult
- Experiences physiologic changes that influence acid-base balance
- May need more time to return to normal after acidosis or alkalosis

Pregnant patient
- Associated with compensated respiratory alkalosis (pH: 7.44)
- $Paco_2$ decreased
- HCO_3^- levels: drop
- Total buffering capacity reduced by renal compensation

– Severe bicarbonate wasting conditions
  - Biliary or pancreatic fistula
  - Poorly functioning ileal loops

DEVELOPMENTAL CONSIDERATIONS

- **Pediatric patient**
  - Neonates: have less homeostatic buffering capacity than older children and adults
    – Tend toward slight metabolic acidosis (may be related to high metabolic acid production and renal immaturity)
    – pH average: 7.30 to 7.35

- **Older adult**
  - Experiences physiologic changes that influence acid-base balance
    – Decreased distal tubule response to vasopressin results in reduced ability to correct acid-base imbalances
    – Decreased chest wall compliance, elasticity of lung tissue, number of alveoli, and strength of expiratory muscles lead to difficulty in regulating pH if patient experiences stress to the body
    – Decreased normal Pao_2 level
  - Can usually maintain acid-base balance under normal conditions; may need more time to return to normal after acidosis or alkalosis
  - Doesn't possess reserves or ability to adapt readily to rapid changes in acid-base status

- **Pregnant patient**
  - Pregnancy associated with compensated respiratory alkalosis; believed to be caused by hyperventilation from stimulating effects of progesterone on the respiratory center
  - $Paco_2$ decreased to approximately 30 mm Hg during pregnancy
  - Arterial pH: approximately 7.44
  - HCO_3^- levels: drop to approximately 20 mEq/L by third trimester
  - Total buffering capacity reduced by renal compensation; hydrogen ion content in the body determines pH

NCLEX CHECKS

It's never too soon to begin your NCLEX preparation. Now that you've reviewed this chapter, carefully read each of the following questions and choose the best answer. Then compare your responses to the correct answers.

1. Understanding acids and bases requires an understanding of pH. What does pH reflect?
- ☐ **1.** Sodium and potassium concentration
- ☐ **2.** Relationship of cations to anions
- ☐ **3.** Hydrogen ion concentration
- ☐ **4.** Oxygen concentration

2. Chemical buffers in the body restore acid-base balance by:
- ☐ **1.** binding or reacting with acids and bases to weaken or neutralize them.
- ☐ **2.** changing breathing pattern.
- ☐ **3.** increasing excretion of acids and bases.
- ☐ **4.** producing bicarbonate.

3. What effect does breathing faster have on arterial pH level?
- ☐ **1.** No effect
- ☐ **2.** Increases arterial pH
- ☐ **3.** Decreases arterial pH
- ☐ **4.** Provides long-term pH regulation

4. An arterial pH of 7.29 indicates blood that:
- ☐ **1.** is electrically neutral.
- ☐ **2.** contains too much acid or not enough base.
- ☐ **3.** contains too much base or not enough acid.
- ☐ **4.** contains an equal ratio of acids and bases.

5. Which is responsible for regulating the metabolic component of acid-base balance?
- ☐ **1.** Chemical buffers
- ☐ **2.** Arterial CO_2 levels
- ☐ **3.** The kidneys
- ☐ **4.** The lungs

6. A client was just placed on mechanical ventilation for a worsening respiratory status. Which ABG parameter indicates the effectiveness of the ventilator breaths?
- ☐ **1.** HCO_3^-
- ☐ **2.** Pa_{CO_2}
- ☐ **3.** Pa_{O_2}
- ☐ **4.** Sa_{O_2}

7. Which are considered regulators of acid-base balance in the body? Select all that apply.
- ☐ **1.** Bicarbonate buffers
- ☐ **2.** Hydrogen buffers
- ☐ **3.** Lungs
- ☐ **4.** Kidneys
- ☐ **5.** Parathyroid glands
- ☐ **6.** Protein buffers

TOP 10

Items to study for your next test on acid-base balance

1. Acid-base values as inversely proportional to the number of H+ ions and measured as pH
2. Very limited margins of acid-base balance
3. Adjustments to and regulation of acid-base balances through several mechanisms that involve the lungs, kidneys, and chemical responses
4. Respiratory system actions that regulate acid-base balance
5. The kidney's role in acid-base balance regulation
6. Sequencing of body responses to imbalances based upon metabolic or respiratory causes (first- and second-line defenses)
7. Diagnostic tests used to measure acid-base balances
8. Normal arterial blood gas parameters
9. Assessment findings that reflect acid-base imbalances
10. Variations of acid-base balance based upon age, gender, maturation, pregnancy, and metabolic rate

8. The anion gap calculation indicates:
- ☐ **1.** the difference in arterial hydrogen and bicarbonate concentrations.
- ☐ **2.** the body's risk of certain alkalotic conditions.
- ☐ **3.** the relationship between arterial CO_2 and O_2 concentrations.
- ☐ **4.** the relationship between the body's cations and anions.

9. An alkalotic condition will cause the kidneys to:
- ☐ **1.** reabsorb bicarbonate.
- ☐ **2.** acidify the urine.
- ☐ **3.** excrete hydrogen.
- ☐ **4.** excrete bicarbonate.

10. Kidney compensation to acid-base imbalances can be expected to occur:
- ☐ **1.** immediately.
- ☐ **2.** within minutes.
- ☐ **3.** within hours or days.
- ☐ **4.** within 1 month.

ANSWERS AND RATIONALES

1. CORRECT ANSWER: 3
pH is a calculation based on the percentage of hydrogen ions in a solution as well as the amount of acids and bases. The anion gap result reflects the relationship of cations to anions. PaO_2 and SaO_2 are indicative of O_2 concentration.

2. CORRECT ANSWER: 1
Chemical buffers neutralize or weaken acids and bases as needed by binding or reacting with them. The respiratory system regulates acid-base balance by changing breathing pattern. The kidneys produce bicarbonate to regulate acid-base balance.

3. CORRECT ANSWER: 2
Because breathing faster or deeper eliminates more CO_2 from the lungs, the level of CO_2 in arterial blood drops and pH rises. A change in breathing pattern provides only temporary pH regulation.

4. CORRECT ANSWER: 2
Normal serum pH ranges from 7.35 to 7.45. A pH of 7.29 indicates a state of acidosis—blood that contains too much acid or not enough base.

5. CORRECT ANSWER: 3
Bicarbonate reflects the metabolic component of acid-base balance. Bicarbonate levels are regulated by the kidneys.

6. CORRECT ANSWER: 2

PaCO_2 allows for evaluation of the effectiveness of ventilation. HCO_3^- reflects the metabolic component of acid-base balance. PaO_2 and SaO_2 yield information about the client's oxygenation status.

7. CORRECT ANSWER: 1, 3, 4, 6

The lungs and kidneys are the major regulators of acid-base balance. Bicarbonate, protein, and phosphate buffers contribute to the maintenance of acid-base balance as well.

8. CORRECT ANSWER: 4

The anion gap calculation reflects the relationship between the body's cations and anions. It's useful in differentiating various acidotic conditions.

9. CORRECT ANSWER: 4

In an alkalotic condition, the kidneys will excrete bicarbonate and retain more hydrogen. This process makes urine more alkaline and lowers blood pH. Reabsorption of bicarbonate, excretion of hydrogen, and acidification of urine occur in response to acidotic conditions.

10. CORRECT ANSWER: 3

Kidney compensation to acid-base imbalances can be expected to occur within hours or days. Chemical buffers function immediately. Respiratory compensation occurs within minutes.

5

Fluid imbalances

LEARNING OBJECTIVES

After studying this chapter, you should be able to:

● Describe the different types of fluid imbalances and how they occur.

● Discuss assessment findings and laboratory results associated with each type of fluid imbalance.

● Identify appropriate nursing care for patients with fluid imbalances.

● Describe patients at greatest risk for fluid imbalances.

CHAPTER OVERVIEW

Fluid imbalances can occur in the extracellular fluid (ECF) and the intracellular fluid (ICF) and are commonly classified as isotonic, hypotonic, or hypertonic. Fluids can also accumulate in an abnormal compartment other than the ECF and ICF; this abnormal accumulation is called *third-space fluid shifting*. Nursing care for a patient with a fluid imbalance involves an accurate assessment, including diagnostic testing. Nursing interventions focus on restoring fluid balance through careful monitoring of intake and output and all body systems.

INTRODUCTION

- **Types of imbalances**
  - Are of three common types
    - Isotonic
    - Hypotonic
    - Hypertonic
  - Can be classified as volume imbalances or osmotic imbalances
  - Volume imbalances
    - Primarily affect ECF
    - Involve relatively equal losses or gains of sodium (Na) and water
  - Osmotic imbalances
    - Primarily affect ICF
    - Involve relatively unequal losses or gains of sodium and water
    - May result in dehydration if water loss is excessive

ECF VOLUME DEFICIT

- **General information**
  - Also known as *hypovolemia*
  - Results from relatively equal losses of sodium and water
  - Volume losses due to ECF
    - Sodium-to-water ratio essentially unchanged; therefore, osmolality unaffected
    - Antidiuretic hormone (ADH) and aldosterone secretion inactive; results in fluid not shifting from ICF to ECF
  - Initial signs and symptoms subtle as the body tries to compensate for the loss of circulating blood volume
    - Can become more serious
    - If not detected and treated early, can progress to *hypovolemic shock*, a common form of shock

- **Causes**
  - Prolonged vomiting or gastric suction
  - Excessive diarrhea
  - Hemorrhage (bleeding may be *frank* [obvious] or *occult* [hidden])
  - Profound urine loss, such as polyuria from diabetic ketoacidosis or diuresis
  - Excessive laxative use
  - Excessive sweating
  - Fever
  - Fistulas
  - Renal failure with increased urination
  - Third-space shifting, such as that which occurs in burns, intestinal obstruction, and peritonitis

- **Assessment findings**
  - Weight loss

Types of fluid imbalances

- Isotonic
- Hypotonic
- Hypertonic

Classifying fluid imbalances

Volume imbalances
- Affect ECF
- Involve equal losses or gains of sodium and water

Osmotic imbalances
- Affect ICF
- Involve unequal losses or gains of sodium and water

Key facts about ECF volume deficit

- Also known as *hypovolemia*
- Results from relatively equal losses of sodium and water
- Volume losses due to the ECF
- If not detected and treated early, can progress to *hypovolemic shock*

Common causes of ECF volume deficit

- Vomiting or gastric suction
- Diarrhea
- Hemorrhage
- Urine loss

Warning signs of hypovolemia

- Cool, pale skin
- Decreased central venous pressure
- Deterioration in mental status
- Flat jugular veins
- Thirst
- Urine output dropping below 10 ml/hour
- Weak or absent peripheral pulses

Common assessment findings in ECF volume deficit

- Weight loss
- Hypotension
- Tachycardia
- Oliguria
- Delayed capillary refill
- Altered LOC
- Hypovolemic shock

Testing for ECF volume deficit

- Increased urine specific gravity
- Increased HCT
- Increased serum osmolality
- Increased BUN level
- Normal or high serum sodium level

Warning signs of hypovolemia

Begin emergency treatment for hypovolemia and impending shock if a patient shows any of these signs and symptoms:

- cool, pale skin over the arms and legs
- decreased central venous pressure
- delayed capillary refill
- deterioration in mental status (from restlessness and anxiety to unconsciousness)
- flat jugular veins
- orthostatic hypotension progressing to marked hypotension
- tachycardia
- thirst
- urine output initially more than 30 ml/minute, then dropping below 10 ml/hour
- weak or absent peripheral pulses
- weight loss.

  - – 5% to 10% drop: mild-to-moderate fluid loss
  - – More than 10% drop: severe fluid loss
- Hypotension
- Orthostatic hypotension
- Tachycardia
- Oliguria
- Decreased skin turgor and cool, pale skin
- Delayed capillary refill
- Dry, furrowed tongue
- Soft eyeballs (can be detected by applying gentle pressure on top of the eyelid)
- Sticky oral mucosa
- Altered level of consciousness (LOC), irritability, and confusion
- Slow-filling jugular veins
- Hypovolemic shock (with prolonged, severe hypovolemia) (see *Warning signs of hypovolemia*)

Diagnostic findings
- Several results increased
  - – Urine specific gravity
  - – Hematocrit (HCT)
  - – Serum osmolality
  - – Blood urea nitrogen (BUN) level
- Normal or high serum sodium level (greater than 145 mEq/L), depending on the amount of fluid and sodium lost
- Normal serum creatinine level in relation to an elevated BUN level

Treatment
- Oral fluids generally inadequate; isotonic fluids given instead
  - – Administered I.V.
  - – Expand circulating volume
  - – Include normal saline and lactated Ringer's solutions
  - – Commonly followed by plasma protein infusion (such as albumin)

Hemodynamic values in hypovolemic shock

Hemodynamic monitoring can help you evaluate your patient's cardiovascular status in hypovolemic shock. Look for these values:

- central venous pressure below the normal range (2 to 8 mm Hg)
- pulmonary artery pressure below the normal mean (10 to 20 mm Hg)
- pulmonary artery wedge pressure below the normal mean (6 to 12 mm Hg)
- cardiac output below the normal range (4 to 8 L/minute).

- Blood transfusion (if patient is hemorrhaging)
- Vasopressors
  - May be needed to support blood pressure until fluid levels normalize
  - Need to be used cautiously to not worsen already inadequate organ perfusion
  - Drugs of choice: norepinephrine or dopamine
- Oxygen therapy (ensures sufficient tissue perfusion)

● **Nursing interventions**
- Monitor fluid intake and output to determine the need for replacement therapy
- Check daily weight, watching for a loss that may indicate fluid deficit (a 1-lb [0.45-kg] weight loss equals a 500-ml fluid loss)
- Monitor vital signs to detect increased pulse or decreased blood pressure
- Monitor hemodynamics (cardiac output, central venous pressure [CVP], pulmonary artery pressure, and pulmonary artery wedge pressure), using arterial cannulation (if available), to judge how well the patient responds to treatment (see *Hemodynamic values in hypovolemic shock*)
- Monitor the quality of peripheral pulses and monitor skin temperature and appearance to assess for continued peripheral vascular constriction
- Assess skin turgor by evaluating resilience and resistance on the forehead or the shoulders; easily pinched skin in these locations may indicate volume deficit (the extremities aren't as useful for assessing skin turgor because of skin changes that normally occur with aging and disease)
- Assess oral mucous membranes; sticky mucous membranes and a dry tongue may indicate fluid volume loss
- Monitor the results of laboratory studies—particularly BUN levels and HCT, which may increase in volume deficit
- Assess LOC; altered LOC may occur in severe volume deficit
- Apply and adjust oxygen therapy as ordered

Key hemodynamic findings in hypovolemic shock

- Central venous pressure below the normal range
- Pulmonary artery pressure below the normal mean
- Pulmonary artery wedge pressure below the normal mean
- Cardiac output below the normal range

Key treatment options for ECF volume deficit

- I.V. isotonic fluids
- Plasma protein infusion
- Blood transfusion
- Vasopressor

Key nursing interventions for a patient with ECF volume deficit

- Monitor fluid intake and output.
- Check daily weight daily.
- Monitor hemodynamic values.
- Assess skin turgor.
- Assess oral mucous membranes.
- Monitor results of laboratory studies.
- Assess LOC.
- Administer I.V. fluids.
- Encourage oral fluids.

- If the patient is bleeding, apply direct, continuous pressure to the area and elevate it if possible; assist with other interventions to stop bleeding
- Maintain patent I.V. access using short, large-bore catheters to allow for faster infusion rates
- Administer I.V. fluids, vasopressors, and blood as prescribed; an auto-transfuser, which allows for reinfusion of the patient's own blood, may be required
- Draw blood for typing and crossmatching as ordered, to prepare for transfusion
- Encourage the patient to drink fluids as appropriate
- Auscultate breath sounds to monitor for signs of fluid overload, a potential complication of I.V. therapy; excess fluid in the lungs may cause a crackling sound on auscultation
- Provide frequent oral care to prevent breakdown of dry mucous membranes
- Turn the patient at least every 2 hours to prevent skin breakdown, a problem of particular concern for a patient with volume deficit

ECF VOLUME EXCESS

● General information
- Also termed *hypervolemia*
- Results from relatively equal gains of sodium and water in the ECF
- Osmolality not significantly affected; fluid and solute gains equally proportioned
- ECF volume: may increase in the interstitial or intravascular compartments
- Body able to compensate and restore fluid balance by fine-tuning several circulating levels, causing kidney release of additional water and sodium
  - Aldosterone
  - ADH
  - Atrial natriuretic peptide
- In severe hypervolemia or with poor heart function: body unable to compensate for extra fluid volume; possibly results in several disorders
  - Pulmonary edema
  - Heart failure
  - Hypertension

● Causes
- Iatrogenic overinfusion of parenteral fluids, particularly normal saline solution
- Administration of hypertonic parenteral fluids, such as 3% or 5% sodium chloride
- Use of plasma proteins such as albumin
- Excessive ingestion of solutes (such as sodium) in foods or medications

---

Key facts about ECF volume excess

- Also termed *hypervolemia*
- Results from relatively equal gains of sodium and water in the ECF
- Body able to compensate and restore fluid balance by fine-tuning circulating levels of aldosterone, ADH, and atrial natriuretic peptide, causing kidney release of additional water and sodium

Key disorders caused by severe hypervolemia or poor heart function

- Pulmonary edema
- Heart failure
- Hypertension

- Excessive administration of saline solution enemas
- Long-term corticosteroid administration
- Heart failure
- Chronic kidney disease that causes accumulation of fluids and solutes between dialysis treatments
- Chronic liver disease
- Hyperaldosteronism
- Hypoalbuminemia, which may be associated with renal disease or malnutrition
- Remobilization of fluids after burn treatment

● **Assessment findings**
- Acute weight gain
  - 5% to 10% increase: mild-to-moderate fluid gain
  - More than 10% increase: more severe fluid gain
- Distended jugular veins
- Polyuria (with normal renal function)
- Elevated blood pressure
- Full, bounding pulse
- Crackles auscultated in lung fields
- Dyspnea
- Tachypnea
- Ascites
- Peripheral edema as fluid is forced into the tissues (see *Evaluating pitting edema*, page 74)
  - May first be visible only in dependent areas
  - May later become generalized

● **Diagnostic findings**
- Decreased HCT (resulting from hemodilution)
- Normal serum sodium level
- Low serum potassium (K) and BUN levels
  - Due to hemodilution
  - Higher levels may indicate renal failure or impaired renal perfusion
- Low oxygen level
  - Accompanies early tachypnea and low partial pressure of arterial carbon dioxide
  - Results from a drop in pH and respiratory alkalosis
- Abnormal chest X-ray
  - Indicates fluid accumulation
  - May reveal pulmonary edema or pleural effusions

● **Treatment**
- Sodium and fluid intake restricted
- Diuretics to promote excess fluid excretion
- Morphine and nitroglycerin (Nitro-Dur) for pulmonary edema

Common causes of ECF volume excess

- Overinfusion of parenteral fluids
- Administration of hypertonic parenteral fluids
- Use of plasma proteins
- Excessive ingestion of solutes in foods or medications
- Heart failure
- Chronic kidney disease
- Chronic liver disease
- Hyperaldosteronism
- Hypoalbuminemia
- Remobilization of fluids after burn treatment

Common assessment findings in ECF volume excess

- Acute weight gain
- Distended jugular veins
- Polyuria
- Elevated blood pressure
- Full, bounding pulse
- Crackles in lung fields
- Dyspnea
- Tachypnea
- Ascites
- Peripheral edema

Testing for ECF volume excess

- Decreased HCT
- Normal serum sodium level
- Low serum potassium
- Low BUN
- Low oxygen level
- Abnormalities on chest X-ray

Evaluating pitting edema

- Evaluated using a scale of +1 to +4
- A slight imprint: indicates +1 pitting edema
- A deep imprint, with the skin slow to return to its original contour: indicates +4 pitting edema
- The skin resists pressure and appears distended: indicates a condition called *brawny edema*

Key treatment options for ECF volume excess

- Fluid intake restrictions
- Sodium restrictions
- Diuretics
- Morphine and nitroglycerin
- Digoxin
- Supportive measures
- Hemodialysis

Evaluating pitting edema

Edema can be evaluated using a scale of +1 to +4. Press your fingertip firmly into the patient's skin over a bony surface for a few seconds. Then note the depth of the imprint your finger leaves on the skin.

A slight imprint indicates +1 pitting edema.

A deep imprint, with the skin slow to return to its original contour, indicates +4 pitting edema.

When the skin resists pressure and appears distended, the condition is called *brawny edema,* which causes the skin to swell so much that fluid can't be displaced.

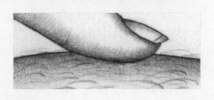

- – Dilate blood vessels
- – Reduce pulmonary congestion and amount of blood returning to the heart
- Digoxin (Lanoxin) for heart failure
  - – Strengthens cardiac contractions
  - – Slows heart rate
- Supportive measures
  - – Oxygen administration
  - – Bed rest
- Hemodialysis or continuous renal replacement therapy for renal dysfunction (see *Continuous venovenous hemofiltration*)

● Nursing interventions

- Monitor fluid intake and output for indications of excess
- Monitor daily weight for increases that may indicate fluid excess; keep in mind that a 1-lb (0.45-kg) weight gain equals 500-ml of fluid gain (approximately 1 kg of weight gain equals 1 L of fluid gain)
- Monitor cardiopulmonary status; assess for increased blood pressure and respiratory rate
- Auscultate breath sounds; note crackles that don't clear with coughing, which may indicate fluid retention (see *How pulmonary edema develops,* page 76)

Continuous venovenous hemofiltration

This illustration shows the standard setup for one type of continuous renal replacement therapy (CRRT) called *continuous venovenous hemofiltration.* In the standard setup for CRRT, a dual-lumen venous catheter provides access to the patient's blood. A pulsatile pump propels the blood through the tubing circuit.

In continuous venovenous hemofiltration (as shown), the patient's blood enters the hemofilter from a line connected to one lumen of the venous catheter, flows through the hemofilter, and returns to the patient through the second lumen of the catheter.

At the first pump, an anticoagulant may be added to the blood. A second pump moves dialysate through the hemofilter. A third pump adds replacement fluid if needed. Finally, the ultrafiltrate (plasma water and toxins) that's removed from the blood drains into a collection bag.

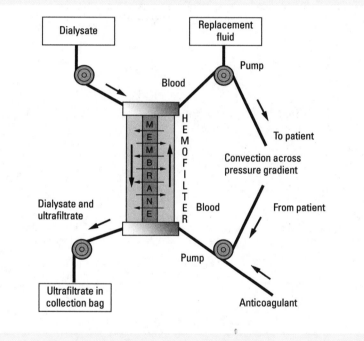

Key facts about continuous venovenous hemofiltration

- One type of continuous renal replacement therapy
- Dual-lumen venous catheter: provides access to the patient's blood
- Pulsatile pump: propels the blood through the tubing circuit
- Blood: flows through the hemofilter, returns to the patient through the second lumen of the catheter
- Ultrafiltrate (plasma water and toxins) removed from the blood

- Assess for subjective complaints of dyspnea, such as complaints of shortness of breath or exertional dyspnea
- Monitor chest X-ray results to detect changes pointing to fluid accumulation
- Monitor laboratory study results for decreased BUN and HCT levels
- Monitor arterial blood gas and watch for a drop in oxygen level or changes in acid-base balance
- Assess for presence and amount of peripheral edema
- Inspect the patient confined to bed rest for sacral edema (the sacrum may be the only place that fluid accumulates in the supine position)

Key nursing interventions for a patient with ECF volume excess

- Monitor fluid intake and output.
- Monitor daily weight.
- Monitor cardiopulmonary status.
- Auscultate breath sounds.
- Assess for complaints of dyspnea.
- Monitor chest X-ray results.
- Monitor laboratory study.
- Monitor arterial blood gas values.
- Assess for peripheral edema.
- Inspect the patient for sacral edema.
- Monitor infusion of I.V. solutions.
- Monitor the effects of prescribed medications.

How pulmonary edema develops

Excess fluid volume in the extravascular spaces of the lung can cause pulmonary edema. It may occur as a chronic condition or develop quickly and rapidly become fatal. These illustrations show how pulmonary edema develops.

NORMAL
Normal pulmonary fluid movement depends on the equal force of two opposing pressures—hydrostatic pressure and plasma osmotic pressure from protein molecules in the blood.

CONGESTION
Abnormally high pulmonary hydrostatic pressure (indicated by increased pulmonary artery wedge pressure) forces fluid out of the capillaries and into the interstitial space, causing pulmonary congestion.

EDEMA
When the amount of interstitial fluid becomes excessive, fluid is forced into the alveoli. Pulmonary edema results. Fluid fills the alveoli and prevents the exchange of gases.

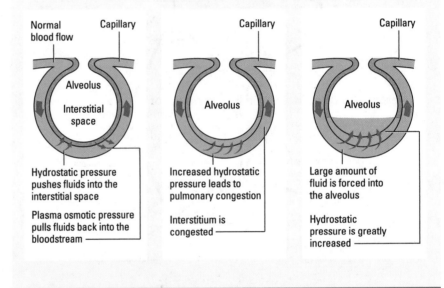

- Make sure the patient turns at least every 2 hours; edematous skin is more prone to breakdown
- Insert a urinary catheter as ordered to more accurately monitor output before starting diuretic therapy
- Monitor infusion of parenteral fluids if ordered; check the rate every hour, and use I.V. controllers (pumps) as necessary to prevent fluid overload
- Monitor the therapeutic and adverse effects of prescribed medications, especially those that may potentiate the imbalance
- Raise the head of the bed (if blood pressure allows) to facilitate breathing and administer oxygen as ordered (see *Patient teaching: Hypervolemia*)

![icon] **TIME-OUT FOR TEACHING**

Patient teaching: Hypervolemia

When teaching a patient with hypervolemia, be sure to cover the following information and then evaluate your patient's learning:

- Teach the patient and his family about hypervolemia, including its causes and associated risks.
- Teach the patient to monitor and record fluid intake and output and daily weight.
- Emphasize the importance of compliance with fluid restrictions if necessary.
- Teach the patient about the effects of sodium intake on fluid balance and about which foods, fluids, medications, and other sodium-containing products to avoid.
- Teach the patient how to safely administer prescribed medications.

ICF VOLUME DEFICIT

● **General information**
- Also known as *dehydration*
- Results from a disproportionately high loss of water in relation to sodium in the ECF
  - Leaves ECF hypertonic, producing several results
    - Water: moves from ICF into ECF, creating hypertonic fluid deficit in ICF
    - Cells: shrink as process continues; can't function without adequate fluid
- Should be considered hypernatremia because sodium is the primary ion affected
- Osmolality of ICF and ECF: eventually reaches equilibrium
  - Creates hypertonicity of both compartments when water has been lost without a corresponding solute loss
  - Serum osmolality increased because of this hypertonicity

● **Causes**
- Excessive insensible water losses from several possible causes
  - Tachypnea
  - Hyperventilation
  - Hyperthermia
  - Severe diaphoresis
- Decreased water intake from several possible causes
  - Dysphagia
  - Debilitating conditions
  - Stroke
  - Coma

Key teaching topics for hypervolemia
- Causes and associated risks
- How to monitor and record fluid intake and output and daily weight
- Importance of compliance with fluid restrictions
- Effect of sodium intake
- Safe administration of medications

Key facts about ICF volume deficit
- Also known as *dehydration*
- Results from a disproportionately high loss of water in relation to sodium in the ECF
- Considered hypernatremia
- Osmolality of ICF and ECF: eventually reaches equilibrium

Common causes of ICF volume deficit
- Excessive insensible water losses
- Decreased water intake
- Prolonged NPO status without adequate parenteral fluid replacement
- Excessive administration of sodium bicarbonate
- Hyperglycemia
- Diabetes insipidus
- Severe gastroenteritis or diarrhea

Common assessment findings in ICF volume deficit

- Weakness
- Thirst
- Fever
- Poor skin turgor
- Tachycardia
- Hypotension

Testing for ICF volume deficit

- Elevated serum sodium level
- Elevated serum osmolality
- Moderately high to normal HCT
- Increased urine specific gravity

Key treatment options for ICF volume deficit

- Oral fluids
- I.V. fluids
- Hypotonic, low-sodium fluids
- Avoidance of hypertonic solutions

- Prolonged nothing-by-mouth (NPO) status without adequate parenteral fluid replacement
- Excessive administration of hypertonic fluids
- Excessive administration of sodium bicarbonate to treat metabolic acidosis
- Administration of tube feedings inadequately diluted with water
- Prolonged total parenteral nutrition therapy
- Hyperglycemia
- Diabetes insipidus
- Severe gastroenteritis or diarrhea

Assessment findings

- Weakness
- Restlessness
- Delirium
- Tetany
- Hyperventilation
- Dry mucous membranes
- Thirst
- Irritability
- Fever
- Flushed skin
- Dry skin
- Poor skin turgor
- Oliguria
- Hyperactive deep tendon reflexes
- Tachycardia
- Hypotension
- Generalized tonic-clonic seizures
- Sudden respiratory arrest

Diagnostic findings

- Elevated serum sodium level (greater than 145 mEq/L)
- Elevated serum osmolality (greater than 300 mOsm/kg)
- Moderately high to normal HCT
- Urine specific gravity greater than 1.030

Treatment

- Oral fluids
  - Encouraged if the patient can tolerate them
  - Must be salt-free because serum sodium level is elevated
- I.V. fluids
  - For severe dehydration
  - Replace lost fluids
  - Should be hypotonic, low-sodium fluids (such as dextrose 5% in water [D_5W])
- Hypertonic solutions avoided
- Vasopressin (Pitressin) possibly used to treat diabetes insipidus

● **Nursing interventions**
  - Monitor vital signs closely to ensure prompt intervention
  - Monitor fluid intake and output; watch for decreased output
  - Obtain daily weight to distinguish weight loss from fluid loss
  - Monitor LOC for changes that may result from excessively rapid infusion of hypotonic fluid
  - Monitor serum sodium level and serum osmolality as well as urine osmolality and urine specific gravity
  - Assess patients who are on NPO status (because of surgery or diagnostic studies) for signs and symptoms of water loss
  - To restore osmolality and lower serum sodium levels, administer fluids as ordered—usually hypotonic I.V. fluids through a volume-control device
    - Give them gradually over 48 hours
    - Hypotonic solutions given too quickly move fluid from veins into cells, making them edematous
    - Swelling brain cells can cause cerebral edema
  - Monitor the patient receiving hypotonic solutions for signs and symptoms of cerebral edema, such as headache, confusion, irritability, lethargy, nausea, vomiting, widening pulse pressure, decreased pulse rate, and seizures
  - Dilute tube feedings with adequate amounts of water to prevent administration of hypertonic fluids
  - Provide a safe environment for any patient who's confused, dizzy, or at risk for a seizure; teach his family to do the same
  - Provide skin and mouth care to maintain the integrity of the skin surface and oral mucous membranes
  - Assess the patient for diaphoresis, which can be the source of major water loss

ICF VOLUME EXCESS

● **General information**
  - Results from a disproportionately high loss of sodium in relation to water in the ECF
    - Sodium loss: occurs initially from ECF; leaves ECF hypotonic
    - Result: cell hypertonic, fluid moves from ECF into ICF to achieve osmotic equilibrium
    - Result: hypotonic fluid excess in ICF (also known as *water intoxication*)
  - May also result from an increase in solute-free fluid in the ECF; for example, from overadministration of D_5W
  - Should be considered hyponatremia
    - Sodium: primary ECF ion
    - Assessment findings essentially the same
  - Serum osmolality affected
    - Results from disproportionately low concentration of sodium in relation to water

Common causes of ICF volume excess

- Prolonged diuretic therapy with low salt intake
- Replacement of lost body fluids with only water or other sodium-free fluids
- Excessive water intake
- Excessive administration of hypotonic fluids
- Heart failure
- Oat cell carcinoma of the lung
- Prolonged use of oral hypoglycemic agents or tricyclic antidepressants
- Alcoholism

Common assessment findings in ICF volume excess

- Confusion and disorientation
- Muscle weakness or twitching
- Headache
- Nausea and vomiting
- Seizures
- Coma
- Late signs of increased ICP

Testing for ICF volume excess

- Decreased serum sodium level
- Decreased serum osmolality
- Hypoproteinemia

– Decreases to below 280 mOsm/kg
- Intracellular edema caused by accumulation of hypo-osmotic fluid in ICF
  - Causes increased intracranial pressure (ICP)
  - Produces the primary signs and symptoms related to the central nervous system, such as confusion and disorientation

● **Causes**
- Prolonged diuretic therapy with low salt intake
- Replacement of lost body fluids (as from severe diaphoresis or hemorrhage) with only water or other sodium-free fluids
- Excessive water intake linked to psychological disturbance
- Irrigation of a nasogastric (NG) tube connected to suction with tap water
- Excessive amounts of ice chips given to patients with NG tubes connected to suction or to patients who are vomiting
- Excessive release of ADH from several causes
  - Stress
  - Surgery
  - Trauma
  - Opioid use
- Excessive I.V. administration of hypotonic fluids
- Excessive administration of tap-water enemas
- Heart failure
- Oat cell carcinoma of the lung (may be associated with syndrome of inappropriate ADH secretion)
- Prolonged use of oral hypoglycemic agents or tricyclic antidepressants
- Alcoholism

● **Assessment findings**
- Confusion and disorientation
- Muscle weakness or twitching
- Hyperirritability
- Mental disturbances such as personality changes
- Headache
- Nausea and vomiting
- Seizures
- Coma
- Polyuria in patients with healthy kidneys
- Late signs of increased ICP
  - Pupillary changes
  - Bradycardia
  - Widened pulse pressure

● **Diagnostic findings**
- Serum sodium level less than 125 mEq/L
- Serum osmolality less than 280 mOsm/kg
- Hypoproteinemia

● **Treatment**
  • Restricted oral and parenteral fluid intake
  • Hypotonic I.V. solutions, such as D_5W, should be avoided until serum sodium levels rise
  • Hypertonic solutions used only in severe situations
    – Draw fluid out of the cells
    – Require close patient monitoring

● **Nursing interventions**
  • Monitor intake and output and vital signs for indications of fluid excess
  • Obtain daily weight to assess for fluid excess; remember that a 1-lb (0.45-kg) weight gain equals a 500-ml fluid gain (approximately 1 kg of weight gain equals 1 L of fluid gain)
  • Assess LOC and mental status for changes in cognitive function, orientation, or personality
  • Monitor laboratory study results for decreasing serum sodium level and serum osmolality
  • Restrict fluids as ordered
  • Irrigate NG tubes connected to suction with normal saline solution
  • If parenteral fluid administration is ordered, monitor infusion carefully to ensure a patent I.V. line and an accurate infusion rate
  • Administer hypotonic parenteral fluids carefully to prevent the development of hypo-osmotic conditions
  • Provide a safe environment for the patient with an alteration in neurologic status; teach his family to do the same
  • Institute seizure precautions in severe cases

THIRD-SPACE FLUID SHIFTING

● **General information**
  • Describes fluid accumulation in a compartment other than ECF or ICF
  • "Third space" creation: requires a cellular membrane that allows water and fluid to enter but not exit
    – Water and fluid unavailable to maintain normal body fluid compartments
    – Result: solute and water imbalances
  • Swelling from inflammation with concurrent loss of fluids involved in accumulation
  • Some third-space fluids due to osmotic changes caused by loss of protein—for example, ascites associated with urine protein loss
  • May be reabsorbed or must be removed mechanically by procedures, such as paracentesis or thoracentesis

● **Causes**
  • Acute bowel obstruction
  • Ascites

Common causes of third-space fluid shifting

- Acute bowel obstruction
- Ascites
- Burns
- Pancreatitis
- Sepsis

Common assessment findings in third-space fluid shifting

- Tachycardia
- Hypotension
- Weight changes (usually gains)

Testing for third-space fluid shifting

- Elevated urine specific gravity
- Elevated HCT

Key treatment options for third-space fluid shifting

- Correction: may occur spontaneously
- Surgery

Key nursing interventions for a patient with third-space fluid shifting

- Monitor extent and severity of shifting.
- Monitor pulse rate and rhythm, blood pressure, and respiratory rate.
- Monitor fluid intake and output.
- Obtain daily weight and assess abdominal girth.
- Monitor urine specific gravity and osmolality.

- Hypoalbuminemia
- Pleural effusion
- Acute peritonitis
- Burns
- Pancreatitis
- Sepsis

● **Assessment findings**
- Hyponatremia
- Tachycardia
- Hypotension
- Oliguria, with urine output less than 30 ml/hour
- Low CVP
- Poor skin turgor
- Weight changes (usually gains)

● **Diagnostic findings**
- Elevated urine specific gravity
- Elevated HCT

● **Treatment**
- Correction: may occur spontaneously
- May require surgery, such as the insertion of a peritoneovenous shunt

● **Nursing interventions**
- Remember that third-space fluid shifting is an acute and serious problem
- Monitor and document several signs to assess the extent and severity of the third-space shift; this helps estimate fluid movement changes from the third space back to normal fluid compartments
    – Pulse rate and rhythm
    – Blood pressure
    – Respiratory rate
    – Fluid intake and output
    – Daily weight
    – Abdominal girth
    – Urine specific gravity and osmolality
- Keep in mind that parenteral fluid administration will provide symptom relief but won't resolve the problem; rather, it will increase the patient's total body weight without making the third-space fluid available to the body

PATIENTS AT RISK FOR FLUID IMBALANCES

- **General information**
  - Several factors that influence susceptibility
    - Certain disease states
    - Medication use
    - Age
  - Factors affecting numerous aspects of fluid balance
    - Routes of water gains or losses
    - Homeostatic regulatory systems
    - Body's ability to compensate for imbalances
  - Four groups at greatest risk
    - Neonates, infants, and children
    - Older adults
    - Pregnant patients
    - Chronically ill patients

- **Neonates, infants, and children**
  - At risk because of immature regulatory mechanisms and physiologic differences in body composition
  - Carry potential for rapid dehydration in disease states due to inefficient urine concentration from immature kidneys
  - Unlike adults, can develop an acute imbalance within hours
  - Have greater ratio of body surface area (BSA) to weight than adults; at greater risk for fluid imbalance from insensible water loss through skin
  - Have a relatively greater GI tract surface area than adults; can experience greater water losses there

- **Older adults**
  - At risk because of physiologic changes, decreased access to fluids caused by compromised mobility, and diminished compensatory reserves
  - After age 65, percentage of total body water progressively decreased to between 30% and 40%
  - Decreased renal function: affects numerous functions
    - Influences excretion of heavy solute loads, such as from tube feedings
    - Increases risk of fluid imbalance from certain medications
      - Diuretics
      - Electrolyte replacement supplements
  - Risk of hyperglycemia and osmotic diuresis: increased because of certain decreases
    - Pancreatic functioning
    - Glucose tolerance
  - Cardiovascular function deterioration: impairs compensation for hypotensive states

Key risk factors for fluid imbalances *(continued)*

Older adults
- Physiologic changes
- Progressive decrease in percentage of total body water
- Decreased renal function
- Decreased pancreatic functioning and glucose tolerance
- Cardiovascular function deterioration
- Decreased mobility and cognition
- Diminished thirst mechanism

Pregnant patients
- Added demands of pregnancy
- Redistribution of fluid between ICF and ECF
- Labor induction with oxytocin

Chronically ill patients
- Increased physiologic stress
- Diminished compensatory reserves
- Major body systems compromised

- Decreased mobility and cognition: may compromise consumption of adequate fluids (and foods), particularly during illness
- Diminished thirst mechanism: increases the risk of dehydration, especially in hot weather
- Decreased skin elasticity: makes skin turgor a poor indicator of hydration status

● **Pregnant patients**
- At risk because of added demands of pregnancy on the body and need for additional fluid
- Redistribution of fluid between ICF and ECF secondary to sodium retention associated with physiologic edema of normal pregnancy
- Excessive intake of dietary sodium: should be avoided because of its relationship to development of hypertension in those at risk
- Labor induction with oxytocin (Pitocin): can lead to water retention and severe hyponatremia

● **Chronically ill patients**
- At risk because of increased physiologic stress and diminished compensatory reserves
- Illness affecting major body systems: may compromise changes in fluid balance
- Diabetes and other endocrine diseases: indirectly affect fluid balance
- Patients with renal insufficiency or chronic kidney disease: must maintain proper fluid balance to prevent acute illness

NCLEX CHECKS

It's never too soon to begin your NCLEX preparation. Now that you've reviewed this chapter, carefully read each of the following questions and choose the best answer. Then compare your responses to the correct answers.

1. Which parameter(s) is an important indicator of rapid fluid changes?
   ☐ **1.** BUN and creatinine
   ☐ **2.** Weight
   ☐ **3.** Skin turgor
   ☐ **4.** Temperature

2. To compensate for decreased fluid volume, the nurse can anticipate which response by the body?
   ☐ **1.** Bradycardia
   ☐ **2.** Tachycardia
   ☐ **3.** Vasodilation
   ☐ **4.** Increased urine output

3. A priority nursing intervention for a client with hypervolemia involves:
- ☐ **1.** establishing I.V. access with a large-bore catheter.
- ☐ **2.** drawing a blood sample for typing and crossmatching.
- ☐ **3.** monitoring respiratory status for signs and symptoms of pulmonary edema.
- ☐ **4.** encouraging the client to consume sodium-free fluids.

4. The nurse can expect to administer normal saline solution (NSS) to a client with:
- ☐ **1.** hypovolemia.
- ☐ **2.** hypervolemia.
- ☐ **3.** water intoxication.
- ☐ **4.** pulmonary edema.

5. Third-space fluid shifting involves the movement of fluid into the:
- ☐ **1.** arteries.
- ☐ **2.** veins.
- ☐ **3.** intracellular space.
- ☐ **4.** abdominal cavity.

6. Which physiologic difference places infants at greater risk for fluid imbalances than adults?
- ☐ **1.** Infants have a diminished thirst mechanism.
- ☐ **2.** Infants have a lower percentage of total body water.
- ☐ **3.** Infants typically retain sodium.
- ☐ **4.** Infants have a greater ratio of BSA to weight.

7. Because diabetes insipidus involves the loss of large amounts of highly dilute urine, a client with this disorder is at risk for which type of fluid imbalance?
- ☐ **1.** Dehydration
- ☐ **2.** Hypovolemia
- ☐ **3.** Hypervolemia
- ☐ **4.** Water intoxication

8. What's the major risk of dehydration?
- ☐ **1.** Excessive circulating blood volume
- ☐ **2.** Low HCT
- ☐ **3.** Cellular shrinkage
- ☐ **4.** Pulmonary edema

9. Rapid administration of hypotonic solutions to a severely dehydrated client should be avoided to prevent which complication?
- ☐ **1.** Pulmonary edema
- ☐ **2.** Cerebral edema
- ☐ **3.** Heart failure
- ☐ **4.** Hypotension

TOP 10

Items to study for your next test on fluid imbalances

1. The pathogenesis of the three types of fluid imbalances

2. The etiology that contributes to the body's compensation responses to each imbalance

3. Nursing assessments, including signs and symptoms found in each imbalance

4. Diagnostic results of each imbalance

5. Nursing management of each imbalance

6. Drug therapy that is impacted by each imbalance

7. Complications that occur with each imbalance

8. Fluid therapy used for replacements needed to correct each imbalance

9. Correlation of osmolarity and albumin levels to fluid restriction for each imbalance

10. Clients at risk for fluid imbalances and a rationale for each risk

10. A client at risk for fluid excess should be weighed daily. A 1-lb weight would be equivalent to how many milliliters of fluid gain? _____

ANSWERS AND RATIONALES

1. CORRECT ANSWER: 2

Acute changes in weight can indicate rapid fluid changes. Keep in mind that a 5% to 10% weight drop can indicate mild-to-moderate loss of fluid volume; a drop of more than 10%, severe loss. Similarly, a 5% to 10% weight increase indicates mild-to-moderate fluid gain, and an increase of more than 10% indicates more severe fluid gain.

2. CORRECT ANSWER: 2

The nurse can expect the client's heart rate to increase (known as *tachycardia*) as the body attempts to improve cardiac output and circulating blood volume despite a fluid volume deficit. Vasoconstriction and decreased urine output can also be expected.

3. CORRECT ANSWER: 3

Pulmonary edema is a potentially serious complication of hypervolemia. Therefore, a priority action for the nurse involves monitoring the client's respiratory status for such signs and symptoms as shortness of breath, tachypnea, dyspnea, and pink, frothy sputum. Establishing I.V. access with a large-bore catheter, drawing a blood sample for typing and crossmatching, and encouraging the consumption of sodium-free fluids are all appropriate actions for the client with hypovolemia.

4. CORRECT ANSWER: 1

NSS, an isotonic solution, helps increase cardiac output, blood pressure, and urine output. The nurse should anticipate administration of NSS to a client with hypovolemia to support blood pressure until decreased fluid levels are back to normal.

5. CORRECT ANSWER: 4

Third-space fluid shifts occur when fluid moves out of the intravascular spaces (arteries, veins, and capillaries), but not into intracellular spaces. Fluid will shift into such sites as the abdominal cavity, the pleural cavity, or the pericardial sac.

6. CORRECT ANSWER: 4

Because the ratio of BSA to weight is several times greater in infants and children than in adults, they're at greater risk for fluid imbalances related to insensible water loss through the skin.

7. CORRECT ANSWER: 1

The loss of large amounts of highly dilute urine (without the loss of solutes), as occurs in diabetes insipidus, leaves the body with an increase in blood solute concentration. This causes water molecules in the ICF to shift into the more concentrated blood in an attempt to regain fluid balance between intracellular and extracellular spaces. This type of fluid imbalance is known as *dehydration*.

8. CORRECT ANSWER: 3

Cellular shrinkage is the major risk of dehydration, as fluids in the cells shift into the more concentrated ECF to regulate fluid balance. Because cells need adequate water to maintain their shape, expel wastes, and obtain nutrients, their function will be impaired.

9. CORRECT ANSWER: 2

Giving a hypotonic solution too quickly to a dehydrated client causes fluid to move from the veins into the cells, possibly resulting in edematous cells. Swelling of the cells in the brain can create cerebral edema. To avoid this potentially devastating problem, give fluids gradually, over a period of about 48 hours.

10. CORRECT ANSWER: 500

It's important to monitor for daily weight increases in a client at risk for fluid excess. A 1-lb (0.45 kg) weight gain equals 500-ml of fluid gain.

6

Electrolyte imbalances

LEARNING OBJECTIVES

After studying this chapter, you should be able to:

- State laboratory test values representative of each electrolyte imbalance.
- Discuss possible causes of each electrolyte imbalance.
- Describe assessment findings for each electrolyte imbalance.
- Describe treatment and nursing care pertinent to each electrolyte imbalance.
- Identify those patients at greatest risk for electrolyte imbalances.

CHAPTER OVERVIEW

Electrolyte imbalances can involve either a deficit or an excess. Nursing care for the patient with an electrolyte deficit commonly includes measures to replace the electrolyte. Nursing care for the patient with an electrolyte excess usually includes restriction of and possible reduction of the excess electrolyte to normal levels. Careful monitoring of serum levels and intake and output, along with patient education, are crucial to preventing life-threatening complications.

INTRODUCTION

● **Basic concepts**
  • Are experienced by many patients who require medical care
  • Can involve either a deficit or an excess
    – Deficits are designated with the prefix *hypo-* (for example, hyponatremia refers to a sodium [Na] deficit)
    – Excesses are designated with the prefix *hyper-* (for example, hypernatremia refers to a sodium excess)

● **Implications**
  • Some gradually developed
    – Example: Sodium imbalances
    – Usually not life-threatening
  • Some, such as those involving potassium (K), life-threatening if not recognized and treated promptly
  • Problems rarely caused by changes in serum concentrations of chloride (Cl) alone
  • Any left untreated: can exacerbate an existing problem or lead to death

SODIUM DEFICIT: HYPONATREMIA

● **General information**
  • Has several causes
    – Excessive sodium loss
    – Excessive water gain in extracellular fluid (ECF) (known as *dilutional hyponatremia*)
    – Inadequate sodium intake (known as *depletional hyponatremia*)
  • ECF osmolality: decreases from sodium deficiency or water excess
    – Sodium: moves out of intracellular fluid (ICF) into ECF
    – Water: moves into ICF
      · Alters ICF osmolality (see *Fluid movement in hyponatremia*, page 90)
      · Causes cellular swelling
      · Eventually causes central nervous system (CNS) changes
  • May be classified according to ECF volume level
    – Abnormally decreased (*hypovolemic hyponatremia*)
      · Sodium and water levels decreased in extracellular area
      · Sodium loss greater than water loss
    – Abnormally increased (*hypervolemic hyponatremia*)
      · Water and sodium levels increased in extracellular area
      · Water gain greater than sodium gain
    – Equal to ICF volume (*isovolumic hyponatremia*)
      · Sodium levels: may appear low because too much fluid is in the body

Key facts about electrolyte imbalances

● Involve either a deficit or an excess
● Can gradually develop
● Can be life-threatening
● If left untreated: can exacerbate an existing problem or lead to death

Key facts about hyponatremia

● Several possible causes: excessive sodium loss, excessive water gain in ECF, or inadequate sodium intake
● ECF osmolality decreased

Classifying electrolyte imbalances

● Abnormally decreased ECF (*hypovolemic hyponatremia*)
● Abnormally increased ECF (*hypervolemic hyponatremia*)
● ECF equal to ICF volume (*isovolumic hyponatremia*)

Fluid movement in hyponatremia

This illustration shows fluid movement in hyponatremia. When serum osmolality decreases because of decreased sodium concentration, fluid moves by osmosis from the extracellular area to the intracellular area.

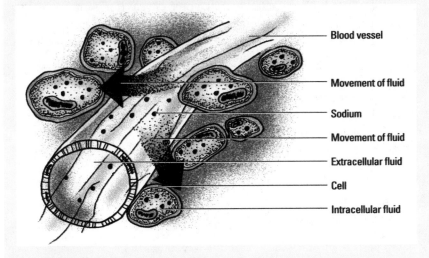

- Blood vessel
- Movement of fluid
- Sodium
- Movement of fluid
- Extracellular fluid
- Cell
- Intracellular fluid

Common causes of hyponatremia

- Prolonged diuretic therapy
- Insufficient sodium intake
- Severe GI fluid loss
- Hypotonic fluid administration
- Compulsive water drinking
- Adrenal insufficiency
- Alcoholism
- SIADH

Common assessment findings in hyponatremia

- Headache
- Nausea and vomiting
- Confusion
- Muscle twitching
- Tremors
- Weakness
- Irritability

· No physical signs of fluid volume excess
· Total body sodium: remains stable

● **Causes**
  • Prolonged diuretic therapy (see *Drugs associated with hyponatremia*)
  • Excessive diaphoresis
  • Insufficient sodium intake
  • Excessive sodium loss from trauma, such as massive burns
  • Severe GI fluid loss due to numerous causes
      – Gastric suctioning or lavage
      – Prolonged vomiting or diarrhea
      – Laxative abuse
  • Hypotonic fluid administration
  • Compulsive water drinking (linked to psychological disturbance)
  • Labor induction with oxytocin (Pitocin)
  • Adrenal insufficiency
  • Salt-losing nephritis
  • Cystic fibrosis
  • Alcoholism
  • Syndrome of inappropriate antidiuretic hormone (SIADH)
  • Repeated tap water enemas

● **Assessment findings**
  • Headache
  • Nausea and vomiting

Drugs associated with hyponatremia

Drugs can cause hyponatremia by potentiating the action of antidiuretic hormone (ADH) or by causing syndrome of inappropriate ADH. Diuretics may also cause hyponatremia by inhibiting sodium reabsorption in the kidney.

Anticonvulsants
- Carbamazepine (Tegretol)

Antidiabetics
- Chlorpropamide (Diabinese)
- Tolbutamide (Orinase) (rarely)

Antineoplastics
- Cyclophosphamide (Cytoxan)
- Vincristine (Oncovin)

Antipsychotics
- Fluphenazine (Prolixin Decanoate)
- Thioridazine (Mellaril)
- Thiothixene (Navane)

Diuretics
- Loop (such as bumetanide [Bumex], furosemide [Lasix], ethacrynic acid [Edecrin])
- Thiazides (such as hydrochlorothiazide [HydroDIURIL])

Sedatives
- Barbiturates
- Morphine (Duramorph)

- Confusion
- Muscle cramps
- Muscle twitching
- Tremors
- Weakness
- Normal or increased weight
- Irritability
- Anxiety
- Hypotension
- Tachycardia
- Decreased urine output
- Decreased skin turgor
- Dry, cracked mucous membranes
- Seizures
- Coma

Diagnostic findings
- Serum sodium level less than 135 mEq/L; serum chloride less than 100 mEq/L
- Urine specific gravity less than 1.010 (greater than 1.012 in SIADH)
- Serum osmolality less than 280 mOsm/kg (dilute blood)

Treatment
- For mild hyponatremia
  - Restricted fluid intake

Key drugs associated with hyponatremia
- Anticonvulsants
- Antidiabetics
- Antineoplastics
- Antipsychotics
- Diuretics
- Sedatives

Testing for hyponatremia

Decreased
- Serum sodium level
- Serum chloride level
- Urine specific gravity
- Serum osmolality

Key treatment options for hyponatremia

Mild
● Restricted fluid intake
● Oral sodium supplements

Related to hypovolemia
● Isotonic I.V. fluids
● High-sodium foods

Severe
● Hypertonic saline solution

Key nursing interventions for a patient with hyponatremia

● Monitor fluid intake and output.
● Restrict fluid intake as ordered.
● Administer parenteral fluids as ordered.
● Monitor vital signs.
● Monitor serum sodium levels.
● Monitor daily weight.
● Provide a safe environment.
● Provide patient teaching.

– Oral sodium supplements
● For hyponatremia related to hypovolemia
  – Isotonic I.V. fluids such as normal saline solution to restore volume
  – High-sodium foods
● For severe hyponatremia (sodium levels less than 120 mEq/L)
  – May require treatment in the intensive care unit
  – Hypertonic saline solution (such as 3% to 5%) infusion
    · Causes water to shift out of cells
    · May lead to intravascular volume overload and brain damage (*osmotic demyelination*), especially in the pons
    · Fluid volume overload prevented with slow infusion of a hypertonic saline solution in small volumes; furosemide usually administered simultaneously
● No hypertonic saline solutions given except in rare instances of severe symptom-producing hyponatremia

● **Nursing interventions**
● Monitor and record fluid intake and output
● Restrict fluid intake as ordered; post a sign about fluid restriction in the patient's room and make sure the staff, the patient, and his family are aware of the restrictions
● Administer parenteral fluids as ordered; sodium should be administered sparingly to prevent increases in total fluid volume
● Be aware that with severe hyponatremia, serum sodium concentrations shouldn't be raised by more than 12 mEq/L during the first 24 hours to avoid serious neurologic problems
● Monitor and record vital signs, particularly blood pressure and pulse rate
● Assess skin integrity at least every 8 hours
● Administer I.V. isotonic or hypertonic saline solutions cautiously to avoid inducing hypernatremia from excessive or too-rapid infusion; use an infusion pump; watch for signs of hypervolemia (dyspnea, crackles, engorged jugular or hand veins) and report them immediately
● Monitor serum sodium levels to determine treatment effectiveness; also monitor other test results, such as urine specific gravity and serum osmolality
● Monitor daily weight for increases linked to water excess or decreases due to the success of fluid restrictions
● Provide a safe environment for a patient who has altered thought processes and reorient him as needed; if seizures are likely, pad the bed's side rails and keep suction equipment and an artificial airway handy
● Provide patient (and his family) teaching to prevent hyponatremia
  – Stress careful diuretic use to avoid excessive sodium loss
  – Stress need to carefully follow any sodium-restricted diet to ensure low but adequate sodium intake

SODIUM EXCESS: HYPERNATREMIA

- **General information**
  - Indicates a water deficit in ECF, which moves water out of ICF to equilibrate; cause could be increased salt intake
  - Usually results in ICF volume deficit; signs of hypervolemia may be present from increased ECF volume in the blood vessels (see *Fluid movement in hypernatremia*)
    - Possible result: cellular shrinkage
    - Impaired neurologic and cognitive function caused by cellular shrinkage in CNS
- **Causes**
  - Significantly deficient water intake
  - Hypertonic parenteral fluid administration
  - Hypertonic tube feedings
  - Excessive salt ingestion
  - Severe watery diarrhea or severe insensible water losses, such as from heat stroke or prolonged high fever
  - Major burns
  - Use of inadequately diluted baby formulas
  - Use of high-protein liquid diets without adequate fluid intake
  - Osmotic diuresis, such as in hyperosmolar hyperglycemic nonketotic syndrome

Fluid movement in hypernatremia

With hypernatremia, the body tries to maintain balance by shifting fluid from the inside of the cells to the outside of the cells. This illustration shows fluid movement in hypernatremia.

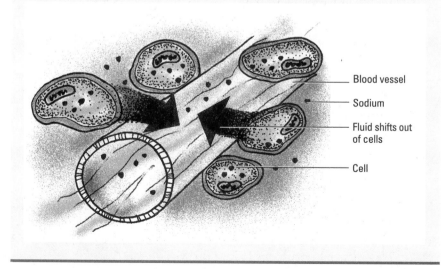

Blood vessel

Sodium

Fluid shifts out of cells

Cell

Key facts about hypernatremia
- Indicates a water deficit in ECF
- May be caused by increased salt intake
- Usually results in ICF volume deficit

Common causes of hypernatremia
- Significantly deficient water intake
- Hypertonic parenteral fluid administration
- Excessive salt ingestion
- Severe watery diarrhea
- Severe insensible water losses
- Major burns
- Medications
- Diabetes insipidus
- Hyperaldosteronism

Key drugs associated with hypernatremia

- Antacids with sodium bicarbonate
- Antibiotics
- Salt tablets
- Sodium bicarbonate
- I.V. sodium chloride preparations
- Sodium polystyrene sulfonate

Common assessment findings in hypernatremia

- Extreme thirst
- Restlessness or agitation
- Anorexia
- Nausea and vomiting

Testing for hypernatremia

Increased
- Serum sodium level
- Serum chloride level
- Urine specific gravity
- Serum osmolality

Key treatment options for hypernatremia

- Oral or I.V. fluid replacement
- Sodium-restricted diet
- Diuretics

Drugs associated with hypernatremia

The drugs listed here can cause high sodium levels. Ask your patient if any of these are a part of his drug therapy:

- antacids with sodium bicarbonate
- antibiotics such as ticarcillin disodium-clavulanate potassium (Timentin)
- salt tablets
- sodium bicarbonate injections (such as those given during cardiac arrest)
- I.V. sodium chloride preparations
- sodium polystyrene sulfonate (Kayexalate).

- Medications, such as sodium polystyrene sulfonate (Kayexalate) (see *Drugs associated with hypernatremia*)
- Diabetes insipidus
- Hyperaldosteronism

Assessment findings
- Extreme thirst
- Restlessness or agitation
- Anorexia
- Nausea and vomiting
- Tachycardia
- Low-grade fever
- Dry, sticky tongue and oral mucosa
- Disorientation
- Hallucinations
- Hyperactive deep tendon reflexes
- Hypertension
- Oliguria or anuria
- Lethargy progressing to coma
- Seizures

Diagnostic findings
- Serum sodium level greater than 145 mEq/L; chloride level elevated
- Urine specific gravity greater than 1.030
- Serum osmolality greater than 300 mOsm/kg

Treatment
- Oral or I.V. fluid replacement to restore fluid volume in the body
  - Fluids given gradually over 48 hours—avoids shifting water into brain cells and causing cerebral edema
  - Sodium-free solutions: should be used
- Sodium-restricted diet
- Diuretic administration accompanied by oral or I.V. fluid replacement to increase sodium excretion

TIME-OUT FOR TEACHING

Patient teaching: Hypernatremia

When teaching a patient with hypernatremia, be sure to cover the following information and then evaluate his learning:

- Teach the patient and his family about hypernatremia, including its causes and associated risks.
- Teach the patient and his family about foods and over-the-counter medications high in sodium to prevent accidental overingestion of sodium.
- Encourage the patient and his family to minimize the use of sodium in cooking and at the table.
- If necessary, instruct the patient and his family about sodium-restricted diets to promote compliance.

Nursing interventions
- Monitor and record fluid intake and output; the patient may have seriously decreased output
- Monitor daily weight for changes
- Assess for changes in mental function and level of consciousness (LOC)
- Monitor and record vital signs, particularly blood pressure, pulse rate, and temperature
- Cautiously administer ordered parenteral fluids (usually hypotonic sodium solution or any hypotonic solution except dextrose 5% in water) to prevent fluid overload and resultant cerebral edema
- Assess skin and mucous membranes for signs of breakdown and infection
- Provide thorough oral hygiene to keep mucous membranes moist and to decrease odor; lubricate the patient's lips frequently with a water-based lubricant and provide mouthwash or gargle if he's alert
- Monitor laboratory test results for trends pointing to hypernatremia
- When a patient is receiving hypertonic fluids, ensure adequate water administration to prevent solute overload; for example, dilute tube feedings and infuse total parenteral nutrition (TPN) at the prescribed rate
- Provide patient teaching as appropriate (see *Patient teaching: Hypernatremia*)

POTASSIUM DEFICIT: HYPOKALEMIA

General information
- Usually results from excessive excretion or inadequate intake of potassium
- Potassium functions
  - The major intracellular cation

Key patient teaching topics for hypernatremia
- Causes and associated risks
- Foods and over-the-counter medications high in sodium
- Use of sodium in cooking and at the table
- Sodium-restricted diets

Key nursing interventions for a patient with hypernatremia
- Monitor fluid intake and output.
- Monitor daily weight.
- Assess for changes in mental function and LOC.
- Monitor vital signs.
- Administer ordered parenteral fluids.
- Assess skin and mucous membranes.
- Monitor laboratory test results.
- Ensure adequate water administration.
- Provide patient teaching.

Key facts about hypokalemia
- Usually results from excessive excretion or inadequate intake of potassium
- May involve increased cellular uptake of potassium

Key drugs associated with hypokalemia

- Adrenergics
- Antibiotics
- Cisplatin
- Corticosteroids
- Diuretics
- Insulin
- Laxatives

Drugs associated with hypokalemia

The drugs listed here can deplete potassium and cause hypokalemia:

- adrenergics, such as albuterol (Proventil) and epinephrine (Bronkaid)
- antibiotics, such as amphotericin B (Fungizone) and gentamicin (Garamycin)
- cisplatin (Platinol-AQ)
- corticosteroids
- diuretics, such as furosemide (Lasix) and thiazides
- insulin
- laxatives (when used excessively).

- Balances sodium in ECF to maintain electroneutrality of body fluids
- Freely excreted by the kidneys; not stored by body
- Exchanged for the hydrogen (H) ion (when changes in body's acid-base balance indicate a need for cation exchange);
- Increased cellular uptake of potassium: occurs in insulin excess and certain disorders, such as chronic kidney disease

Causes

- Prolonged diuretic therapy with thiazides, furosemide, or other drugs (see *Drugs associated with hypokalemia*)
- Inadequate dietary potassium intake
- Administration of potassium-deficient parenteral fluids or TPN
- Severe diaphoresis
- Severe GI fluid losses from gastric suctioning or lavage, prolonged vomiting or diarrhea, or laxative abuse without potassium replacement
- Excessive secretion of endogenous insulin or administration of exogenous insulin
- Excessive stress (corticosteroid release results in sodium retention and potassium excretion)
- Alkalosis
- Hepatic disease
- Hyperaldosteronism
- Renal tubular defect (tubular acidosis)
- Malabsorption syndrome
- Acute alcoholism
- Cushing's syndrome or tumors of the adrenal cortex

Assessment findings

- Anorexia
- Nausea and vomiting
- Drowsiness and lethargy
- Leg cramps
- Muscle weakness, especially in legs

Common causes of hypokalemia

- Prolonged diuretic therapy
- Inadequate dietary potassium intake
- Administration of potassium-deficient parenteral fluids or TPN
- Severe GI fluid losses
- Excessive insulin
- Hepatic disease
- Renal tubular defect
- Cushing's syndrome or tumors of the adrenal cortex

Common assessment findings in hypokalemia

- Leg cramps
- Muscle weakness, especially in legs
- Paresthesia
- Cardiac arrhythmias

ECG changes in hypokalemia

Lab values: Serum potassium <3.5 mEq/L

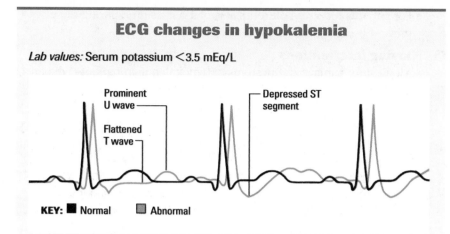

Prominent
U wave

Flattened
T wave

Depressed ST
segment

KEY: ■ Normal   ▢ Abnormal

- Decreased or absent deep tendon reflexes
- Paresthesia
- Decreased bowel sounds
- Constipation
- Decreased bowel motility (known as *ileus*)
- Hypotension
- Cardiac arrhythmias
  - Premature atrial contractions
  - Premature ventricular contractions
- Coma

● **Diagnostic findings**
- Electrocardiogram (ECG) changes
  - Depressed ST segment
  - Flattened or inverted T waves
  - Characteristic U waves (see *ECG changes in hypokalemia*)
- Serum potassium level less than 3.5 mEq/L
- Elevated pH and bicarbonate level
- Increased 24-hour urine level
- Slightly elevated serum glucose level
- Decreased serum magnesium (Mg) level

● **Treatment**
- A high-potassium, low-sodium diet
- Oral potassium supplementation
  - Uses potassium salts
  - Potassium chloride preferred
- I.V. potassium replacement therapy for certain patients
  - Those with severe hypokalemia
  - Those who can't take oral supplements

Testing for hypokalemia
- ECG changes
- Decreased serum potassium level
- Elevated pH and bicarbonate level

Key treatment options for hypokalemia
- High-potassium, low-sodium diet
- Oral potassium supplementation
- I.V. potassium replacement therapy
- Potassium-sparing diuretic

- For patients requiring diuretics, use of a potassium-sparing diuretic to prevent excessive loss of potassium in urine

● **Nursing interventions**
- Monitor for signs and symptoms of hypokalemia in patients who are at risk
- Observe patients receiving diuretics closely because they're more susceptible to hypokalemia; closely observe patients taking digoxin (Lanoxin), especially if they're also taking a diuretic, because hypokalemia can potentiate the action of digoxin and cause digoxin toxicity
- Check heart rate and rhythm and ECG tracings in a patient with a serum potassium level less than 3 mEq/L (severe hypokalemia) because hypokalemia is commonly associated with hypovolemia, which may create tachyarrhythmias; also monitor these parameters closely if the patient is receiving a potassium infusion of more than 5 mEq/hour or a concentration of more than 40 mEq/L of fluid.
- Assess the patient's respiratory rate, depth, and pattern
  – Hypokalemia may weaken or paralyze respiratory muscles; notify physician immediately if respirations become shallow and rapid
  – Keep a handheld resuscitation bag at the bedside of a severe hypokalemia patient
- Monitor fluid intake and output closely; because 40 mEq of potassium is lost per 1 L of urine output, diuresis puts the patient at risk for serious potassium loss
- Monitor serum potassium levels carefully; keep in mind that relatively minor changes in serum potassium levels can cause serious cardiac complications
- Monitor for signs of hypokalemia-related metabolic alkalosis, such as irritability and confusion
- Check for signs of constipation, such as abdominal distention and decreased bowel sounds; although medication may be prescribed to combat constipation, don't use laxatives that promote potassium loss
- Administer oral potassium replacements in at least 4 oz of fluid or with food to prevent gastric irritation
- To prevent a quick load of potassium from entering the body, don't crush slow-release tablets
- Administer I.V. potassium supplement infusions cautiously; always dilute and mix thoroughly in adequate amounts of fluid (see *Guidelines for I.V. potassium administration*)
- Never administer potassium as I.V. push or as a bolus, which could prove fatal
- Assess the I.V. infusion site for signs and symptoms of infiltration or pain; high-concentration solutions may cause discomfort and irritation
- Provide patient (and his family) teaching as appropriate

Key nursing interventions for a patient with hypokalemia

- Monitor patients who are at risk.
- Monitor heart rate and rhythm.
- Assess respiratory rate, depth, and pattern.
- Monitor fluid intake and output.
- Monitor serum potassium levels.
- Monitor for signs of hypokalemia-related metabolic alkalosis.
- Administer potassium replacements.
- Provide patient teaching.

Guidelines for I.V. potassium administration

When administering I.V. potassium (K), there are several guidelines and monitoring points you should follow. Remember, potassium only needs to be replaced using an I.V. line if hypokalemia is severe or if the patient can't take oral potassium supplements.

ADMINISTRATION

- Use premixed potassium solution.
- To prevent or reduce toxic effects, I.V. infusion concentrations shouldn't exceed 60 mEq/L. Rates are usually 10 mEq/hour. More rapid infusions may be used in severe cases; however, rapid infusion requires closer monitoring of cardiac status. A rapid rise in serum potassium levels can lead to hyperkalemia, resulting in cardiac complications. The maximum adult dose generally shouldn't exceed 200 mEq/24 hours unless prescribed.
- Use infusion devices when administering potassium solutions to control flow rate.
- Never administer potassium by I.V. push or bolus; doing so can cause arrhythmias and cardiac arrest.

PATIENT MONITORING

- Monitor the patient's cardiac rhythm during rapid I.V. potassium administration to prevent toxic effects from hyperkalemia. Report irregularities immediately.
- Evaluate the results of treatment by checking serum potassium levels and assessing the patient for signs and symptoms of toxic reaction, such as muscle weakness and paralysis.
- Watch the I.V. site for signs and symptoms of infiltration, phlebitis, or tissue necrosis.
- Monitor the patient's urine output and notify the physician if volume is inadequate. Urine output should exceed 30 ml/hour to avoid hyperkalemia.
- Repeat potassium level measurements every 1 to 3 hours.

Key guidelines for I.V. potassium administration

Administration
- Use premixed potassium solution.
- Concentrations shouldn't exceed 60 mEq/L. Rates are usually 10 mEq/hour.
- Use infusion devices.
- Never administer potassium by I.V. push or bolus.

Patient monitoring
- Monitor cardiac rhythm.
- Check serum potassium levels.
- Watch the I.V. site for infiltration, phlebitis, or tissue necrosis.
- Monitor urine output.
- Repeat potassium level measurements every 1 to 3 hours.

– Teach measures to increase dietary intake of potassium, especially if patient is taking a diuretic
– Instruct in proper use of oral potassium supplements

POTASSIUM EXCESS: HYPERKALEMIA

● **General information**
- Results from impaired renal excretion of potassium or excessive potassium intake
- Can also occur in metabolic acidosis
  - Potassium moves into serum as hydrogen moves into cells
  - pH lowered
- When associated with acidosis, involves a movement of potassium from cells into serum, rather than an increase in total body potassium levels

Key facts about hyperkalemia

- Results from impaired renal excretion of potassium or excessive potassium intake
- Can occur in metabolic acidosis
- When associated with acidosis, involves a movement of potassium from cells into serum, rather than an increase in total body potassium levels
- Affects cardiac function

Key drugs associated with hyperkalemia

- Angiotensin-converting enzyme inhibitors
- Antibiotics
- Beta-adrenergic blockers
- Chemotherapeutic drugs
- Digoxin
- Heparin
- Nonsteroidal anti-inflammatory drugs
- Potassium supplements
- Potassium-sparing diuretics

Common causes of hyperkalemia

- Increased dietary potassium intake, especially with decreased urine output
- Excessive administration of potassium supplements
- Use of potassium-sparing diuretics
- Severe, widespread cell damage
- Administration of large volumes of blood
- Acute renal failure or chronic kidney disease

Drugs associated with hyperkalemia

The drugs listed here can cause increased potassium (K) levels. Ask your patient if any of these are a part of his drug therapy:

- angiotensin-converting enzyme inhibitors (such as captopril [Capoten], enalapril [Vasotec], and lisinopril [Zestril])
- antibiotics (such as penicillin G [Pfizerpen], sulfamethoxazole, and trimethoprim [Bactrim])
- beta-adrenergic blockers (such as propranolol [Inderal])
- chemotherapeutic drugs (such as cyclophosphamide [Cytoxan])
- digoxin (Lanoxin)
- heparin
- nonsteroidal anti-inflammatory drugs (such as indomethacin [Indocin])
- potassium supplements (in excessive amounts)
- potassium-sparing diuretics (such as spironolactone [Aldactone]).

- Excessive serum potassium levels: act as a myocardial depressant
    - Decreases heart rate and cardiac output
    - Causes possible cardiac arrest
- Causes skeletal muscle weakness, usually the initial symptom that prompts patients to seek health care assistance
- Also causes smooth-muscle hyperactivity
    - Happens particularly in the GI tract
    - Can result in colic and diarrhea

Causes
- Increased dietary potassium intake, especially with decreased urine output
- Excessive administration of potassium supplements
- Excessive use of salt substitutes; some form of potassium used in most as a sodium substitute
- Use of potassium-sparing diuretics, such as spironolactone (Aldactone) (see *Drugs associated with hyperkalemia*)
- Severe, widespread cell damage from several possible causes
    - Burns
    - Trauma
    - Crush injuries
    - Intravascular hemolysis
    - Increased catabolism
- Administration of large volumes of blood nearing its expiration date
    - "Old" blood: undergoes increased cell hemolysis
    - Result: potassium released as cells die
- Lysis of tumor cells from chemotherapy (potassium released from dying cells into ECF)
- Hyponatremia
- Hypoaldosteronism
- Metabolic or respiratory acidosis

ECG changes in hyperkalemia

Lab values: Serum potassium >5 mEq/L

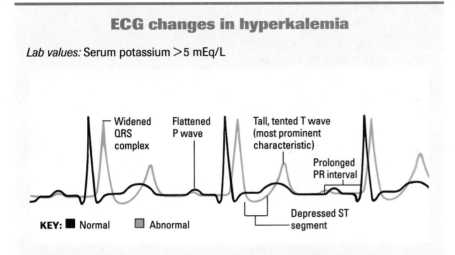

Widened QRS complex

Flattened P wave

Tall, tented T wave (most prominent characteristic)

Prolonged PR interval

Depressed ST segment

KEY: ■ Normal   ▨ Abnormal

- Acute renal failure or chronic kidney disease, which diminishes potassium excretion
- Any disease that can cause kidney damage
  - Diabetes
  - Sickle cell disease
  - Systemic lupus erythematosus

● **Assessment findings**
  - Irritability
  - Confusion
  - Paresthesia and numbness in extremities
  - Skeletal muscle weakness
  - Abdominal cramps
  - Nausea
  - Flaccid muscle paralysis
  - Diarrhea
  - Oliguria
  - Bradycardia
  - Idioventricular cardiac arrhythmias
  - Hypotension
  - Cardiac arrest

● **Diagnostic findings**
  - Serum potassium level greater than 5 mEq/L
  - Decreased arterial pH, indicating acidosis
  - ECG abnormalities that can lead to asystole if not reversed
    - Tall, tented T waves
    - Widened QRS complex
    - Prolonged PR interval
    - Depressed ST segment
    - Flattened or absent P wave (see *ECG changes in hyperkalemia*)

Key treatment options for hyperkalemia

- Administration of sodium polystyrene sulfonate
- Administration of loop diuretics
- Dietary potassium intake restricted
- Medications readjusted or stopped
- Hemodialysis

Key emergency treatment options for hyperkalemia

- Cardiac monitoring
- Used for severe cases (serum potassium level greater than 7 mEq/L)
- 10% calcium gluconate or 10% calcium chloride I.V.
- Sodium bicarbonate I.V.
- Regular insulin I.V.; used with I.V. hypertonic dextrose

Treatment

- Administration of sodium polystyrene sulfonate (Kayexalate)
  - Is a cation-exchange resin
  - Aids potassium excretion
  - Onset of action possibly delayed several hours; duration of action 4 to 6 hours
  - Numerous results as medication sits in intestines
    - Sodium: moves across bowel wall into blood
    - Potassium: moves out of blood into intestines
    - Loose stools: remove potassium from body
  - Should be accompanied by sorbitol or another osmotic substance to promote medicine's excretion
- Loop diuretic may be given
  - Increases potassium loss
  - Resolves any acidosis present
- Dietary potassium intake restricted
- Medications associated with a high potassium level readjusted or stopped
- Hemodialysis for acute symptom-producing cases
- Emergency treatment in severe cases (serum potassium level greater than 7 mEq/L)
  - Cardiac monitoring
  - Possible administration of several drugs
    - 10% calcium gluconate or 10% calcium chloride I.V. to counteract myocardial effects of hyperkalemia
    - Sodium bicarbonate I.V. to an acidosis patient; decreases serum potassium level by temporarily shifting potassium into cells
    - Regular insulin I.V. to move potassium into cells and lower serum potassium levels; used with I.V. hypertonic dextrose (10% to 50% glucose)

Nursing interventions

- Monitor patients at risk for hyperkalemia, specifically those in acidosis and those receiving potassium or potassium-sparing diuretics
- Before administering I.V. potassium supplements, determine whether the patient has a urine output greater than 30 ml/hour; inability to adequately excrete potassium may lead to dangerously high potassium levels
- Assess vital signs; monitor cardiovascular status closely by following pulse rate and rhythm and blood pressure
- Anticipate cardiac monitoring and a 12-lead ECG, which are indicated with elevated serum potassium levels; a patient with ECG changes may need aggressive treatment to prevent cardiac arrest
- Monitor bowel sounds and the number and character of bowel movements; hyperactive bowel sounds result from the body's attempt to

maintain homeostasis by causing significant potassium excretion through the bowels
- Monitor serum potassium levels to determine treatment effectiveness; a serum potassium level exceeding 6 mEq/L requires cardiac monitoring because asystole may occur as hyperkalemia makes depolarization of cardiac muscle easier and shortens repolarization times
- Assess motor and sensory function, especially of the extremities, for changes that may indicate changes in serum potassium levels
- Monitor neurologic status for changes; loss of consciousness may not occur with severe hyperkalemia until cardiac arrest occurs
- Be prepared to give calcium gluconate by slow I.V. infusion in acute cases to counteract the myocardial depressant effects of hyperkalemia; the patient must be on a cardiac monitor during administration
    - Patients not receiving digoxin may receive calcium gluconate
    - Hyperkalemic patients taking digoxin may not receive calcium; administering calcium gluconate with digoxin may exacerbate digoxin's effects, leading to acute digoxin toxicity and possible cardiac arrest
- If the patient is receiving insulin and glucose infusion therapy, monitor him for signs and symptoms of hypoglycemia, including muscle weakness, syncope, hunger, and diaphoresis
- Prepare the patient for the possibility of dialysis, either peritoneal or hemodialysis, which may be ordered in acute cases (in acute symptom-producing hyperkalemia, only hemodialysis is used)
- Administer sodium polystyrene sulfonate—orally or rectally—as ordered to decrease serum potassium levels
    - Administer oral form with sorbitol or another osmotic substance to enhance sodium polystyrene sulfonate's potassium-removing action
        - Patient should have a bowel movement after each oral dose to prevent bowel perforation; administer soapsuds enemas as necessary to promote excretion
    - Administer rectal sodium polystyrene sulfonate as a retention enema
        - Use of indwelling urinary drainage catheter with balloon inflated helps enema administration and retention
        - Cramps or diarrhea are common, making enema administration and retention difficult
        - Encourage patient to retain enemas for 30 to 60 minutes
    - Monitor patient for hypokalemia when administering drug for 2 or more consecutive days
    - Monitor for signs of hypernatremia in patient receiving sodium polystyrene sulfonate; watch for signs of heart failure
- Administer sodium bicarbonate as ordered to a patient with acidosis; this decreases serum potassium levels by creating alkalosis

Key nursing interventions for a patient with hyperkalemia
- Monitor patients at risk.
- Assess vital signs.
- Anticipate cardiac monitoring and a 12-lead ECG.
- Monitor serum potassium levels.
- Assess motor and sensory function.
- Monitor neurologic status.
- Administer insulin and glucose as ordered.
- Prepare the patient for the possibility of dialysis.
- Administer sodium polystyrene sulfonate.
- Administer sodium bicarbonate as ordered.
- Implement safety measures.
- Provide patient teaching.

Key patient teaching topics for hyperkalemia

- Causes and associated risks
- Foods and fluids high in potassium
- Avoiding salt substitutes
- Signs and symptoms of hyperkalemia
- Signs and symptoms of hypokalemia

TIME-OUT FOR TEACHING

Patient teaching: Hyperkalemia

When teaching a patient with hyperkalemia, be sure to cover the following information and then evaluate your patient's learning:

- Teach the patient and his family about hyperkalemia, including its causes and associated risks.
- Teach patients, particularly those with renal failure or renal insufficiency, about foods and fluids high in potassium (K) and the importance of avoiding them to prevent hyperkalemia.
- Remind patients that most salt substitutes are high in potassium and should be avoided if the patient is at risk for or has hyperkalemia.
- Explain the signs and symptoms of hyperkalemia, including muscle weakness, diarrhea, and pulse irregularities. Urge the patient to report such signs and symptoms to his physician.
- Describe the signs and symptoms of hypokalemia to the patient if he's taking medication to lower his serum potassium level.

- If the patient has hyperkalemia and needs a transfusion, obtain fresh blood
- If the patient has muscle weakness, implement safety measures; continue to evaluate muscle strength and advise him to ask for help before attempting to get out of bed and walk
- Be aware that hemolysis of blood samples, either from too tight a tourniquet or too rapidly pulling blood into a vial or syringe, may cause falsely elevated potassium levels (pseudohyperkalemia); a sample should be redrawn if no clinical symptoms exist
- Provide patient teaching as appropriate (see *Patient teaching: Hyperkalemia*)

CALCIUM DEFICIT: HYPOCALCEMIA

Key facts about hypocalcemia

- Results from abnormalities of PTH secretion or from inadequate dietary intake or excessive losses of bound, ionized (unbound), or total body calcium
- Usually reflects decreased circulating ionized calcium levels

● **General information**
- Results from abnormalities of parathyroid hormone (PTH) secretion or from inadequate dietary intake or excessive losses of bound, ionized (unbound), or total body calcium
- Usually reflects decreased circulating ionized calcium levels
- Can cause skeletal and neuromuscular abnormalities
- Impairs clotting mechanisms
- Affects cell membrane integrity and permeability (calcium helps maintain cellular integrity)
- One-half of ingested calcium bound to protein (serum protein abnormalities influence serum calcium levels)
- One-half of ionized calcium absorbed in the gut with vitamin D (GI tract or vitamin D abnormalities decrease serum calcium levels)

- Increased neural excitability and spontaneous stimulation of sensory and motor fibers reflected in symptoms

● **Causes**
- Surgically induced or primary hypoparathyroidism
- Acute renal failure or chronic kidney disease
- Chronic malabsorption syndrome
- Vitamin D deficiency
- Inadequate exposure to ultraviolet light
- Chronic, insufficient dietary intake of calcium
  - Alcoholics particularly at risk
    · Poor nutritional intake
    · Poor calcium absorption
    · Low magnesium level (affects PTH secretion)
- Hyperphosphatemia (interferes with calcium absorption)
- Acute pancreatitis or pancreatic insufficiency
- Administration of large amounts of citrated blood
- Alkalosis
- Hypoalbuminemia
- Hypomagnesemia
- Anticonvulsants
  - Phenobarbital (Luminal)
  - Phenytoin (Dilantin)
- Diuretics, especially loop diuretics
  - Furosemide
  - Ethacrynic acid (Edecrin)
- Antineoplastic drugs
  - Mithramycin (Mithracin)
  - Cisplatin (Platinol-AQ)

● **Assessment findings**
- Muscle cramps or tremors
- Hyperactive deep tendon reflexes
- Paresthesia of the fingers, toes, and face
- Tetany
- Positive Trousseau's sign
- Positive Chvostek's sign (see *Checking for Trousseau's and Chvostek's signs*, page 106)
- Spasms
  - Laryngeal and bronchial muscles
  - Abdominal muscles
- Brittle nails or dry skin and hair
- Increased risk of fractures
- Confusion
- Irritability and anxiety
- Memory loss
- Seizures

Common causes of hypocalcemia
- Hypoparathyroidism
- Kidney disease
- Vitamin D deficiency
- Inadequate exposure to ultraviolet light
- Chronic, insufficient dietary intake of calcium
- Hyperphosphatemia
- Acute pancreatitis or pancreatic insufficiency
- Administration of large amounts of citrated blood

Common assessment findings in hypocalcemia
- Muscle cramps or tremors
- Tetany
- Positive Trousseau's sign
- Positive Chvostek's sign
- Irritability and anxiety
- Seizures
- Arrhythmias
- Angina, bradycardia, and hypotension

Common indications of Trousseau's and Chvostek's signs

Trousseau's sign
- Adducted thumb
- Flexed wrist and metacarpophalangeal joints
- Extended interphalangeal joints
- Carpal spasm indicating tetany

Chvostek's sign
- Brief contraction of the upper lip, nose, or side of the face

Testing for hypocalcemia

- ECG: prolonged QT interval and ST segment
- Decreased serum calcium level
- Decreased ionized calcium level
- Low albumin level

Key treatment options for hypocalcemia

- Dietary adjustments
- Aluminum hydroxide antacids

Acute
- I.V. calcium gluconate
- I.V. calcium chloride

Chronic
- Vitamin D supplements
- Oral calcium supplements

Checking for Trousseau's and Chvostek's signs

Testing for Trousseau's and Chvostek's signs can aid in the diagnosis of tetany and hypocalcemia. Use these guidelines to check for these important signs.

TROUSSEAU'S SIGN
To check for Trousseau's sign, apply a blood pressure cuff to the patient's upper arm and inflate it to a pressure 20 mm Hg above the systolic pressure. Trousseau's sign may appear after 1 to 4 minutes. The patient will experience an adducted thumb, flexed wrist and metacarpophalangeal joints, and extended interphalangeal joints (with fingers together)—carpal spasm—indicating tetany, a major sign of hypocalcemia.

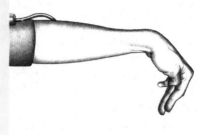

CHVOSTEK'S SIGN
You can induce Chvostek's sign by tapping the patient's facial nerve adjacent to the ear. A brief contraction of the upper lip, nose, or side of the face indicates Chvostek's sign.

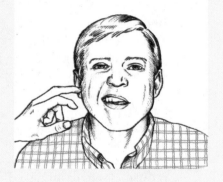

- Arrhythmias
- Angina, bradycardia, and hypotension

● **Diagnostic findings**
- ECG: prolonged QT interval and ST segment (see *ECG changes in hypocalcemia*)
- Serum calcium level less than 8.5 mg/dl
- Ionized calcium level less than 4.5 mg/dl
- Low albumin level
- Prolonged prothrombin time and partial thromboplastin time

● **Treatment**
- For acute hypocalcemia
  - Immediate correction necessary
  - I.V. calcium gluconate
  - I.V. calcium chloride

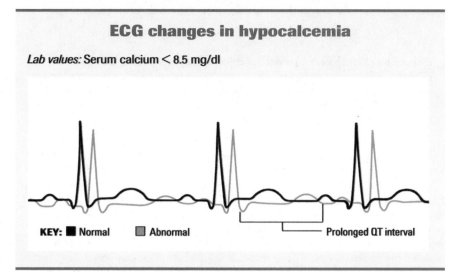

ECG changes in hypocalcemia

Lab values: Serum calcium < 8.5 mg/dl

KEY: ■ Normal   ▨ Abnormal   Prolonged QT interval

   – Magnesium replacement may also be needed
- For chronic hypocalcemia
   – Vitamin D supplements
   – Oral calcium supplements
- Dietary adjustments made to allow for an adequate intake of many elements
   – Calcium
   – Vitamin D
   – Protein
- Aluminum hydroxide antacids used to bind with excess phosphorus (P) in patients with high phosphorus levels

● **Nursing interventions**
- Carefully assess patients at increased risk for hypocalcemia, especially after parathyroidectomy or massive transfusions; be especially alert for the coexistence of other electrolyte imbalances, such as hypokalemia and hypomagnesemia
- Monitor vital signs, and assess the patient frequently
- Monitor respiratory status, including rate, depth, and rhythm; watch for stridor, dyspnea, and crowing
- If patient shows signs of hypocalcemia, keep tracheotomy tray and handheld resuscitation bag at bedside in case of laryngospasm
- Place patient on a cardiac monitor, and observe for changes in heart rate and rhythm; notify physician if patient develops arrhythmias, such as ventricular tachycardia or heart block
- Check the patient for Chvostek's and Trousseau's signs
- Monitor pertinent laboratory test results, including calcium levels and albumin levels, and those of other electrolytes such as magnesium; re-

Key nursing interventions for a patient with hypocalcemia

- Monitor patients at risk.
- Monitor vital signs.
- Monitor respiratory status.
- Observe for changes in heart rate and rhythm.
- Check for Chvostek's and Trousseau's signs.
- Monitor laboratory test results.
- Take precautions for seizures.
- Reorient a confused patient.
- Administer oral replacements as ordered.
- Administer I.V. calcium replacement therapy.
- Assess the patient's nutritional intake.
- Provide patient teaching.

Key facts about administering I.V. calcium safely

- Always clarify whether physician has ordered calcium gluconate or calcium chloride.

Preparing
- Dilute in dextrose 5% in water.

Administering
- Administer I.V. slowly.
- Initially, calcium may be given as a slow I.V. bolus.
- Bolus may be followed by a slow I.V. drip using an infusion pump.

Monitoring
- Watch for signs and symptoms of hypercalcemia.
- Observe the I.V. site for signs of infiltration.
- Closely monitor serum calcium levels.

Administering I.V. calcium safely

Be prepared to administer parenteral calcium (Ca) to a patient who has symptom-producing hypocalcemia. Always clarify whether the physician has ordered calcium gluconate or calcium chloride. Doses vary according to the specific drug. Note the type and dosage of each calcium preparation carefully, and follow these steps when administering it.

PREPARING
Dilute the prescribed I.V. calcium preparation in dextrose 5% in water. Never dilute calcium in solutions containing bicarbonate because precipitation will occur. Avoid giving the patient calcium diluted in normal saline solution because the sodium chloride will increase renal calcium loss.

ADMINISTERING
Always administer I.V. calcium slowly, according to the physician's order or established protocol. Never give it rapidly because it may result in syncope, hypotension, or cardiac arrhythmias. Initially, calcium may be given as a slow I.V. bolus. If hypocalcemia persists, the initial bolus may be followed by a slow I.V. drip using an infusion pump.

MONITORING
Overcorrection may lead to hypercalcemia. Watch for signs and symptoms of hypercalcemia, including anorexia, nausea, vomiting, lethargy, and confusion. Institute cardiac monitoring, and observe the patient for cardiac arrhythmias, especially if the patient is receiving digoxin (Lanoxin). Observe the I.V. site for signs of infiltration; calcium can cause tissue sloughing and necrosis. Closely monitor serum calcium levels.

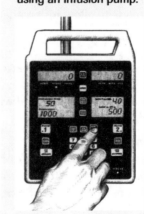
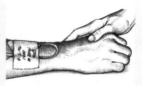

---

member to check the ionized calcium level after every four units of blood transfused
- Take precautions for seizures such as padding bed side rails
- Reorient a confused patient; provide a calm, quiet environment
- Administer oral replacements as ordered
  - Give calcium supplements 1 to 1½ hours after meals
  - Give supplement with milk if GI upset occurs
- Administer I.V. calcium replacement therapy carefully; ensure patency of the I.V. line because infiltration can cause tissue necrosis and sloughing (see *Administering I.V. calcium safely*)

TIME-OUT FOR TEACHING

Patient teaching: Hypocalcemia

When teaching a patient with hypocalcemia, be sure to cover the following information and then evaluate your patient's learning:

- Teach the patient and family about hypocalcemia, including its causes and associated risks.
- Encourage the older patient to take a calcium (Ca) supplement as ordered, and to exercise as much as he can to prevent calcium loss from bones.

- Teach the patient about foods and fluids high in calcium, such as dairy products and green, leafy vegetables. Emphasize the importance of a high-calcium diet.
- Teach the patient that exercise enhances calcium mobilization from bones to replenish extracellular fluid levels.

- Keep calcium gluconate at the bedside of a patient recovering from parathyroid or thyroid surgery to allow prompt administration if a rapid drop in serum calcium level occurs
- Assess the patient's nutritional intake for calcium or vitamin D deficiencies; adjust dietary intake to increase calcium
- Provide patient teaching as appropriate (see *Patient teaching: Hypocalcemia*)

CALCIUM EXCESS: HYPERCALCEMIA

● General information

- Occurs when rate of calcium entry into ECF exceeds rate of renal calcium excretion
  - Bone resorption and formation: normally occur at same rate
  - Mobilization of calcium from bone: results in increased serum calcium levels
- Symptoms directly related to degree of serum calcium elevation; severe symptoms may occur with levels greater than 14 mg/dl
  - Stem from effects of excess calcium in cells
  - Causes a decrease in cell membrane excitability
  - Especially affects the tissues of skeletal muscle, the heart muscle, and the nervous system
- Increased intestinal absorption of calcium from several possible sources: results in increased serum calcium levels
  - Increased availability
  - Increased vitamin D absorption
  - Altered GI metabolism
- Renal abnormalities (particularly of the tubules) that interfere with calcium secretion and excretion: can cause increased serum calcium levels

Common causes of hypercalcemia

- Primary hyperparathyroidism
- Excessive intake of calcium supplements
- Excessive use of calcium-containing antacids
- Prolonged immobility
- Excessive vitamin D intake

Common assessment findings in hypercalcemia

- Lethargy
- Muscle weakness or flaccidity
- Hyporeflexia and decreased muscle tone
- Urinary calculi
- Arrhythmias and cardiac arrest

Testing for hypercalcemia

- Increased serum calcium level
- Increased ionized calcium level
- ECG changes

- Patients with metastatic cancer at especially high risk
  - Cancer: causes bone destruction as malignant cells invade bones; may cause release of substance similar to PTH (increases serum calcium levels)
  - Kidneys: can become overwhelmed and unable to excrete excess calcium when serum calcium levels increase; keeps calcium levels elevated
  - Prognosis poor for hypercalcemia associated with cancer; 1-year survival rate of only 10% to 30%

Causes
- Primary hyperparathyroidism (most common cause)
- Excessive intake of calcium supplements
- Excessive use of calcium-containing antacids (phosphate-binding gels)
- Prolonged immobility
- Excessive vitamin D intake
- Use of lithium (Lithobid) or thiazide diuretics
- Metastatic carcinoma
- Thyrotoxicosis
- Hypophosphatemia
- Renal tubular acidosis
- Milk-alkali syndrome

Assessment findings
- Lethargy (may progress to coma in severe cases)
- Altered mental status, depression, or personality changes
- Muscle weakness or flaccidity
- Hyporeflexia and decreased muscle tone
- Hypertension
- Nausea and vomiting
- Extreme thirst
- Anorexia
- Constipation
- Polyuria
- Urinary calculi
- Pathologic fractures and bone pain
- Metastatic calcifications, particularly in the cornea and skin (causes itching)
- Arrhythmias and cardiac arrest

Diagnostic findings
- Serum calcium level greater than 10.5 mg/dl
- Ionized calcium level above 5.1 mg/dl
- Bone changes on X-ray such as pathologic fractures
- ECG changes
  - Shortened QT interval

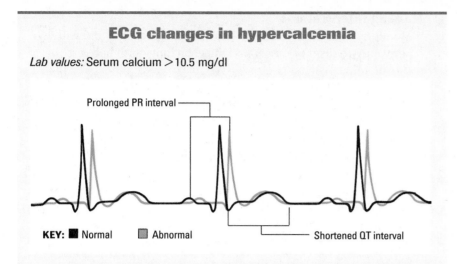

ECG changes in hypercalcemia

Lab values: Serum calcium >10.5 mg/dl

Prolonged PR interval

KEY: ■ Normal ■ Abnormal   Shortened QT interval

– Prolonged PR interval
– Flattened T waves
– Heart block (see *ECG changes in hypercalcemia*)

● **Treatment**
• Dietary calcium intake reduced
• Discontinued use of medications or infusions containing calcium
• Calcium excretion measures
  – Hydration: encourages diuresis and aids calcium excretion
  – Normal saline solution typically used (renal tubular reabsorption of calcium inhibited by sodium in solution)
  – Loop diuretics to promote calcium excretion
    • Furosemide
    • Ethacrynic acid
• Hemodialysis or peritoneal dialysis
  – Uses a solution that contains little or no calcium
  – May be used for patients with severe conditions
    • Life-threatening hypercalcemia
    • Renal failure
• Measures to inhibit bone resorption
  – Corticosteroids
    • Administered I.V. and then orally
    • Decrease calcium absorption from GI tract
  – Zoledronate (Zometa) administration
  – Etidronate disodium (Didronel) administration
  – Pamidronate disodium (Aredia) administration
  – Calcitonin (Miacalcin) administration
    • Naturally occurring hormone
    • Effects short-lived

Key treatment options for hypercalcemia

• Dietary calcium intake reduced
• Discontinued use of medications or infusions containing calcium
• Calcium excretion measures (hydration and diurectics)
• Hemodialysis or peritoneal dialysis
• Measures to inhibit bone resorption

Key nursing interventions for a patient with hypercalcemia

- Monitor patients at risk.
- Monitor vital signs.
- Monitor cardiac rhythm.
- Assess neurologic and neuromuscular function.
- Monitor fluid intake and output.
- Monitor serum electrolyte levels.
- Encourage the patient to drink 3 to 4 L of fluids daily (if not contraindicated).
- In acute moderate-to-severe hypercalcemia, administer I.V. isotonic normal saline solution.
- Administer loop diuretics.
- Provide a safe environment.
- Provide patient teaching.

● **Nursing interventions**
- Monitor patients at risk for hypercalcemia, especially those with hyperparathyroidism or cancer and those on long-term bed rest
- Ambulate the patient as soon as possible to prevent bones from releasing calcium
- Monitor vital signs and assess the patient frequently
- Place the patient on a cardiac monitor to detect arrhythmias
- Assess neurologic and neuromuscular function and report changes
- Monitor the patient's fluid intake and output
- Monitor serum electrolyte levels (especially calcium) to determine the effectiveness of treatment and detect new imbalances that might result from therapy
- Encourage the patient to drink 3 to 4 L of fluids daily (if not contraindicated) to stimulate calcium excretion from the kidneys and decrease the risk of calculi formation
- Strain the urine for calculi; also check for flank pain, which can indicate the presence of renal calculi
- In a patient with acute moderate-to-severe (levels greater than 13 mg/dl) hypercalcemia, administer I.V. isotonic normal saline solution, usually at a rate of 200 to 500 ml/hour, to reverse dehydration and promote urinary calcium excretion; monitor the patient for signs of pulmonary edema during therapy, such as crackles and dyspnea
- Administer loop diuretics, such as furosemide, to prevent volume overload with I.V. normal saline solution and to increase urinary calcium excretion; make sure the patient is properly hydrated first so he doesn't experience volume depletion
- If the patient is receiving digoxin, watch for signs and symptoms of a toxic reaction, such as anorexia, nausea, vomiting, or an irregular heart rate
- Handle a chronic hypercalcemia patient gently to prevent pathologic fractures; reposition bedridden patients frequently; perform active or passive range-of-motion exercises to prevent complications from immobility
- Provide a safe environment
  - Keep the bed in its lowest position, with side rails raised as needed and wheels locked
  - Keep the patient's belongings and call bell within reach
  - Reorient the patient if he's confused
- Offer emotional support to the patient and his family throughout treatment; overt signs of hypercalcemia can be emotionally distressing for all involved
- Provide patient (and his family) teaching
  - Teach them to recognize signs and symptoms
    · Personality changes
    · Muscle weakness

- Pathologic fractures
  – Stress importance of avoiding calcium-containing foods and fluids
    - Dairy products
    - Other supplements or products containing calcium

PHOSPHORUS DEFICIT: HYPOPHOSPHATEMIA

● **General information**
  - Commonly results from decreased intestinal absorption of phosphorus
  - May result from renal wasting of phosphorus as a method of controlling acid-base balance or during diuresis
  - May result from phosphorus redistribution from ECF to ICF, such as from I.V. glucose administration
  - Severe cases (serum phosphorus levels less than 1 mg/dl): body can't support its energy needs, leading to possible organ failure
  - Affects the musculoskeletal, central nervous, cardiac, and hematologic systems

● **Causes**
  - Inadequate dietary phosphorus intake such as in malnutrition
  - Severe, prolonged vomiting
  - Excessive administration of phosphate-binding gels
  - Thiazides, loop diuretics, and acetazolamide (Diamox)
  - Alcoholism and alcohol withdrawal
  - Administration of carbohydrates or TPN without phosphorus to malnourished patients
  - Hyperglycemia or insulin administration
    – Insulin: transports glucose and phosphorus into cells
    – Reduces serum phosphorus levels
  - Malabsorption syndromes
  - Hyperparathyroidism
  - Severe metabolic acidosis such as in diabetic ketoacidosis
  - Respiratory alkalosis
    – Causes phosphorus to shift into the cells
    – Reduces serum phosphorus levels
  - Thermal burns
  - Hypokalemia
  - Hypomagnesemia
  - Acute gout
  - Aldosteronism
  - Pancreatitis
  - Renal disease
  - High calcium intake

Key facts about hypophosphatemia

- Commonly results from decreased intestinal absorption of phosphorus
- May result from renal wasting of phosphorus
- May result from phosphorus redistribution from ECF to ICF
- May lead to organ failure

Common causes of hypophosphatemia

- Inadequate dietary phosphorus
- Severe, prolonged vomiting
- Excessive administration of phosphate-binding gels
- Thiazides, loop diuretics, and acetazolamide
- Alcoholism
- Hyperparathyroidism
- High calcium intake

Common assessment findings in hypophosphatemia

- Paresthesia
- Profound muscle weakness
- Rapid, shallow respirations
- Potential for respiratory depression
- Altered LOC

Testing for hypophosphatemia

- Decreased serum phosphorus level
- Decreased magnesium levels
- Increased calcium levels

Key treatment options for hypophosphatemia

- Diet high in phosphorus-rich foods
- Oral phosphorus supplements
- I.V. phosphorus replacement

Assessment findings

- Paresthesia
- Profound muscle weakness
- Muscle pain and tenderness
- Anorexia
- Malaise
- Rapid, shallow respirations
- Potential for respiratory depression
- Altered LOC
- Seizures
- Diplopia
- Nystagmus and unequal pupils
- Rhabdomyolysis (with severe hypophosphatemia)
- Heart failure
- Hemolytic anemia
- Platelet dysfunction
- Increased susceptibility to infection
- Skeletal abnormalities
    - Loss of bone density
    - Osteomalacia
    - Bone pain
    - Fractures

Diagnostic findings

- Serum phosphorus level less than 2.5 mg/dl (or 1.8 mEq/L); severe hypophosphatemia less than 1 mg/dl
- Elevated creatine kinase levels with rhabdomyolysis
- X-rays revealing skeletal changes typical of osteomalacia or bone fractures
- Abnormal electrolytes
    - Decreased magnesium levels
    - Increased calcium levels

Treatment

- A diet high in phosphorus-rich foods
    - Eggs
    - Nuts
    - Whole grains
    - Meat
    - Fish
    - Poultry
    - Milk products
- Oral phosphorus supplements if calcium is contraindicated or for patients who can't tolerate milk
    - Neutra-Phos
    - Neutra-Phos-K

- I.V. phosphorus replacement for patients with severe hypophosphatemia or a nonfunctioning GI tract

● **Nursing interventions**
- Monitor patients at risk for hypophosphatemia, especially those receiving TPN without phosphorus replacement
- Monitor vital signs and intake and output; remember, hypophosphatemia can lead to respiratory failure, low cardiac output, confusion, seizures, or coma
- Assess the patient's LOC and neurologic status each time you check his vital signs
- If the patient has severe hypophosphatemia, monitor the rate and depth of respirations; report signs and symptoms of hypoxia, such as confusion, restlessness, increased respiratory rate and, in later stages, cyanosis
- Assess for paresthesia, particularly in the circumoral area—an early sign of hypophosphatemia
- Monitor for evidence of heart failure related to reduced myocardial functioning; such evidence includes crackles, shortness of breath, decreased blood pressure, and elevated heart rate
- Monitor the patient's temperature at least every 4 hours; check white blood cell counts; follow strict sterile technique in changing dressings and report signs of infection
- Assess frequently for evidence of decreasing muscle strength, such as weak hand grasps or slurred speech
- Carefully monitor serum electrolyte levels, especially calcium and phosphorus levels, as well as other pertinent laboratory test results, and be sure to report abnormalities
- Administer prescribed phosphorus supplements
  - Diarrhea is possible with oral supplements
  - Mixing with juice improves taste of phosphorus supplements
  - Vitamin D may be used with oral phosphorus supplements to increase absorption
- Infuse I.V. phosphorus solutions slowly, using an infusion device to control the rate
  - During infusions, watch for signs of hypocalcemia, hyperphosphatemia, and I.V. infiltration
  - Be aware that potassium phosphate can cause tissue sloughing and necrosis if infiltrated
  - Monitor serum phosphorus levels every 6 hours
- Be aware of adverse effects of I.V. replacement for hypophosphatemia
  - Hyperphosphatemia
  - Hypocalcemia
- Initiate safety precautions for a patient with confusion or decreased LOC
  - Ensure maintained bed rest if ordered

Key nursing interventions for a patient with hypophosphatemia

- Monitor patients at risk.
- Monitor vital signs and intake and output.
- Assess LOC and neurologic status.
- Monitor respiratory status.
- Assess for paresthesia.
- Monitor for evidence of heart failure.
- Assess muscle strength.
- Monitor serum electrolyte levels.
- Administer prescribed phosphorus supplements.
- Initiate safety precautions.
- Provide patient teaching.

Key facts about hyperphosphatemia

- Most commonly results from the kidney's inability to excrete excess phosphorus
- Also results from increased release of phosphorus from damaged cells
- May lead to hypocalcemia

Common causes of hyperphosphatemia

- Kidney disease
- Excessive dietary phosphorus intake
- Excessive vitamin D use
- Hypoparathyroidism

Common assessment findings in hyperphosphatemia

- Tetany
- Circumoral paresthesia
- Muscle spasms, cramps, pain, and weakness
- Positive Trousseau's and Chvostek's signs
- Decreased mental function, delirium, and seizures

– Keep the bed in lowest position with wheels locked and side rails raised
– For a patient at risk for seizures, keep side rails padded and artificial airway at the bedside
– Reorient the patient as needed; keep clocks, calendars, and familiar personal objects within sight
– Assist the patient with ambulation and activities of daily living (ADLs) if needed; keep essential objects near him
- Provide patient (and his family) teaching as needed
  – Instruct in measures to increase dietary phosphorus intake
  – Reassure patient and his family that confusion caused by low phosphorus level is temporary and will most likely decrease with therapy

PHOSPHORUS EXCESS: HYPERPHOSPHATEMIA

General information
- Most commonly results from the kidney's inability to excrete excess phosphorus along with an increased release of phosphorus from damaged cells
- Severe cases: when serum phosphorus levels reach 6 mg/dl or higher
- Causes few clinical problems by itself, but may lead to hypocalcemia, which can be life-threatening
- Signs and symptoms usually caused by hypocalcemia effects

Causes
- Acute renal failure or chronic kidney disease
- Excessive dietary phosphorus intake
- Excessive vitamin D use (results in increased phosphorus absorption)
- Hypoparathyroidism
- Cancer chemotherapy
- Excessive use of laxatives and phosphorus-based enemas
- Ruptured abdominal viscera (increased phosphorus level a critical sign in a patient with acute pain)

Assessment findings
- Tetany
- Circumoral paresthesia
- Muscle spasms, cramps, pain, and weakness
- Positive Trousseau's and Chvostek's signs
- Decreased mental function, delirium, and seizures
- Soft tissue calcification (with long-standing hyperphosphatemia)

Diagnostic findings
- Serum phosphorus level greater than 4.5 mg/dl (or 2.6 mEq/L)
- Serum calcium level less than 8.5 mg/dl
- Skeletal changes revealed in X-ray studies
  – Due to osteodystrophy (defective bone development)

– Applies to chronic cases
- Increased blood urea nitrogen (BUN) and creatinine levels, which reflect worsening renal function
- ECG changes characteristic of hypocalcemia (prolonged QT interval and ST segment)

Treatment
- Reduced phosphorus intake
  – Dietary phosphorus reduced
  – Use of phosphorus-based laxatives and enemas eliminated
- Drug therapy
  – Used to decrease absorption of phosphorus in the GI system
  – Includes use of several medications
    · Aluminum
    · Magnesium
    · Calcium gel
    · Phosphate-binding antacids
    · Calcium salts such as calcium carbonate (Caltrate 600) and calcium acetate (PhosLo)
    · Polymeric phosphate binders, such as sevelamer hydrochloride (Renagel)
- I.V. saline solution administration for severe cases
  – Promotes renal excretion of phosphorus
  – Patient: must have functional kidneys
- Acetazolamide to increase renal excretion of phosphorus
- Hemodialysis or peritoneal dialysis
  – Used for chronic kidney disease
  – Also used for extreme acute case with symptom-producing hypocalcemia

Nursing interventions
- Monitor patients at risk, particularly those with hypocalcemia and those receiving phosphorus in I.V. infusions, enemas, or laxatives
- Monitor vital signs, keeping in mind the signs and symptoms of hypocalcemia
  – Notify physician promptly if signs or symptoms of worsening hypocalcemia are noted, such as paresthesia in fingers or around mouth, hyperactive reflexes, or muscle cramps
  – Notify physician if signs or symptoms of calcification are detected, including oliguria, vision impairment, conjunctivitis, irregular heart rate or palpitations, and papular eruptions
- Monitor fluid intake and output; decreased urine output can seriously affect renal clearance of excess serum phosphorus
- Monitor for neuromuscular irritability, which accompanies high phosphorus levels
- Carefully monitor serum electrolyte levels, especially calcium and phosphorus; also monitor BUN and serum creatinine levels because

---

Testing for hyperphosphatemia

- Increased serum phosphorus level
- Decreased serum calcium level
- ECG changes characteristic of hypocalcemia

Key treatment options for hyperphosphatemia

- Reduced phosphorus intake
- Drug therapy: to decrease absorption of phosphorus in the GI system
- I.V. saline solution administration for severe cases
- Acetazolamide
- Hemodialysis or peritoneal dialysis

Key nursing interventions for a patient with hyperphosphatemia

- Monitor patients at risk.
- Monitor vital signs.
- Monitor fluid intake and output.
- Monitor for neuromuscular irritability.
- Monitor serum electrolyte levels.
- Administer prescribed medications.
- Prepare the patient for possible dialysis.
- Initiate seizure precautions.
- Provide patient teaching.

Key patient teaching topics for hyperphosphatemia

- Causes and associated risks
- Avoiding preparations that contain phosphorus
- Avoiding foods and fluids high in phosphorus

TIME-OUT FOR TEACHING

Patient teaching: Hyperphosphatemia

When teaching a patient with hyperphosphatemia, be sure to cover the following information and then evaluate your patient's learning:

- Teach the patient and his family about hyperphosphatemia, including its causes and associated risks.
- Instruct the patient to avoid preparations that contain phosphorus, such as laxatives, enemas, and supplements.
- Teach the patient to avoid foods and fluids high in phosphorus, such as cheeses, nuts, whole-grain cereals, dried fruits, peanuts, and vegetables.

hyperphosphatemia can impair renal tubules when calcification occurs

- Administer prescribed medications, monitor their effectiveness, and assess the patient for possible adverse reactions; give antacids with meals to increase their effectiveness in binding phosphorus
- Prepare the patient for possible dialysis if hyperphosphatemia is severe
- If a patient's condition results from chronic kidney disease or if his treatment includes a low-phosphorus diet, consult a dietitian to assist him in complying with dietary restrictions
- Initiate seizure precautions in patients with elevated phosphorus levels
- Provide patient teaching as necessary (see *Patient teaching: Hyperphosphatemia*)

MAGNESIUM DEFICIT: HYPOMAGNESEMIA

General information
- Has several possible causes
  - Poor dietary intake of magnesium
  - Poor magnesium absorption by the GI tract
  - Excessive magnesium loss from the GI tract
  - Excessive magnesium excretion by the kidneys
- Increases muscle cell irritability and contractility
- Causes decreased blood pressure and may result in ventricular arrhythmias
- Produces signs and symptoms similar to hypokalemia (conditions commonly occur simultaneously)

Causes
- Excessive dietary intake of calcium or vitamin D

Key facts about hypomagnesemia

- May result from poor dietary intake of magnesium or excessive excretion by kidneys
- May be caused by poor magnesium absorption by the GI tract or excessive magnesium loss from the GI tract
- Causes increased muscle cell irritability and contractility

- Severe GI fluid losses (can result from numerous conditions)
  - Gastric suctioning or lavage
  - Prolonged vomiting or diarrhea
  - Laxative abuse
- Prolonged, excessive diuretic therapy
- Administration of I.V. fluids or TPN without magnesium replacement
- Prolonged malnutrition or starvation
- Malabsorption syndromes
- Ulcerative colitis
- Hypercalcemia
- Hypoparathyroidism
- Hypoaldosteronism
- High-dose steroid use
- Cancer chemotherapy
- Use of specific drugs
  - Amphotericin B (Fungizone)
  - Cisplatin
  - Cyclosporine (Sandimmune)
  - Pentamidine isethionate (NebuPent)
  - Aminoglycoside antibiotics
    · Tobramycin (Tobrex)
    · Gentamicin (Garamycin)
- Burns and debridement therapy
- Sepsis
- Pancreatitis
- Diabetic ketoacidosis
- Chronic alcoholism and alcohol withdrawal
- Pregnancy-induced hypertension

Assessment findings
- Tachycardia and other arrhythmias and hypotension
- Tremors
- Tetany
- Hyperactive deep tendon reflexes, positive Babinski's reflex (see *Grading deep tendon reflexes,* page 120)
- Positive Chvostek's and Trousseau's signs
- Memory loss
- Emotional lability
- Confusion
- Dizziness
- Anorexia
- Dysphagia
- Nausea
- Hallucinations
- Seizures
- Coma

Common causes of hypomagnesemia
- Excessive dietary intake of calcium or vitamin D
- Severe GI fluid losses
- Diuretic therapy
- Administration of I.V. fluids or TPN without magnesium replacement
- Hypercalcemia
- Medication
- Burns and debridement therapy
- Alcoholism

Common assessment findings in hypomagnesemia
- Tachycardia and other arrhythmias and hypotension
- Hyperactive deep tendon reflexes, positive Babinski's reflex
- Positive Chvostek's and Trousseau's signs
- Emotional lability
- Confusion
- Dizziness
- Seizures

Grading deep tendon reflexes

- 0: Absent
- ++: Normal
- +++: Increased but not necessarily abnormal
- ++++: Hyperactive, clonic

Testing for hypomagnesemia

- Decreased serum magnesium level
- Hypocalcemia
- Hypokalemia
- ECG changes

Treatment options for hypomagnesemia

- Dietary magnesium intake increased
- Oral magnesium supplements
- I.V. or deep I.M. injections of magnesium sulfate

Grading deep tendon reflexes

If you suspect your patient has hypomagnesemia, you'll want to test his deep tendon reflexes to determine whether his neuromuscular system is irritable—an indication that his magnesium level is too low. When grading your patient's deep tendon reflexes, use the following scale:

0	Absent
++	Normal
+++	Increased but not necessarily abnormal
++++	Hyperactive, clonic

To record the patient's reflex activity, draw a stick figure and mark the strength of the response at the proper locations. This figure indicates normal deep tendon reflex activity.

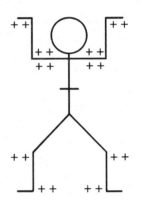

Diagnostic findings
- Serum magnesium level less than 1.8 mg/dl (signs and symptoms occur at about 1 mg/dl)
- Hypocalcemia
- Hypokalemia
- ECG changes
  - Flattened T wave
  - Slightly widened QRS complex
  - Diminished voltage of P waves and QRS complex
  - Prominent U wave (see *ECG changes in hypomagnesemia*)

Treatment
- Dietary magnesium intake increased
- Oral magnesium supplements encouraged
- I.V. or deep I.M. injections of magnesium sulfate used for more severe cases

Nursing interventions
- Monitor patients at risk for hypomagnesemia, particularly those with hypokalemia and those receiving TPN without magnesium replacement
- Closely monitor a patient with hypomagnesemia who's also taking digoxin for signs and symptoms of digoxin toxicity
  - Low magnesium level may increase body's retention of digoxin
  - Suspect digoxin toxicity if patient has anorexia, arrhythmias, nausea, vomiting, or yellow-tinged vision
- Monitor the patient's vital signs closely
- Monitor the patient's respiratory status; a magnesium deficiency can cause laryngeal stridor and compromise the airway

ECG changes in hypomagnesemia

Lab values: Serum magnesium < 1.5 mg/dl

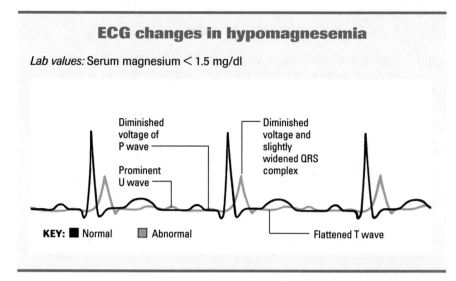

Diminished voltage of P wave

Prominent U wave

Diminished voltage and slightly widened QRS complex

Flattened T wave

KEY: ■ Normal   ■ Abnormal

Key nursing interventions for a patient with hypomagnesemia

- Monitor patients at risk.
- Monitor vital signs.
- Monitor respiratory status.
- Monitor for cardiac arrhythmias.
- Assess mental status.
- Evaluate neuromuscular status.
- Monitor serum electrolyte levels.
- Initiate seizure precautions.
- Administer magnesium supplements.
- Provide patient teaching.

- Connect the patient to a cardiac monitor if his magnesium level is below 1 mg/dl; watch the rhythm strip closely for arrhythmias
- Assess the patient's mental status and report changes
- Evaluate the patient's neuromuscular status regularly by checking for hyperactive deep tendon reflexes, tremors, and tetany; check for Chvostek's and Trousseau's signs if hypocalcemia is also suspected
- Monitor the patient's urine output at least every 4 hours; magnesium generally isn't administered if urine output is less than 10 ml in 4 hours
- Monitor the patient's serum electrolyte levels, and notify the physician if the serum potassium level or calcium level is low; both hypocalcemia and hypokalemia can cause hypomagnesemia
- Check the patient for dysphagia before giving food, oral fluids, or oral medications; hypomagnesemia may impair his ability to swallow
- Initiate seizure precautions to prevent patient injury; if a seizure occurs, report the type of seizure, its length, and the patient's behavior during the seizure; reorient him as needed
- Keep emergency equipment nearby for airway protection
- Establish I.V. access and maintain a patent I.V. line in case your patient needs I.V. magnesium replacement or I.V. fluids
- When preparing an infusion of magnesium sulfate, keep in mind that I.V. magnesium sulfate comes in various concentrations (such as 10%, 12.5%, and 50%), so read the order carefully (see *Infusing magnesium sulfate,* page 122)
- When administering magnesium I.M., inject the dose into the deep gluteal muscle
- I.M. injections of magnesium are painful; if giving more than one injection, alternate injection sites
- Administer magnesium supplements as needed and ordered

Key precautions for infusing magnesium sulfate

- Using an infusion pump, administer slowly—no faster than 150 mg/minute.
- Monitor vital signs and deep tendon reflexes.
- Check serum magnesium level after each bolus dose or at least every 6 hours if using a continuous I.V. drip.
- Place on continuous cardiac monitoring.
- Monitor urine output.
- Keep calcium gluconate on hand to counteract adverse reactions.

Key patient teaching topics for hypomagnesemia

- Causes and associated risks
- Dangers of diuretic and laxative abuse
- Foods high in magnesium

Infusing magnesium sulfate

If the physician prescribes magnesium sulfate to raise your patient's serum magnesium level, you'll need to take some special precautions, such as those listed here:

- Using an infusion pump, administer magnesium sulfate slowly—no faster than 150 mg/minute. Injecting a bolus dose too rapidly can trigger cardiac arrest.
- Monitor your patient's vital signs and deep tendon reflexes during magnesium sulfate therapy. Every 15 minutes, check for signs and symptoms of magnesium excess, such as hypotension and respiratory distress.
- Check the patient's serum magnesium level after each bolus dose or at least every 6 hours if he has a continuous I.V. drip.
- Stay especially alert for an above-normal serum magnesium level if your patient's renal function is impaired.
- Place the patient on continuous cardiac monitoring. Observe him closely, especially if he's also receiving digoxin (Lanoxin).
- Monitor urine output before, during, and after magnesium sulfate infusion. Notify the physician if output measures less than 100 ml over 4 hours.
- Keep calcium gluconate on hand to counteract adverse reactions. Have resuscitation equipment nearby and be prepared to use it if the patient goes into cardiac or respiratory arrest.

TIME-OUT FOR TEACHING

Patient teaching: Hypomagnesemia

When teaching a patient with hypomagnesemia, be sure to cover the following information and then evaluate your patient's learning:

- Teach the patient and his family about hypomagnesemia, including its causes and associated risks.
- Teach the patient about the dangers of diuretic and laxative abuse and explain the link to hypomagnesemia.
- Teach the patient about foods high in magnesium, such as green vegetables, nuts, beans, and fruits.

- During magnesium replacement, check the cardiac monitor frequently and assess the patient closely for signs of magnesium excess, such as hypotension and respiratory distress; keep calcium gluconate at the bedside in case such signs occur
- When hypomagnesemia is suspected as the cause of an arrhythmia, also assess the patient for signs of hypokalemia
  - Remember that hypokalemia isn't easily corrected in the presence of hypomagnesemia
  - Check serum magnesium levels with persistently decreased potassium levels
- Provide patient teaching as appropriate (see *Patient teaching: Hypomagnesemia*)

MAGNESIUM EXCESS: HYPERMAGNESEMIA

● **General information**
- Usually results from acute renal failure or chronic kidney disease
- Produces a sedative effect on the neuromuscular junction
- Inhibits acetylcholine release
- Diminishes muscle cell excitability
- Can cause hypotension and possibly cardiac arrest

● **Causes**
- Acute renal failure or chronic kidney disease (most common causes)
- Excessive use of magnesium-containing antacids or laxatives (see *Drugs associated with hypermagnesemia*)
- Excessive administration of I.V. magnesium sulfate to treat specific conditions
  - Seizures
  - Gestational hypertension
  - Preterm labor (higher serum magnesium level possibly developed in patient's fetus)
- Untreated diabetic ketoacidosis
- Hypoadrenalism
- Hemodialysis with a magnesium-rich dialysate

● **Assessment findings**
- Lethargy and drowsiness
- Depressed neuromuscular activity
- Depressed respirations
- Sensation of warmth throughout the body (see *Signs and symptoms of hypermagnesemia,* page 124)
- Hypoactive deep tendon reflexes
- Hypotension
- Bradycardia
- Cardiac arrest
- Coma

● **Diagnostic findings**
- Serum magnesium level greater than 2.5 mg/dl
- ECG changes
  - Widened QRS complex

Drugs associated with hypermagnesemia

Closely monitor your patient's serum magnesium level if he's receiving:

- an antacid (Gaviscon, Maalox)
- a laxative (Milk of Magnesia, Haley's M-O, magnesium citrate)
- a magnesium supplement (magnesium oxide, magnesium sulfate).

Key facts about hypermagnesemia

- May result from kidney disease
- Diminishes muscle cell excitability
- Can cause cardiac arrest

Common causes of hypermagnesemia

- Acute renal failure or chronic kidney disease
- Excessive use of magnesium-containing antacids or laxatives
- Excessive administration of I.V. magnesium sulfate
- Untreated diabetic ketoacidosis
- Hypoadrenalism

Common assessment findings in hypermagnesemia

- Lethargy and drowsiness
- Depressed neuromuscular activity
- Sensation of warmth throughout the body
- Hypoactive deep tendon reflexes
- Hypotension

Key drugs associated with hypermagnesemia

- Antacids
- Laxatives
- Magnesium supplements

Testing for hypermagnesemia

- Increased serum magnesium level
- ECG changes

Key treatment options for hypermagnesemia

- Oral or I.V. fluids
- Loop diuretics
- For magnesium toxicity, 10% calcium gluconate
- Mechanical ventilation
- Hemodialysis with a magnesium-free dialysate

Signs and symptoms of hypermagnesemia

Use this chart to compare total serum magnesium levels with the typical signs and symptoms that may appear.

TOTAL SERUM MAGNESIUM LEVEL	SIGNS AND SYMPTOMS
3 mg/dl	• Feelings of warmth • Flushed appearance • Mild hypotension • Nausea and vomiting
4 mg/dl	• Diminished deep tendon reflexes • Facial paresthesia • Muscle weakness
5 mg/dl	• Bradycardia • Drowsiness • Electrocardiogram changes • Worsening hypotension
7 mg/dl	• Loss of deep tendon reflexes
8 mg/dl	• Respiratory compromise
12 mg/dl	• Coma • Heart block
15 mg/dl	• Respiratory arrest
20 mg/dl	• Cardiac arrest

– Prolonged PR interval
– Elevated T wave (see *ECG changes in hypermagnesemia*)

● **Treatment**
- Oral or I.V. fluids
    - Applies to patients with normal renal function
    - Increases urine output
    - Rids body of excess magnesium
- Loop diuretics to promote magnesium excretion
- For magnesium toxicity, 10% calcium gluconate (a magnesium antagonist)
- Mechanical ventilation, if necessary to relieve respiratory depression
- Hemodialysis with a magnesium-free dialysate for patients with severe renal dysfunction

● **Nursing interventions**
- Monitor patients at risk, especially those with conditions predisposing to hypermagnesemia, such as acute renal failure and chronic kidney disease
- Monitor vital signs, particularly blood pressure (which can drop sharply) and respirations (which may be depressed and can progress to apnea)

ECG changes in hypermagnesemia

Lab values: Serum magnesium > 2.5 mg/dl

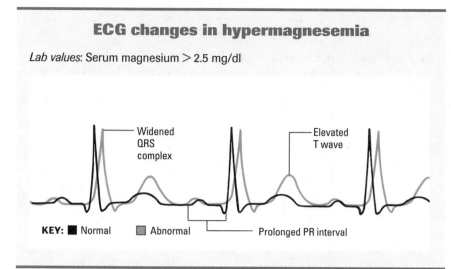

Widened QRS complex

Elevated T wave

KEY: ■ Normal   ▨ Abnormal   Prolonged PR interval

- Prepare the patient for continuous cardiac monitoring; assess ECG tracings for pertinent changes
- Check for flushed skin and diaphoresis
- Monitor urine output; the kidneys excrete most of the body's magnesium
- Assess for changes in mental status
  - Institute safety measures if LOC decreases
  - Reorient the patient if he's confused
- Assess neuromuscular status for deficits; evaluate reflexes, grip strength, and respiratory muscle function (see *Testing the patellar reflex,* page 126)
- Monitor laboratory tests and report abnormal results
  - Monitor serum electrolyte levels and other laboratory test results that reflect renal function, such as BUN and creatinine levels
  - Monitor patient for hypocalcemia (may accompany hypermagnesemia), because low serum calcium level suppresses PTH secretion
- Provide adequate fluids—both I.V. and oral—if prescribed, to help the patient's kidneys excrete excess magnesium
  - Be aware that accurate intake and output records are needed when giving large volumes of fluids
  - Observe the patient closely for signs of fluid overload and kidney failure
- Avoid giving the patient medications that contain magnesium
- Teach the patient and his family to minimize intake of foods high in magnesium
  - Green vegetables
  - Nuts
  - Beans
  - Fruits

Key nursing interventions for a patient with hypermagnesemia

- Monitor patients at risk.
- Monitor vital signs.
- Monitor cardiac rhythm.
- Monitor urine output.
- Assess mental status.
- Institute safety measures.
- Assess neuromuscular status.
- Monitor laboratory tests results.
- Administer I.V. and oral fluids as ordered.
- Avoid medications that contain magnesium.
- Provide patient teaching.

Testing the patellar reflex

- Strike the patellar tendon just below the patella with the patient sitting or lying in a supine position.
- Look for leg extension or contraction of the quadriceps muscle in the front of the thigh.

Testing the patellar reflex

To gauge your patient's magnesium (Mg) status, test the patellar reflex, one of the deep tendon reflexes that serum magnesium levels affect. To test this reflex, strike the patellar tendon just below the patella with the patient sitting or lying in a supine position, as shown. Look for leg extension or contraction of the quadriceps muscle in the front of the thigh.

If the patellar reflex is absent, notify the physician immediately. This finding may mean your patient's serum magnesium level is 7 mg/dl or higher.

SITTING POSITION
Have the patient sit on the side of the bed with his legs dangling freely, as shown. Then test the reflex.

SUPINE POSITION
With the patient in the supine position, flex the knee at a 45-degree angle, and place your nondominant hand behind it for support. Then test the reflex.

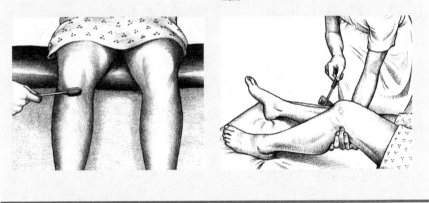

CHLORIDE DEFICIT: HYPOCHLOREMIA

Key facts about hypochloremia

- Commonly associated with hyponatremia
- May lead to hypochloremic alkalosis if chloride loss is significantly higher than sodium loss
- May cause respiratory depression or seizures

- **General information**
  - Serum chloride level: less than 98 mEq/L
  - Commonly associated with hyponatremia
  - May lead to hypochloremic alkalosis if chloride loss is significantly higher than sodium loss (see *How hypochloremic metabolic alkalosis develops*)
  - May cause tetany or respiratory depression, leading to respiratory arrest
  - May lead to seizures or coma if accompanied by significant sodium loss

- **Causes**
  - Decreased chloride intake or absorption
  - Sodium deficiency, potassium deficiency, or metabolic alkalosis
  - Prolonged I.V. dextrose administration without electrolytes
  - Excessive chloride loss (such as from prolonged diarrhea or diaphoresis)

How hypochloremic metabolic alkalosis develops

A dangerous development, hypochloremia can lead to hypochloremic metabolic alkalosis. This illustration shows how this happens.

Nasogastric suctioning can deplete chloride ions (Cl⁻).

Kidneys retain sodium ions (Na⁺) and bicarbonate ions (HCO₃⁻) to balance chloride loss.

HCO₃⁻ accumulate in extracellular fluid.

Excess HCO₃⁻ raises the pH level and leads to hypochloremic metabolic alkalosis.

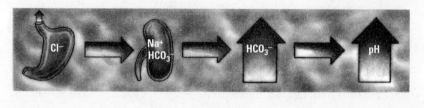

- Loss of hydrochloric acid in gastric secretions due to several causes
  - Prolonged vomiting or diaphoresis
  - Gastric suctioning
  - Gastric surgery
- Rapid removal of sodium-containing ascitic fluid (as in paracentesis)
- Addison's disease
- Untreated diabetic ketoacidosis
- Chronic respiratory acidosis
- Heart failure (dilutional hypochloremia)

Assessment findings
- Muscle weakness
- Muscle cramps
- Agitation
- Irritability
- History of specific disorders
  - Prolonged diarrhea or diaphoresis
  - Vomiting
  - Gastric suctioning
  - Gastric surgery
- Tetany
- Shallow, depressed breathing
- Hyperactive deep tendon reflexes
- Muscle hypertonicity
- Cardiac arrhythmias

Diagnostic findings
- Serum chloride level less than 98 mEq/L
- Serum sodium level less than 135 mEq/L (indicates hyponatremia)

Common causes of hypochloremia
- Decreased chloride intake or absorption
- Sodium deficiency
- Prolonged I.V. dextrose administration without electrolytes
- Loss of hydrochloric acid in gastric secretions
- Chronic respiratory acidosis

Common assessment findings in hypochloremia
- Muscle weakness
- Muscle cramps
- Agitation
- Irritability
- Shallow, depressed breathing
- Hyperactive deep tendon reflexes
- Muscle hypertonicity

Testing for hypochloremia

Increased
- Serum pH
- HCO_3^-
- Total carbon dioxide content

Decreased
- Serum chloride level
- Serum sodium level

Key treatment options for hypochloremia

- Oral chloride supplements
- Normal saline solution given I.V.

Key nursing interventions for a patient with hypochloremia

- Monitor patients at risk.
- Monitor vital signs.
- Monitor cardiac rhythm.
- Monitor LOC, muscle strength, and movement.
- Monitor fluid intake and output.
- Check serum electrolyte and ABG levels.
- Provide foods high in chloride.
- Administer oral or I.V. chloride supplements.
- Provide a safe environment.
- Provide patient teaching.

- Serum pH greater than 7.45, bicarbonate (HCO_3^-) greater than 26 mEq/L, and a total carbon dioxide content greater than 32 mEq/L (indicates metabolic alkalosis)

Treatment
- Oral chloride supplements such as a salty broth
- Normal saline solution given I.V.; alternatively, to avoid hypernatremia or to treat hypokalemia, potassium chloride given I.V.

Nursing interventions
- Monitor patients at risk for hypochloremia, especially those with hyponatremia and those receiving diuretic therapy or nasogastric (NG) suctioning
- Monitor vital signs, especially respiratory rate and pattern, and observe for worsening respiratory function
- Place the patient on a cardiac monitor because hypokalemia may be present with hypochloremia; have emergency equipment handy in case the patient's condition deteriorates
- Monitor LOC, muscle strength, and movement
- Monitor and record the patient's fluid intake and output, and check the results of his serum electrolyte and arterial blood gas (ABG) levels
- Provide foods high in chloride, such as salty broth and tomato juice; don't give plain water (it will only worsen hyponatremia)
- Administer oral or I.V. chloride supplements, as prescribed
- Use normal saline solution, not tap water, to flush the patient's NG tube if it's connected to suction
- Monitor the patient's response to therapy, especially neuromuscular, respiratory, and cardiac status; be especially alert for respiratory difficulty
- Provide a safe environment; assist the patient with ambulation, and keep his personal articles and call bell within easy reach
- Reduce environmental stimuli to avoid agitating the patient
- Provide patient teaching as necessary
  - Explain all prescribed medication therapies, including the importance of compliance and possible adverse reactions
  - Discuss nutritional sources of sodium, potassium, and chloride; reinforce teaching with written guidelines

CHLORIDE EXCESS: HYPERCHLOREMIA

General information
- Refers to excess chloride in the ECF
- Serum chloride level: greater than 106 mEq/L
- Because chloride regulation closely linked to sodium regulation, possibly associated with hypernatremia
- May be associated with metabolic acidosis
  - Results from inverse relationship between chloride and bicarbonate

– Called *hyperchloremic metabolic acidosis* when related to a high chloride level (see *Anion gap and metabolic acidosis*, page 130)
- Clinical signs: usually reflect metabolic acidosis
- Severe cases: coma may occur

Causes
- Excessive chloride intake
- Renal tubular acidosis
- Dehydration
- Excessive reabsorption of chloride from GI tract
- Excessive intake of sodium chloride with water loss
- Respiratory alkalosis
- Administration of ion exchange resins that contain sodium (such as polystyrene sulfonate) or of carbonic anhydrase inhibitors (such as acetazolamide)
- Hyperparathyroidism
- Metabolic acidosis
- Head injury
- Hypernatremia
- Cardiac decompensation
- Acute renal failure or chronic kidney disease

Assessment findings
- Lethargy
- Drowsiness
- Weakness
- Dyspnea, tachypnea
- Headache
- Metabolic acidosis
- Kussmaul's respirations (with pH less than 7.2)
- Diminished cognitive ability
- Arrhythmias
- Coma

Diagnostic findings
- Serum chloride level greater than 106 mEq/L
- Serum sodium level greater than 145 mEq/L (indicates hypernatremia)
- Serum pH less than 7.35, a normal anion gap (8 to 14 mEq/L), and HCO_3^- less than 22 mEq/L (indicates metabolic acidosis)

Treatment
- Fluid administration
  - Dilutes chloride
  - Speeds renal excretion of chloride ions
- Diuretics administration to help eliminate chloride
- Restricted sodium and chloride intake
- I.V. sodium bicarbonate administration
  - For severe cases

Key facts about hyperchloremia
- Refers to excess chloride in the ECF
- Possibly associated with hypernatremia
- May be associated with metabolic acidosis

Common causes of hyperchloremia
- Excessive chloride intake
- Dehydration
- Excessive intake of sodium chloride with water loss
- Hyperparathyroidism
- Kidney disease

Common assessment findings in hyperchloremia
- Lethargy
- Drowsiness
- Weakness
- Dyspnea, tachypnea
- Kussmaul's respirations (with pH less than 7.2)
- Diminished cognitive ability

Testing for hyperchloremia

- Increased serum chloride level
- Increased serum sodium level
- Decreased serum pH
- Normal anion gap (8 to 14 mEq/L)
- Decreased HCO_3^-

Key treatment options for hyperchloremia

- Fluid administration
- Diuretics
- Restricted sodium and chloride intake
- I.V. sodium bicarbonate

Key nursing interventions for a patient with hyperchloremia

- Monitor patients at risk.
- Monitor vital signs.
- Monitor cardiac rhythm.
- Assess respiratory pattern.
- Monitor serum electrolyte levels and ABG values.
- Monitor fluid intake and output.
- Institute safety precautions.
- Provide patient teaching.

Anion gap and metabolic acidosis

Hyperchloremia increases the likelihood that a patient will develop hyperchloremic metabolic acidosis. This illustration shows the relationship between chloride and bicarbonate in the development of hyperchloremic metabolic acidosis.

A normal anion gap in a patient with metabolic acidosis indicates that the acidosis is most likely caused by a loss of bicarbonate ions by the kidneys or the GI tract. In such cases, a corresponding increase in chloride ions also occurs.

Acidosis can also result from an accumulation of chloride ions in the form of acidifying salts. A corresponding decrease in bicarbonate ions occurs at the same time. In this illustration, the chloride level is high (>106 mEq/L) and the bicarbonate level is low (<22 mEq/L).

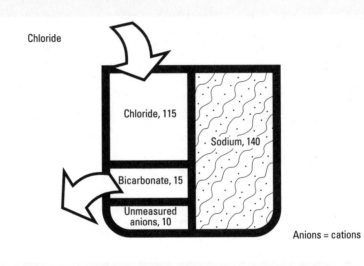

- Raises serum HCO_3^- levels
- Promotes renal excretion of chloride ions
- Promotes acidosis correction

● **Nursing interventions**
- Monitor patients at risk for hyperchloremia, including those with hypernatremia and metabolic acidosis
- Monitor vital signs, including cardiac rhythm
- Look for changes in respiratory pattern that may indicate a worsening of the acid-base imbalance
- Carefully monitor serum electrolyte levels and ABG values; report changes immediately
- Monitor fluid intake and output
- If the patient is receiving high doses of sodium bicarbonate, watch for signs and symptoms of overcompensation, such as metabolic alkalosis and CNS and peripheral nervous system overstimulation

- Continue to assess the patient's neurologic, cardiac, and respiratory status, and note his response to therapy
- Institute safety precautions to prevent injury
- Reassure the patient and his family that altered LOC is usually temporary and will probably improve with treatment
- For the patient with muscle weakness, assist with his ADLs as needed and continue to monitor his strength
- Teach the patient which foods to avoid, such as salty broth, processed meats, and canned soups. Encourage the patient not to use a salt shaker and to read labels of salt substitutes; many contain calcium chloride or potassium chloride

PATIENTS AT RISK FOR ELECTROLYTE IMBALANCES

● General information
- Because of age- and illness-related physiologic changes, possess bodies with impaired abilities to compensate for imbalance
- At risk for fluid imbalances because of close association between fluids and electrolytes
- Four groups at highest risk
  - Neonates, infants, and children
  - Older adults
  - Pregnant patients
  - Chronically ill patients

● Neonates, infants, and children
- At high risk for elevated electrolyte levels from electrolyte replacement therapy
- Infants fed improperly diluted infant formula: can experience renal damage from a hypertonic solute load
- Infants fed cow's milk rather than formula or breast milk: may develop hyperphosphatemia (higher phosphorus level in cow's milk)

● Older adults
- At particular risk for electrolyte imbalances, especially hypokalemia, if taking diuretics or digoxin
- Predisposing conditions
  - Digoxin toxicity (because of potassium, calcium, and magnesium imbalances)
  - Excessive solute loads (because of inadequate water intake)
  - Electrolyte deficits (because of inadequate nutrition)
    - Diuretic therapy: may aggravate
    - Diet: should be assessed and monitored closely
- Experience risk factors related to deteriorated renal function
  - Decreased renal blood flow and urine flow rates
  - Impaired excretion of many electrolytes
  - Possible electrolyte imbalances

Groups at highest risk for electrolyte imbalances

- Neonates, infants, and children
- Older adults
- Pregnant patients
- Chronically ill patients

Key risk factors for electrolyte imbalances

Neonates, infants, and children
- Improperly diluted infant formula
- Use of cow's milk rather than formula or breast milk

Older adults
- Use of diuretics or digoxin
- Predisposing conditions
  -Digoxin toxicity
  -Inadequate water intake
  -Inadequate nutrition
  -Deteriorated renal function

Key risk factors for electrolyte imbalances
(continued)

Pregnant patients
- Hypermagnesemia: if therapeutic use of magnesium sulfate in gestational hypertension
- Hyponatremia: if Pitocin administered for labor induction
- Hypernatremia and hypokalemia: if preterm labor is treated with tocolytic drugs

Chronically ill patients
- Renal failure
- Diabetes mellitus
- Endocrine disorders
- Impaired ability to compensate for imbalances

● **Pregnant patients**
- May be predisposed to hypermagnesemia due to therapeutic use of magnesium sulfate in gestational hypertension
- May develop severe hyponatremia if administered Pitocin for labor induction
- May be predisposed to hypernatremia and hypokalemia if preterm labor is treated with tocolytic drugs
  - Ritodrine hydrochloride (Yutopar)
  - Terbutaline sulfate (Brethine)

● **Chronically ill patients**
- May have diseases considered to be electrolyte imbalance etiologic factors
  - Renal failure
  - Diabetes mellitus
  - Endocrine disorders
- Have impaired ability to compensate for imbalances; should be closely monitored

NCLEX CHECKS

It's never too soon to begin your NCLEX preparation. Now that you've reviewed this chapter, carefully read each of the following questions and choose the best answer. Then compare your responses to the correct answers.

1. The nurse is administering I.V. fluids to a client with hyponatremia. During routine assessment, the nurse auscultates crackles bilaterally over the lungs, and the client complains of dyspnea. Which is the most appropriate response by the nurse?
- ☐ **1.** Obtain a blood sample to check serum sodium level.
- ☐ **2.** Notify the physician to stop the infusion.
- ☐ **3.** Weigh the client and record the result on the bedside flow sheet.
- ☐ **4.** Maintain the present rate of I.V. infusion and continue to monitor respiratory status.

2. When taken by a client with an electrolyte imbalance, levels of which drug should be monitored closely?
- ☐ **1.** Acetazolamide (Diamox)
- ☐ **2.** Morphine
- ☐ **3.** Digoxin (Lanoxin)
- ☐ **4.** Furosemide (Lasix)

3. The most appropriate method to administer I.V. potassium chloride involves:
- ☐ **1.** infusing it at a rate no faster then 10 mEq/hour.
- ☐ **2.** pushing the dose over 3 to 5 minutes.
- ☐ **3.** preparing the final concentration to be 100 mEq/L or less.
- ☐ **4.** calculating the appropriate drip rate.

4. The nurse has placed her client with hyperkalemia on a cardiac monitor. For which associated ECG abnormalities should the nurse be alert? Select all that apply.

- ☐ **1.** Widened QRS complex
- ☐ **2.** Prominent U wave
- ☐ **3.** Shortened QT interval
- ☐ **4.** Tall, tented T waves
- ☐ **5.** Prolonged PR interval
- ☐ **6.** Lengthened QT interval

5. Positive Chvostek's and Trousseau's signs indicate which electrolyte imbalance?

- ☐ **1.** Hypernatremia
- ☐ **2.** Hyperkalemia
- ☐ **3.** Hypercalcemia
- ☐ **4.** Hypocalcemia

6. A tracheotomy tray should be readily available for a client with hypocalcemia because of the potential for:

- ☐ **1.** bronchodilation.
- ☐ **2.** vasoconstriction.
- ☐ **3.** laryngospasm.
- ☐ **4.** cardiac arrhythmias.

7. Which nursing intervention is most appropriate for a client with hypercalcemia?

- ☐ **1.** Ambulate the client as soon as possible.
- ☐ **2.** Encourage compliance with fluid restrictions.
- ☐ **3.** Maintain the client on strict bed rest.
- ☐ **4.** Encourage the consumption of green, leafy vegetables.

8. Signs and symptoms of acute hyperphosphatemia are usually caused by the effects of which electrolyte imbalance?

- ☐ **1.** Hypokalemia
- ☐ **2.** Hypocalcemia
- ☐ **3.** Hypomagnesemia
- ☐ **4.** Hypochloremia

9. Which signs and symptoms indicate hypermagnesemia?

- ☐ **1.** Edema, tachycardia, and hypertension
- ☐ **2.** Decreased mental function, muscle spasms, and seizures
- ☐ **3.** Emotional lability, laryngeal stridor, and hyperactive deep tendon reflexes
- ☐ **4.** Lethargy; slow, shallow respirations; and bradycardia

TOP 10

Items to study for your next test on electrolyte imbalances

1. Electrolyte imbalances that are life-threatening
2. Diagnostics and laboratory values related to electrolyte imbalances
3. Specific causes and contributing factors for each electrolyte imbalance
4. Nursing assessments of each electrolyte imbalance, especially those that are life-threatening
5. Correlation of electrolytes to fluid status and hydration of body
6. Treatments, including fluids, diet, and drug therapy, related to electrolyte imbalances
7. Drugs that must be modified due to therapy used to regulate electrolyte imbalance
8. Nursing care of each electrolyte imbalance
9. Nursing care for clients receiving TPN, including care for laboratory and diagnostic testing
10. Clients at risk for electrolyte imbalances, including a rationale for each risk

10. Which electrolyte should be kept readily available for a client with hypermagnesemia?

- ☐ **1.** Potassium
- ☐ **2.** Calcium
- ☐ **3.** Sodium
- ☐ **4.** Phosphorus

ANSWERS AND RATIONALES

1. CORRECT ANSWER: 2

Because the client is displaying signs of hypervolemia, the nurse should notify the physician to stop the present infusion. The client may be receiving fluids too quickly, or the volume may have exceeded the client's needs. Maintaining the present I.V. rate could worsen his respiratory status and place him in a state of respiratory distress.

2. CORRECT ANSWER: 3

Because many conditions of electrolyte imbalances can potentiate the effects of digoxin, serum digoxin levels should be monitored closely.

3. CORRECT ANSWER: 1

I.V. potassium chloride should be administered slowly, usually no faster than 10 mEq/hour. An infusion device should be used to control flow rate, and the infusion concentration shouldn't exceed 60 mEq/L. Potassium should never be administered by I.V. push or bolus.

4. CORRECT ANSWER: 1, 4, 5

Tall, tented T waves are a prominent ECG characteristic of a client with hyperkalemia. Other ECG abnormalities may include a widened QRS complex, a prolonged PR interval, a depressed ST segment, and a flattened or absent P wave. A prominent U wave is characteristic of hypomagnesemia; a shortened QT interval is characteristic of hypercalcemia; and a lengthened QT interval is characteristic of hypocalcemia.

5. CORRECT ANSWER: 4

Because hypocalcemia increases nerve excitability, the client may display positive Chvostek's and Trousseau's signs.

6. CORRECT ANSWER: 3

Laryngeal muscles are particularly prone to spasm in a client with hypocalcemia; therefore, a tracheotomy tray should be readily available in case an airway needs to be established. Although cardiac arrhythmias are also likely to occur, a tracheotomy tray wouldn't prevent or relieve them.

7. CORRECT ANSWER: 1

The client with hypercalcemia should be ambulated as soon as possible to prevent bones from releasing calcium and increasing serum levels. The client should increase fluid intake to promote calcium excretion from the kidneys and to prevent the risk of calculi formation. Green, leafy vegetables are calcium-rich foods and should be avoided by the client with hypercalcemia.

8. CORRECT ANSWER: 2

Hyperphosphatemia alone causes few clinical problems. However, because phosphorus and calcium have an inverse relationship, calcium levels are low when phosphorus levels are high. Signs and symptoms are reflective of hypocalcemia.

9. CORRECT ANSWER: 4

Because an abnormally high magnesium level depresses the neuromuscular system, signs and symptoms may include drowsiness and lethargy; slow, shallow, depressed respirations; and bradycardia.

10. CORRECT ANSWER: 2

Calcium is a magnesium-antagonist and can be administered to reverse the effects of a toxic serum magnesium level.

Acid-base imbalances

LEARNING OBJECTIVES

After studying this chapter, you should be able to:

● Describe the four major types of acid-base imbalances.
● List causes of each acid-base imbalance.
● Identify nursing interventions for each acid-base imbalance.
● Analyze arterial blood gas values for acid-base imbalances.
● Identify patients at risk for acid-base imbalances.

CHAPTER OVERVIEW

Acid-base balance is essential to life. The two major types of acid-base imbalances are alkalosis and acidosis. Each type can be respiratory or metabolic in origin, and primary or compensated. Additionally, an acid-base imbalance is classified as mixed (or combined) when both a metabolic imbalance and a respiratory imbalance occur at the same time. A thorough assessment, including careful evaluation of arterial blood gas (ABG) values, is essential for determining which type of imbalance a patient has. Nursing care focuses on monitoring the patient and correcting the imbalance.

INTRODUCTION

● **Description**
- Are common clinical conditions that can accompany any disorder
- Electrolyte balance and acid-base balance both influenced by hydrogen ion (H^+)
- ABG measurements: remain the major diagnostic tool for evaluating acid-base states
  - Degree of acidity and alkalinity measured by pH
    - pH levels inversely proportional to hydrogen ion concentration
    - Hydrogen ion concentration increases, pH decreases; results in acidosis
    - Hydrogen ion concentration decreases, pH increases; results in alkalosis
  - Partial pressure of arterial carbon dioxide ($Paco_2$): reflects adequacy of lung ventilation (see *Using ABG values to assess respiratory acid-base imbalances,* page 138)
  - Bicarbonate (HCO_3^-) level: reflects activity of kidneys in retaining or excreting bicarbonate (see *Using ABG values to assess metabolic acid-base imbalances,* page 139)

● **Forms**
- Categorized into four major types
  - Respiratory acidosis
  - Respiratory alkalosis
  - Metabolic acidosis
  - Metabolic alkalosis
- Each type has three possible forms
  - Primary: originate from acute condition (such as respiratory alkalosis resulting from hyperventilation syndrome)
  - Mixed (combined): involve both metabolic and respiratory imbalance occurring at same time
  - Compensated: involve body's attempt to bring pH back to normal after a primary imbalance has occurred; usually associated with chronic disorders (such as chronic obstructive pulmonary disease [COPD])
- Body responds with a physiologic process known as *compensation*
  - Renal system compensates for respiratory imbalances; can take hours or days to compensate
  - Respiratory system compensates for metabolic imbalances; is efficient and can compensate quickly

Key facts about acid-base imbalances

- Can accompany any disorder
- Influenced by H^+
- ABG measurements: major diagnostic tool for evaluating acid-base states
- Body responds with physiologic process known as *compensation*

Types of acid-base imbalances

- Respiratory acidosis
- Respiratory alkalosis
- Metabolic acidosis
- Metabolic alkalosis
- Can be classified as primary, mixed, or compensated

GO WITH THE FLOW

Using ABG values to assess respiratory acid-base imbalances

To help determine if a patient is experiencing a respiratory acid-base imbalance, follow these decision-tree steps to interpret his arterial blood gas (ABG) values.

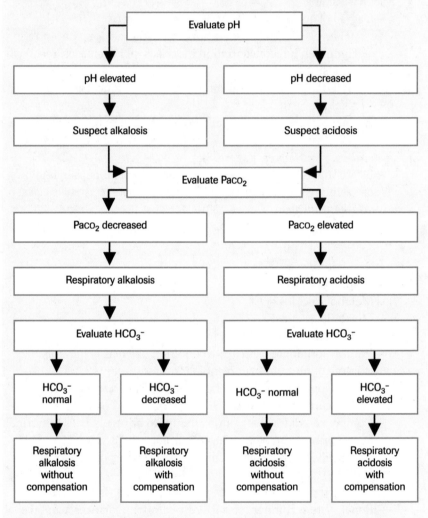

GO WITH THE FLOW

Using ABG values to assess metabolic acid-base imbalances

To help determine if a patient is experiencing a metabolic acid-base imbalance, follow these decision-tree steps to interpret his arterial blood gas (ABG) values.

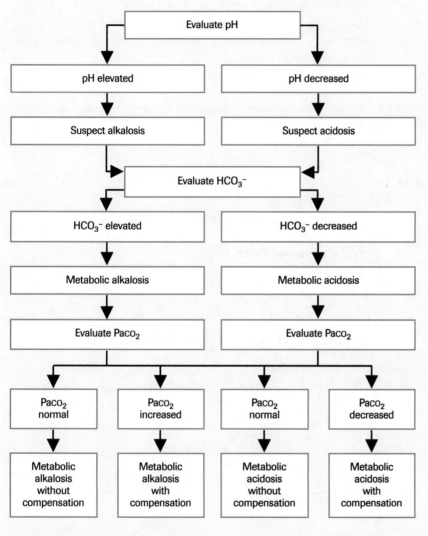

Key facts about respiratory acidosis

- Results from altered alveolar ventilation leading to CO_2 retention
- Alveolar hypoventilation: most common cause
- May be acute or chronic
- Body: attempts to compensate by increasing renal reabsorption of bicarbonate

Common causes of respiratory acidosis

- Alveolar hypoventilation
- Respiratory arrest
- Pulmonary edema
- Pneumonia
- Chest wall injury

RESPIRATORY ACIDOSIS

● **General information**
- Primary acid-base imbalance resulting from altered alveolar ventilation leading to CO_2 retention (see *Respiratory acidosis: ABG findings*)
- Constituted by low arterial pH and elevated serum CO_2 levels (hypercapnia)
- Alveolar hypoventilation is most common cause
  - Abnormally slow or shallow respirations or poor alveolar ventilation: results in inadequate gas exchange, causes CO_2 to accumulate in lungs and serum
  - Increases levels of circulating carbonic acid (H_2CO_3) and lowers pH
- May be acute (as in sudden ventilatory failure) or chronic (as in emphysema)
- Body attempts to compensate by increasing renal reabsorption of bicarbonate (see *How respiratory acidosis develops*)

● **Causes**
- Alveolar hypoventilation
- Acute abdominal distention (inhibits pulmonary excursion)
- Respiratory arrest
- Overdose of sedatives or anesthetic
- Airway obstruction

Respiratory acidosis: ABG findings

To help determine if a patient is experiencing respiratory acidosis, use this chart to interpret his arterial blood gas (ABG) values.

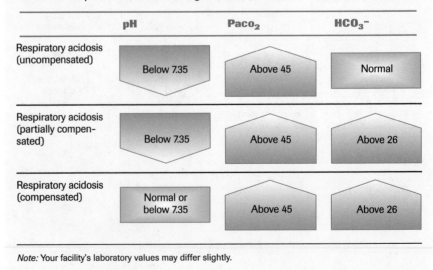

	pH	Paco$_2$	HCO$_3$$^-$
Respiratory acidosis (uncompensated)	Below 7.35	Above 45	Normal
Respiratory acidosis (partially compensated)	Below 7.35	Above 45	Above 26
Respiratory acidosis (compensated)	Normal or below 7.35	Above 45	Above 26

Note: Your facility's laboratory values may differ slightly.

How respiratory acidosis develops

This series of illustrations shows how respiratory acidosis develops at the cellular level.

STEP 1

- When pulmonary ventilation decreases, retained carbon dioxide (CO_2) combines with water (H_2O) to form carbonic acid (H_2CO_3) in larger-than-normal amounts.
- The carbonic acid dissociates to release free hydrogen ions (H^+) and bicarbonate ions (HCO_3^-).
- The excessive carbonic acid causes a drop in pH.
- *Look for a partial pressure of carbon dioxide ($Paco_2$) level above 45 mm Hg and a pH level below 7.35.*

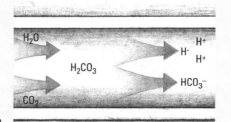

STEP 2

- As the pH level falls, 2,3 diphosphoglycerate (2,3-DPG) increases in the red blood cells and causes a change in hemoglobin (Hb) that makes the Hb release oxygen (O_2).
- The altered Hb, now strongly alkaline, picks up hydrogen ions and CO_2, thus eliminating some of the hydrogen ions and excess CO_2.
- *Look for decreased arterial oxygen saturation.*

STEP 3

- Whenever $Paco_2$ increases, CO_2 builds up in all tissues and fluids, including cerebrospinal fluid and the respiratory center in the medulla.
- The CO_2 reacts with water to form carbonic acid, which then breaks into hydrogen ions and bicarbonate ions.
- The increased amount of CO_2 and free hydrogen ions stimulates the respiratory center to increase the respiratory rate.
- An increased respiratory rate expels more CO_2 and helps to reduce the CO_2 level in the blood and other tissues.
- *Look for rapid, shallow respirations and a decreasing $Paco_2$.*

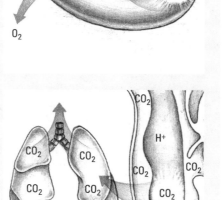

(continued)

Key steps in development of respiratory acidosis

Step 1
- When pulmonary ventilation decreases, retained carbon dioxide combines with water to form carbonic acid.
- The excessive carbonic acid causes a drop in pH.

Step 2
- As the pH level falls, hemoglobin releases oxygen.

Step 3
- Carbon dioxide builds up in all tissues and fluids.
- The carbon dioxide reacts with water to form carbonic acid, which then breaks into hydrogen ions and bicarbonate ions.
- The increased amount of carbon dioxide and hydrogen ions stimulates the respiratory center to increase the respiratory rate to reduce the carbon dioxide level.

Step 4
- Cerebral blood vessels dilate, which can cause cerebral edema and depress central nervous system activity.

Step 5
- The increasing $Paco_2$ stimulates the kidneys to conserve bicarbonate ions and sodium ions, and to excrete hydrogen ions.

Step 6
- As the concentration of hydrogen ions overwhelms the body's compensatory mechanisms, hydrogen ions move into the cells, and potassium ions move out.
- A concurrent lack of oxygen causes an increase in the anaerobic production of lactic acid, which critically depresses neurologic and cardiac functions.

How respiratory acidosis develops *(continued)*

STEP 4

- Eventually, CO_2 and hydrogen ions cause cerebral blood vessels to dilate, which increases blood flow to the brain.
- That increased flow can cause cerebral edema and depress central nervous system activity.
- *Look for headache, confusion, lethargy, nausea, or vomiting.*

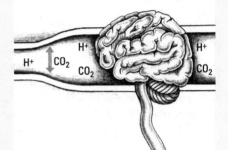

STEP 5

- As respiratory mechanisms fail, the increasing $Paco_2$ stimulates the kidneys to conserve bicarbonate ions and sodium ions (Na^+), and to excrete hydrogen ions (some in the form of ammonium [NH_4]).
- The additional bicarbonate ions and sodium ions combine to form extra sodium bicarbonate ($NaHCO_3^-$), which can then buffer more free hydrogen ions.
- *Look for increased acid content in the urine, increasing serum pH and bicarbonate levels, and shallow, depressed respirations.*

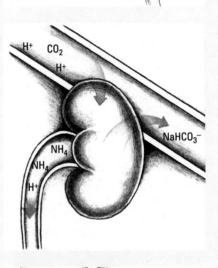

STEP 6

- As the concentration of hydrogen ions overwhelms the body's compensatory mechanisms, hydrogen ions move into the cells, and potassium ions (K^+) move out.
- A concurrent lack of oxygen causes an increase in the anaerobic production of lactic acid, which further skews the acid-base balance and critically depresses neurologic and cardiac functions.
- *Look for hyperkalemia, arrhythmias, increased $Paco_2$, decreased arterial oxygen pressure, decreased pH, and decreased level of consciousness.*

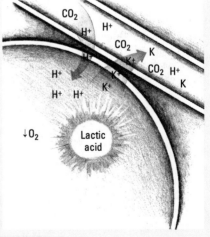

- COPD
- Heart failure
- Pulmonary edema
- Pneumonia
- Cardiac arrest
- Pneumothorax or hydrothorax
- Chest wall injury, such as fractured ribs
- Amyotrophic lateral sclerosis
- Pulmonary fibrosis
- Pickwickian syndrome
- Cystic fibrosis
- Myasthenia gravis
- Cerebral trauma
- Guillain-Barré syndrome

Assessment findings
- Dyspnea
- Tachycardia
- Slow, shallow respirations
- Diminished or absent breath sounds over the affected area
- Confusion
- Headache
- Tremors
- Dizziness
- Seizures
- Warm, flushed skin
- Asterixis (a fine, flapping tremor)
- Altered level of consciousness (LOC)
- Cyanosis (a late sign)

Diagnostic findings (uncompensated)
- Arterial pH less than 7.35
- $Paco_2$ greater than 45 mm Hg
- HCO_3^- level 22 to 26 mEq/L

Diagnostic findings (compensated)
- Arterial pH borderline (7.35 or lower)
- $Paco_2$ greater than 45 mm Hg
- HCO_3^- level greater than 26 mEq/L

Treatment
- When underlying cause is pulmonary: correcting or improving ventilation, lowering $Paco_2$ level
- When underlying cause is nonpulmonary (such as neuromuscular disorders or drug overdose): correcting or improving underlying cause
- Multiple measures may be taken to correct pulmonary causes
  - Bronchodilators to open constricted airways
  - Supplemental oxygen as needed
  - Drug therapy to treat hyperkalemia

Common assessment findings in respiratory acidosis
- Dyspnea
- Slow, shallow respirations
- Headache
- Altered LOC

Testing for respiratory acidosis

Uncompensated
- Arterial pH less than 7.35
- $Paco_2$ greater than 45 mm Hg
- HCO_3^- level 22 to 26 mEq/L

Compensated
- Arterial pH borderline (7.35 or lower)
- $Paco_2$ greater than 45 mm Hg
- HCO_3^- level greater than 26 mEq/L

Key treatment options for respiratory acidosis
- Pulmonary: correcting or improving ventilation, lowering $Paco_2$ level
- Nonpulmonary: correcting or improving underlying cause

– Antibiotics to treat infection
– Chest physiotherapy to remove secretions from the lungs
– Removal of a foreign body from the airway, if needed
– Artificial airway insertion and mechanical ventilation if hypoventilation can't be corrected with above measures

● **Nursing interventions**
- Encourage the patient to turn, cough, and breathe deeply every 2 hours, which improves ventilation; chest physiotherapy may also be ordered
- Maintain a patent airway through the use of measures such as suctioning to prevent CO_2 retention
- Monitor ABG levels for changes in pH and CO_2
- Monitor vital signs, particularly respiratory rate and depth, for changes that may indicate worsening acidosis
- Assist with endotracheal (ET) intubation if the patient remains unable to ventilate adequately
- Monitor neurologic status and report significant changes
- Position the patient in the semi-Fowler's or orthopneic position to ease breathing
- Ensure that the patient drinks 2 to 3 qt (2 to 3 L) of fluids daily (unless contraindicated) to help liquefy secretions, aid their expulsion, and promote adequate CO_2 exchange
- Administer supplemental oxygen as ordered; do so cautiously in a patient with COPD because excessive oxygen decreases or completely depresses the ventilatory drive and may worsen acidosis
- Monitor serum potassium (K) levels for hyperkalemia because potassium moves out of the cell during respiratory acidosis
- Administer medications as ordered to treat the underlying respiratory dysfunction—for example, bronchodilators for bronchospasms and antibiotics for respiratory infection
- Administer sedatives cautiously; many of them depress the respiratory drive, which can lead to CO_2 accumulation
- Provide emotional support and reassurance to the patient, who likely will be quite anxious
- Institute safety measures as needed to protect a confused patient
- Provide patient teaching as necessary
    – Preventive measures, including coughing and deep-breathing techniques
    – Need for supplemental oxygen therapy or home oxygen therapy, if indicated
    – Proper technique for using bronchodilators
    – Need for repeated ABG analyses

Key nursing interventions for a patient with respiratory acidosis

- Maintain patent airway.
- Monitor ABG levels.
- Monitor vital signs, particularly respiratory rate and depth.
- Administer supplemental oxygen; assist with ET intubation if necessary.
- Monitor serum potassium level.
- Administer sedatives cautiously.
- Provide patient teaching as necessary.

RESPIRATORY ALKALOSIS

● **General information**
- Occurs when alveolar hyperventilation results in decreased serum CO_2 levels (hypocapnia), causing excessive CO_2 exhalation (see *Respiratory alkalosis: ABG findings*)
- Decreased serum CO_2 levels: lead to decreased carbonic acid production; in turn, leads to increased arterial pH
- Hyperventilation: most common cause
- May be acute (resulting from sudden increase in ventilation) or chronic (which may be difficult to identify because of renal compensation)
- Body: attempts to compensate by increasing renal excretion of bicarbonate (can take 24 to 48 hours) (see *How respiratory alkalosis develops*, pages 146 and 147)

● **Causes**
- Psychogenic conditions such as hysteria or acute anxiety
- Hyperventilation syndrome
- Overventilation with mechanical ventilator
- Aspirin overdose
- Hypermetabolic states such as fever or sepsis
- Severe pain
- Central nervous system (CNS) trauma or lesions
- Hepatic failure
- Hypoxia

(Text continues on page 148.)

Key facts about respiratory alkalosis

- Alveolar hyperventilation results in decreased serum CO_2 levels, causing excessive CO_2 exhalation
- Hyperventilation: most common cause
- May be acute or chronic
- Body: attempts to compensate by increasing renal excretion of bicarbonate

Common causes of respiratory alkalosis

- Acute anxiety
- Hyperventilation syndrome
- Overventilation with mechanical ventilator
- CNS trauma or lesions
- Hypoxia

Respiratory alkalosis: ABG findings

To help determine if a patient is experiencing respiratory alkalosis, use this chart to interpret his arterial blood gas (ABG) values.

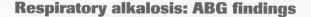

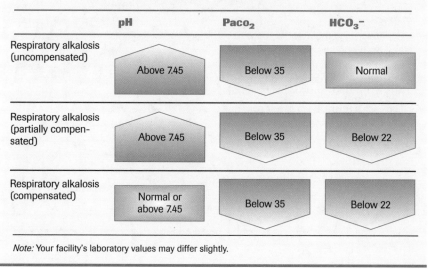

	pH	Paco$_2$	HCO$_3^-$
Respiratory alkalosis (uncompensated)	Above 7.45	Below 35	Normal
Respiratory alkalosis (partially compensated)	Above 7.45	Below 35	Below 22
Respiratory alkalosis (compensated)	Normal or above 7.45	Below 35	Below 22

Note: Your facility's laboratory values may differ slightly.

Key steps in development of respiratory alkalosis

Step 1
- When pulmonary ventilation increases, excessive amounts of CO_2 are exhaled.
- Hypocapnia occurs, which leads to a reduction in carbonic acid production, a loss of hydrogen and bicarbonate ions, and a subsequent rise in pH.

Step 2
- Hydrogen ions are pulled out of the cells and into the blood in exchange for potassium ions.
- The hydrogen ions entering the blood combine with bicarbonate ions to form carbonic acid, which lowers the pH.

Step 3
- Hypocapnia causes an increase in heart rate without an increase in blood pressure.

Step 4
- Hypocapnia produces cerebral vasoconstriction.
- Hypocapnia also overexcites the autonomic nervous system.

Step 5
- The kidneys increase secretion of bicarbonate ions and reduce excretion of hydrogen ions.

Step 6
- Continued low $Paco_2$ increases cerebral and peripheral hypoxia.
- Eventually, the alkalosis overwhelms the central nervous system and the heart.

How respiratory alkalosis develops

This series of illustrations shows how respiratory alkalosis develops at the cellular level.

STEP 1
- When pulmonary ventilation increases above the amount needed to maintain normal carbon dioxide (CO_2) levels, excessive amounts of CO_2 are exhaled.
- This causes hypocapnia (a fall in partial pressure of arterial carbon dioxide [$Paco_2$]), which leads to a reduction in carbonic acid (H_2CO_3) production, a loss of hydrogen ions (H^+) and bicarbonate ions (HCO_3^-), and a subsequent rise in pH.
- *Look for a pH level above 7.45, a $Paco_2$ level below 35 mm Hg, and a bicarbonate level below 22 mEq/L.*

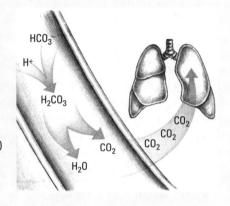

STEP 2
- In defense against the rising pH, hydrogen ions are pulled out of the cells and into the blood in exchange for potassium ions (K^+).
- The hydrogen ions entering the blood combine with bicarbonate ions to form carbonic acid, which lowers the pH.
- *Look for a further decrease in bicarbonate levels, a fall in pH, and a fall in serum potassium levels (hypokalemia).*

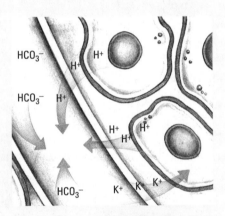

STEP 3
- Hypocapnia stimulates the carotid and aortic bodies and the medulla, which causes an increase in heart rate without an increase in blood pressure.
- *Look for angina, electrocardiogram changes, restlessness, and anxiety.*

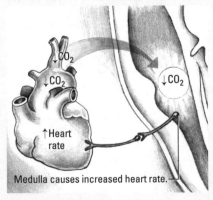

Medulla causes increased heart rate.

How respiratory alkalosis develops *(continued)*

STEP 4

- Simultaneously, hypocapnia produces cerebral vasoconstriction, which prompts a reduction in cerebral blood flow.
- Hypocapnia also overexcites the medulla, pons, and other parts of the autonomic nervous system.
- *Look for increasing anxiety, diaphoresis, dyspnea, alternating periods of apnea and hyperventilation, dizziness, and tingling in the fingers or toes.*

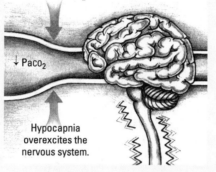

Decreased $Paco_2$ causes vasoconstriction.

↓ $Paco_2$

Hypocapnia overexcites the nervous system.

STEP 5

- When hypocapnia lasts more than 6 hours, the kidneys increase secretion of bicarbonate ions and reduce excretion of hydrogen ions.
- Periods of apnea may result if the pH remains high and the $Paco_2$ remains low.
- *Look for slowing of the respiratory rate, hypoventilation, and Cheyne-Stokes respirations.*

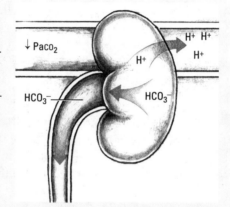

↓ $Paco_2$

H^+ H^+

H^+

H^+

HCO_3^-

HCO_3^-

STEP 6

- Continued low $Paco_2$ increases cerebral and peripheral hypoxia from vasoconstriction.
- Severe alkalosis inhibits calcium (Ca^{++}) ionization, which in turn causes increased nerve excitability and muscle contractions.
- Eventually, the alkalosis overwhelms the central nervous system and the heart.
- *Look for decreasing level of consciousness, hyperreflexia, carpopedal spasm, tetany, arrhythmias, seizures, and coma.*

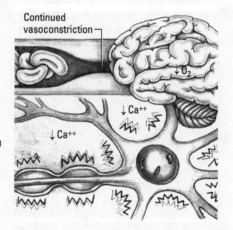

Continued vasoconstriction

↓ O_2

↓ Ca^{++}

↓ Ca^{++}

Common assessment findings in respiratory alkalosis

- Rapid, deep respirations
- Tachycardia
- Light-headedness
- Decreased concentration and attention span
- Syncope

Testing for respiratory alkalosis

Uncompensated
- Arterial pH greater than 7.45
- $Paco_2$ level less than 35 mm Hg
- HCO_3^- level: 22 to 26 mEq/L

Compensated
- Arterial pH borderline (7.45 or slightly higher)
- $Paco_2$ level less than 35 mm Hg
- HCO_3^- level less than 22 mEq/L

Key treatment options for respiratory alkalosis

- Discontinuation of causative agent
- Oxygen therapy
- Teaching patient to breathe into paper bag or cupped hands
- For intubated patients: adjusting mechanical ventilator settings

- Pregnancy
- Hyperventilation during labor and delivery

● **Assessment findings**
- Rapid, deep respirations
- Tachycardia
- Light-headedness
- Headache
- Vertigo
- Decreased concentration and attention span
- Paresthesia
- Tetany
- Carpopedal spasm (Trousseau's sign)
- Tinnitus
- Palpitations
- Dry mouth
- Blurred vision
- Syncope
- Seizures and coma
- Hyperactive deep tendon reflexes
- Twitching
- Arrhythmias

● **Diagnostic findings (uncompensated)**
- Arterial pH greater than 7.45
- $Paco_2$ level less than 35 mm Hg
- Partial pressure of arterial oxygen (Pao_2) normal or elevated (80 to 100)
- HCO_3^- level: 22 to 26 mEq/L

● **Diagnostic findings (compensated)**
- Arterial pH borderline (7.45 or slightly higher)
- $Paco_2$ level less than 35 mm Hg
- HCO_3^- level less than 22 mEq/L
- Serum K level less than 3.8 mEq/L
- Urine pH alkaline (greater than 8.0)
- Serum calcium (Ca) level less than 7 mg/dl

● **Treatment**
- Several measures taken to correct underlying disorder
  - Discontinuation of causative agent (such as salicylate or other drug)
  - Steps to reduce fever, eliminate source of sepsis
  - Oxygen therapy to treat acute hypoxemia
  - Sedative or anxiolytic to treat anxiety
- Further measures taken to counteract hyperventilation
  - Teaching patient to breathe into paper bag or cupped hands (forces patient to breathe exhaled CO_2; raises CO_2 level)

– For intubated patients: adjusting mechanical ventilator settings as needed by decreasing tidal volume or number of breaths per minute

● Nursing interventions

- Monitor vital signs, specifically respiratory rate and depth
- Instruct the patient to breathe slowly and less deeply to decrease CO_2 loss; as necessary, have the patient breathe into a paper bag or use a rebreather mask to rebreathe CO_2
- If the patient is intubated, adjust mechanical ventilator settings to decrease ventilatory rate and depth
- Administer sedatives as ordered to slow the respiratory rate; monitor the patient carefully to guard against respiratory depression and CO_2 retention
- Intervene as necessary to correct the underlying cause of hyperventilation, such as pain or anxiety
- Monitor ABG values, particularly $Paco_2$ levels, to evaluate the effectiveness of interventions
- Monitor laboratory results for values indicating compensation, such as decreased bicarbonate levels and normalization of pH; such values won't appear until at least 24 hours after onset of hyperventilation
- Monitor for low serum potassium levels in a patient with chronic hyperventilation, because potassium is exchanged for hydrogen ions and moves from the extracellular to the intracellular space
- Provide undisturbed rest periods after the patient's respiratory rate returns to normal (hyperventilation may result in severe fatigue)
- Stay with the patient during periods of extreme stress and anxiety; offer reassurance and maintain a calm, quiet environment
- Provide patient teaching as appropriate
  - Anxiety-reducing techniques
  - Controlled-breathing exercises

METABOLIC ACIDOSIS

● General information

- Results from loss of bicarbonate from extracellular fluid, accumulation of metabolic acids, or combination of the two (see *Metabolic acidosis: ABG findings,* page 150)
  - Anion gap (difference between amount of sodium [Na] and bicarbonate in blood) greater than 14 mEq/L: condition due to accumulation of metabolic acids or unmeasured anions
  - Normal anion gap (8 to 14 mEq/L): condition may be due to bicarbonate loss
- Metabolic acids, such as hydrochloric acid (HCl), produced by metabolism or ingested foods
- Chloride (Cl): component of hydrochloric acid, competes with bicarbonate for combination with sodium

---

Key nursing interventions for a patient with respiratory alkalosis

- Monitor vital signs, specifically respiratory rate and depth.
- Instruct the patient to breathe slowly and less deeply.
- If the patient is intubated, adjust mechanical ventilator settings.
- Administer sedatives as ordered.
- Monitor ABG values.
- Monitor serum potassium levels.
- Provide patient teaching as appropriate.

Key facts about metabolic acidosis

- Results from loss of bicarbonate from extracellular fluid, accumulation of metabolic acids, or combination of the two
- Major sign: decreased arterial pH accompanied by decreased arterial bicarbonate levels
- Body: attempts to compensate through hyperventilation

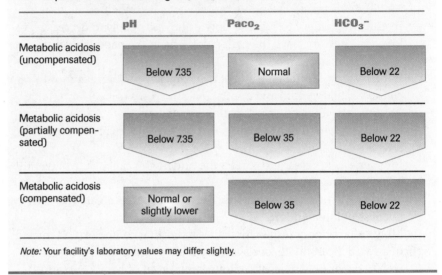

Metabolic acidosis: ABG findings

To help determine if a patient is experiencing metabolic acidosis, use this chart to interpret his arterial blood gas (ABG) values.

	pH	Paco$_2$	HCO$_3^-$
Metabolic acidosis (uncompensated)	Below 7.35	Normal	Below 22
Metabolic acidosis (partially compensated)	Below 7.35	Below 35	Below 22
Metabolic acidosis (compensated)	Normal or slightly lower	Below 35	Below 22

Note: Your facility's laboratory values may differ slightly.

Common causes of metabolic acidosis

- Diabetic ketoacidosis
- Excessive acid accumulation
- Excessive loss of bicarbonate from the intestines
- Hypoxia
- Anaerobic carbohydrate metabolism

– Increased metabolic acid production caused by excessive chloride retention or ingestion
– Kidneys: can't retain sufficient bicarbonate to compensate; results in excess of hydrogen ions and, eventually, metabolic acidosis
- Major sign: decreased arterial pH accompanied by decreased arterial bicarbonate levels
- Never results from respiratory problem with exception of lactic acidosis from anaerobic metabolism (lack of available oxygen at the cellular level) (see *Understanding lactic acidosis*)
- Body: attempts to compensate through hyperventilation
  – Increased circulating hydrogen ions levels: result in rapid stimulation of peripheral chemoreceptors; increases respiratory rate within minutes of acidosis onset
  – Results in decreased Paco$_2$ levels
  – Respiratory compensation: begins within minutes but takes several hours to reach full effect (see *How metabolic acidosis develops,* pages 152 and 153)

● **Causes**
- Diabetic ketoacidosis
- Excessive acid accumulation, as from renal failure or salicylate toxicity
- Diuretic therapy resulting in excessive bicarbonate loss through the kidneys
- Excessive loss of bicarbonate from the intestines, such as from prolonged, severe diarrhea; malabsorption; or fistula drainage

Understanding lactic acidosis

Lactate, produced as a result of carbohydrate metabolism, is metabolized by the liver. The normal lactate level is 0.93 to 1.65 mEq/L. With tissue hypoxia, however, cells are forced to switch to anaerobic metabolism and more lactate is produced. When lactate accumulates in the body faster than it can be metabolized, lactic acidosis occurs. It can happen any time the demand for oxygen in the body is greater than its availability. Causes of lactic acidosis include septic shock, cardiac arrest, pulmonary disease, seizures, and strenuous exercise; the latter two cause transient lactic acidosis. Hepatic disorders can also cause lactic acidosis because the liver can't metabolize lactate.

TREATMENT

Treatment focuses on eliminating the underlying cause. If the pH is below 7.1, sodium bicarbonate may be given. Use caution when administering sodium bicarbonate, however, because it may cause alkalosis.

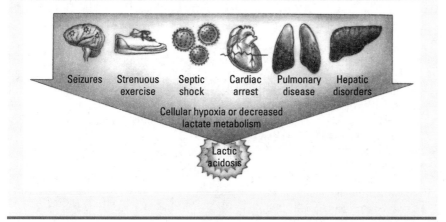

- Use of carbonic anhydrase inhibitors such as acetazolamide (Diamox)
- Chronic alcoholism
- Starvation
- Hypoxia
- Decreased tissue perfusion, such as from trauma or burns
- Anaerobic carbohydrate metabolism
- Excessive gain of chloride, such as from the administration of ammonium chloride

● **Assessment findings**
  - Kussmaul's respirations
  - Lethargy
  - Drowsiness
  - Confusion
  - Headache
  - Flushed, warm, dry skin
  - Fruity-smelling breath

(Text continues on page 154.)

Key steps in development of metabolic acidosis

Step 1
- Hydrogen ions bind with chemical buffers.

Step 2
- Excess hydrogen ions decrease pH and increase the respiratory rate.
- $Paco_2$ decreases, allowing more hydrogen ions to bind with bicarbonate ions.

Step 3
- Healthy kidneys try to compensate for acidosis by secreting excess hydrogen ions into the renal tubules.
- Those ions are buffered by phosphate or ammonia, and then are excreted into the urine in the form of a weak acid.

Step 4
- Each time a hydrogen ion is secreted into the renal tubules, a sodium ion and bicarbonate ion are absorbed from the tubules and returned to the blood.

Step 5
- Excess hydrogen ions in the ECF diffuse into cells.
- The cells release potassium ions into the blood.

Step 6
- Excess hydrogen ions lead to reduced excitability of nerve cells, causing CNS depression.

How metabolic acidosis develops

This series of illustrations shows how metabolic acidosis develops at the cellular level.

STEP 1
- As hydrogen ions (H^+) start to accumulate in the body, chemical buffers (plasma bicarbonate [HCO_3^-] and proteins) in the cells and extracellular fluid (ECF) bind with them.
- *No signs are detectable at this stage.*

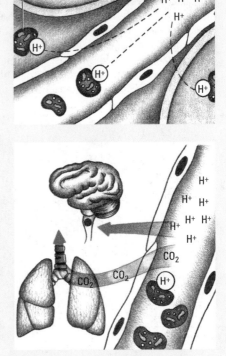

STEP 2
- Excess hydrogen ions that don't bind with the buffers decrease pH to increase the respiratory rate.
- The increased respiratory rate lowers partial pressure of arterial carbon dioxide ($Paco_2$), which allows more hydrogen ions to bind with bicarbonate ions.
- Respiratory compensation occurs within minutes but isn't sufficient to correct the imbalance.
- *Look for a pH level below 7.35, a bicarbonate level below 22 mEq/L, a decreasing $Paco_2$ level, and rapid, deeper respirations.*

STEP 3
- Healthy kidneys try to compensate for acidosis by secreting excess hydrogen ions into the renal tubules.
- Those ions are buffered by phosphate or ammonia, and then are excreted into the urine in the form of a weak acid.
- *Look for acidic urine.*

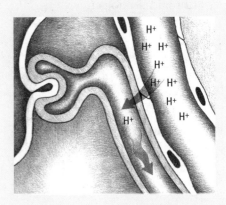

How metabolic acidosis develops *(continued)*

STEP 4

- Each time a hydrogen ion is secreted into the renal tubules, a sodium ion (Na^+) and bicarbonate ion are absorbed from the tubules and returned to the blood.
- *Look for pH and bicarbonate levels that return slowly to normal.*

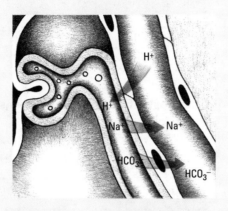

STEP 5

- Excess hydrogen ions in the ECF diffuse into cells.
- To maintain the balance of the charge across the membrane, the cells release potassium ions (K^+) into the blood.
- *Look for signs and symptoms of hyperkalemia, including colic and diarrhea, weakness or flaccid paralysis, tingling and numbness in the extremities, bradycardia, a tall T wave, a prolonged PR interval, and a wide QRS complex.*

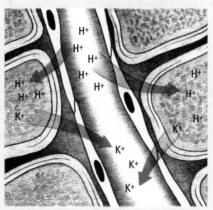

STEP 6

- Excess hydrogen ions alter the normal balance of potassium ions, sodium ions, and calcium ions (Ca^{++}), leading to reduced excitability of nerve cells.
- *Look for signs and symptoms of progressive central nervous system depression, including lethargy, dull headache, confusion, stupor, and coma.*

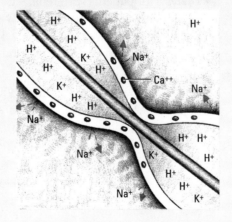

Testing for metabolic acidosis

Uncompensated
- Arterial pH level less than 7.35
- $Paco_2$ level 35 to 45 mm Hg
- Arterial HCO_3^- level less than 22 mEq/L

Compensated
- Arterial pH borderline (7.35 or slightly lower)
- $Paco_2$ level less than 35 mm Hg
- Arterial HCO_3^- level less than 22 mEq/L

Key treatment options for metabolic acidosis

- Mechanical ventilation
- Sodium bicarbonate I.V.
- Dialysis for patients with renal failure
- Insulin for patients with diabetes

- Peripheral vasodilation
- Nausea and vomiting
- Twitching
- Hypotension
- Arrhythmias
- Seizures
- Stupor
- Coma

● **Diagnostic findings (uncompensated)**
- Arterial pH level less than 7.35
- $Paco_2$ level 35 to 45 mm Hg
- Arterial HCO_3^- level less than 22 mEq/L
- Base excess negative
- Serum CO_2 level less than 18 mEq/L

● **Diagnostic findings (compensated)**
- Arterial pH borderline (7.35 or slightly lower)
- $Paco_2$ level less than 35 mm Hg
- Arterial HCO_3^- level less than 22 mEq/L
- Base excess negative
- Serum K level greater than 5.5 mEq/L
- Urine pH less than or equal to 4.5

● **Treatment**
- Mechanical ventilation, if needed to assist respiratory compensation
- Sodium bicarbonate ($NaHCO_3^-$) I.V. to neutralize blood acidity in patients with a pH lower than 7.1 and bicarbonate loss
- Parenteral fluid replacement as needed to maintain fluid balance
- Dialysis for patients with renal failure or a toxic reaction to a drug
- Rapid-acting insulin for patients with diabetes, to reverse diabetic ketoacidosis and drive potassium back into the cell
- Antidiarrheals to treat diarrhea-induced bicarbonate loss

● **Nursing interventions**
- Monitor patients at risk for metabolic acidosis, especially those with diabetes mellitus, sepsis, or shock
- Monitor vital signs, particularly respiratory rate and depth
- Monitor neurologic status closely because changes can occur rapidly
- Monitor ABG values, particularly pH, because small decreases in pH indicate large increases in hydrogen ion concentration
- Monitor bicarbonate and potassium levels; low bicarbonate and high potassium levels may be early indicators of acidosis
- Institute cardiac monitoring for a patient with elevated serum potassium levels
- Insert an I.V. line as ordered, and maintain patent I.V. access; have a large-bore catheter in place for emergency situations
- Administer sodium bicarbonate cautiously through an existing I.V. line in a large vein

– Flush line with normal saline solution before and after administering sodium bicarbonate; it's incompatible with many drugs, and may inactivate or cause precipitation if administered with incompatible drugs

– Be aware that too much bicarbonate can cause metabolic alkalosis and pulmonary edema

- Position the patient to promote chest expansion and facilitate breathing; if the patient is stuporous, turn him frequently
- Intervene to correct the underlying cause of acidosis as necessary; in many cases, correction of the underlying problem will resolve acidosis, averting the need for more aggressive intervention, such as sodium bicarbonate administration
- Administer I.V. fluids containing lactate as ordered, unless contraindicated; lactate is converted to bicarbonate in the liver
- Administer insulin and normal saline solution to correct hyperglycemia in a diabetic patient with metabolic acidosis linked to hyperglycemia; remember that insulin administration will also lower serum potassium levels
- Administer oxygen to correct lactic acidosis linked to overexertion by decreasing hypoxemia and triggering a conversion to aerobic metabolism
- Expect to assist with peritoneal dialysis or hemodialysis to correct pH in renal failure, drug overdose, or poisoning
- Provide a high-carbohydrate, low-fat diet for a patient with chronic acidosis; this will decrease metabolic waste products and, therefore, ameliorate acidosis
- Orient the patient as needed; if he's confused, take steps to ensure his safety, such as keeping his bed in the lowest position
- Investigate reasons, as appropriate, for the patient's ingestion of toxic substances
- Provide patient teaching as necessary
  – Need for blood glucose testing if indicated
  – Need for strict adherence to antidiabetic therapy if appropriate

METABOLIC ALKALOSIS

● **General information**
- Results from loss of hydrogen (acids), gain in bicarbonate, or both (see *Metabolic alkalosis: ABG findings,* page 156)
- Major cause is loss of an acid, such as hydrochloric acid, from the stomach, through nasogastric (NG) suctioning or excessive vomiting
- Loss of a metabolic acid: increases pH level
- pH: increases as hydrogen ion concentration decreases
- Hydrogen ion concentration decreased, more carbonic acid dissociated and bicarbonate concentration increased through renal reabsorption

---

Key nursing interventions for a patient with metabolic acidosis

- Monitor vital signs, particularly respiratory rate and depth.
- Monitor neurologic status.
- Monitor ABG values.
- Monitor bicarbonate and potassium levels.
- Administer sodium bicarbonate cautiously.
- Intervene to correct the underlying cause as necessary.
- Provide patient teaching as necessary.

Key facts about metabolic alkalosis

- Results from loss of hydrogen (acids), gain in bicarbonate, or both
- Major cause is loss of an acid from the stomach
- pH: increases as hydrogen ion concentration decreases
- Body: attempts to compensate for metabolic alkalosis through hypoventilation

Metabolic alkalosis: ABG findings

To help determine if a patient is experiencing metabolic alkalosis, use this chart to interpret his arterial blood gas (ABG) values.

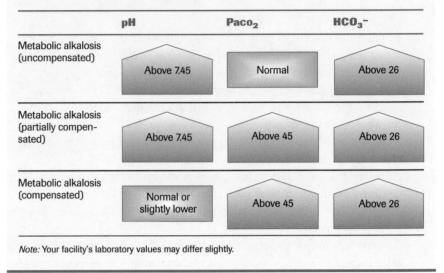

	pH	Paco$_2$	HCO$_3^-$
Metabolic alkalosis (uncompensated)	Above 7.45	Normal	Above 26
Metabolic alkalosis (partially compensated)	Above 7.45	Above 45	Above 26
Metabolic alkalosis (compensated)	Normal or slightly lower	Above 45	Above 26

Note: Your facility's laboratory values may differ slightly.

Common causes of metabolic alkalosis

- Excessive administration or ingestion of bicarbonate
- Excessive loss of hydrogen
- Prolonged diuretic therapy
- Hypokalemia

Common assessment findings in metabolic alkalosis

- Decreased respiratory rate and depth
- Hypotension
- Paresthesia in fingers and toes
- Circumoral paresthesia
- Confusion

- Process: results in increased renal excretion of hydrogen, chloride, and potassium
- Chloride: competes with bicarbonate for combination with sodium; chloride levels fall, bicarbonate levels rise (compensate to balance sodium)
- Body: attempts to compensate for metabolic alkalosis through hypoventilation (see *How metabolic alkalosis develops*)
- Stimulation of chemoreceptors: decreases; slows respiratory rate and conserves CO_2

● **Causes**
- Excessive administration or ingestion of bicarbonate, such as from antacids or carbonated soda
- Excessive loss of hydrogen from NG suctioning or vomiting
- Prolonged diuretic therapy, particularly potassium-wasting diuretics such as furosemide (Lasix), ethacrynic acid (Edecrin), and thiazides such as hydrochlorothiazide (HydroDIURIL)
- Sodium bicarbonate administration during cardiopulmonary resuscitation
- Hypokalemia
- Cushing's syndrome
- Hyperaldosteronism
- Renal artery stenosis

● **Assessment findings**
- Decreased respiratory rate and depth

How metabolic alkalosis develops

This series of illustrations shows how metabolic alkalosis develops at the cellular level.

STEP 1
- As bicarbonate ions (HCO_3^-) start to accumulate in the body, chemical buffers in extracellular fluid (ECF) and cells bind with the ions.
- *No signs are detectable at this stage.*

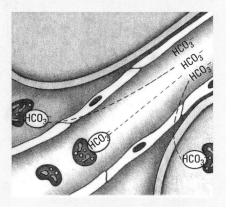

STEP 2
- Excess bicarbonate ions that don't bind with chemical buffers elevate serum pH levels which, in turn, depresses chemoreceptors in the medulla.
- Depression of those chemoreceptors causes a decrease in respiratory rate, which increases the partial pressure of arterial carbon dioxide ($Paco_2$).
- The additional carbon dioxide (CO_2) combines with water (H_2O) to form carbonic acid (H_2CO_3).
- *Note:* Lowered oxygen levels limit respiratory compensation. *Look for a serum pH level above 7.45, a bicarbonate level above 26 mEq/L, a rising $Paco_2$, and slow, shallow respirations.*

STEP 3
- When the bicarbonate level exceeds 28 mEq/L, the renal glomeruli can no longer reabsorb excess bicarbonate ions.
- That excess bicarbonate is excreted in the urine; hydrogen ions (H^+) are retained.
- *Look for alkaline urine and pH, and HCO_3^- levels that return slowly to normal.*

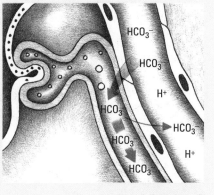

(continued)

Key steps in development of metabolic alkalosis

Step 1
- As bicarbonate ions accumulate, chemical buffers bind with the ions.

Step 2
- Excess bicarbonate ions that don't bind with chemical buffers elevate serum pH levels, depressing chemoreceptors in the medulla.
- Respiratory rate decreases, which increases $Paco_2$.

Step 3
- That excess bicarbonate is excreted in the urine; hydrogen ions are retained.

Step 4
- The kidneys excrete excess sodium ions, water, and bicarbonate ions.

Step 5
- Lowered hydrogen ion levels in the ECF cause the ions to diffuse out of the cells.
- Extracellular potassium ions move into the cells.

Step 6
- As levels of hydrogen ions decline, calcium ionization makes nerve cells more permeable to sodium ions.
- Sodium ion movement produces overexcitability of the peripheral and central nervous systems.

How metabolic alkalosis develops *(continued)*

STEP 4

- To maintain electrochemical balance, the kidneys excrete excess sodium ions (Na^+), water, and bicarbonate ions.
- Look for polyuria initially, then signs and symptoms of hypovolemia, including thirst and dry mucous membranes.

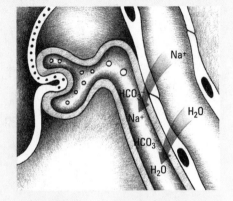

STEP 5

- Lowered hydrogen ion levels in the ECF cause the ions to diffuse out of the cells.
- To maintain the balance of charge across the cell membrane, extracellular potassium ions (Ka^+) move into the cells.
- *Look for signs and symptoms of hypokalemia, including anorexia, muscle weakness, loss of reflexes, and others.*

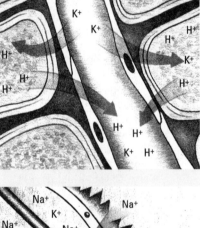

STEP 6

- As levels of hydrogen ions decline, calcium ionization (Ca^{++}) decreases.
- That decrease in ionization makes nerve cells more permeable to sodium ions.
- Sodium ions moving into nerve cells stimulate neural impulses and produce overexcitability of the peripheral and central nervous systems.
- *Look for tetany, belligerence, irritability, disorientation, and seizures.*

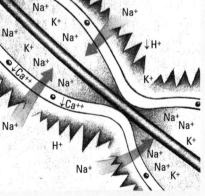

- Hypotension
- Dizziness
- Paresthesia in fingers and toes
- Circumoral paresthesia
- Carpopedal spasm
- Muscle hypertonicity
- Nausea and vomiting
- Confusion
- Irritability
- Agitation
- Seizures
- Coma

Diagnostic findings (uncompensated)
- Arterial pH greater than 7.45
- $Paco_2$ level 35 to 45 mm Hg
- Arterial HCO_3^- level greater than 26 mEq/L
- Base excess positive
- Serum CO_2 level greater than 28 mEq/L

Diagnostic findings (compensated)
- Arterial pH borderline (7.45 or slightly higher)
- $Paco_2$ level greater than 45 mm Hg
- Arterial HCO_3^- levels greater than 26 mEq/L
- Base excess positive
- Serum potassium and chloride levels (relative to sodium) decreased

Treatment
- Discontinuation of thiazide diuretics, such as hydrochlorothiazide or other diuretics, and NG suctioning
- Antiemetic to treat underlying nausea and vomiting
- Acetazolamide to increase renal excretion of bicarbonate

Nursing interventions
- Monitor patients at risk for metabolic alkalosis, particularly those with gastric fluid losses from long-term NG suctioning or vomiting
- Assess fluid intake and output to determine the amount of gastric fluid loss
- Monitor vital signs, especially respirations, which will usually decrease as the body attempts to conserve CO_2
- Monitor heart rate and rhythm to detect hypokalemia; a 12-lead electrocardiogram may be indicated
- Assess the patient's LOC; watch for apathy and confusion, which may be evident in a patient's conversation
- Watch closely for signs of muscle weakness, tetany, or decreased activity
- Intervene as necessary to correct the underlying cause of the imbalance; for example, control vomiting by administering an antiemetic
- Monitor ABG values

Testing for metabolic alkalosis

Uncompensated
- Arterial pH greater than 7.45
- $Paco_2$ level 35 to 45 mm Hg
- Arterial HCO_3^- level greater than 26 mEq/L

Compensated
- Arterial pH borderline (7.45 or slightly higher)
- $Paco_2$ level greater than 45 mm Hg
- Arterial HCO_3^- levels greater than 26 mEq/L

Key treatment options for metabolic alkalosis
- Discontinuation of thiazide diuretics
- Antiemetic
- Acetazolamide

Key nursing interventions for a patient with metabolic alkalosis
- Monitor patients at risk.
- Monitor vital signs, especially respirations.
- Monitor heart rate and rhythm.
- Assess the patient's LOC.
- Monitor ABG values.
- Administer I.V. fluid and electrolyte supplements as ordered.
- Provide patient teaching as necessary.

TIME-OUT FOR TEACHING

Patient teaching: Metabolic alkalosis

When teaching a patient with metabolic alkalosis, be sure to cover this information and then evaluate the patient's learning.

- Teach the patient and his family about metabolic alkalosis, including its causes and associated risks.
- Warn the patient and his family about the dangers of excessive bicarbonate ingestion; explain that alkalosis can develop from overuse of antacids or sodium bicarbonate.
- Teach the patient taking a potassium-wasting diuretic to watch for and report symptoms of hypokalemia, such as weakness and excessive urine output.
- Teach the patient how to replace potassium by increasing dietary intake or taking oral supplements.

- Administer I.V. fluid and electrolyte supplements as ordered to replace fluid volume, potassium, and chloride losses; monitor electrolyte studies to prevent overreplacement
- Administer diluted potassium solutions with an infusion device
- Supply sufficient chloride to enable renal absorption of sodium with chloride and subsequent renal excretion of excessive bicarbonate
- Irrigate an NG tube connected to suction with normal saline solution instead of tap water to prevent loss of gastric electrolytes
- Provide patient teaching as necessary (see *Patient teaching: Metabolic alkalosis*)

MIXED (COMBINED) IMBALANCES

● **General information**
- Two primary acid-base imbalances occurring simultaneously in one of several circumstances
  - One disturbance results in acidosis, other in alkalosis
  - Acidosis: result of both disturbances
  - Alkalosis: result of both disturbances

● **Examples**
- Metabolic acidosis with respiratory acidosis
  - Seen with cardiac arrest
  - Decreased bicarbonate from lactic acidosis that results from hypoxemia
  - CO_2 retention from respiratory arrest
- Metabolic acidosis with respiratory alkalosis
  - Seen with salicylate intoxication
  - Decreased bicarbonate from overproduction of organic acids resulting from altered peripheral metabolism by the salicylate

---

Key facts about mixed imbalances

- Two primary acid-base imbalances occurring simultaneously
- Metabolic acidosis examples: with respiratory acidosis, with respiratory alkalosis, with metabolic alkalosis, with respiratory alkalosis, and with respiratory acidosis

    – Decreased CO_2 from stimulation of the respiratory centers by the salicylate
- Metabolic acidosis with metabolic alkalosis
    – Seen with renal failure and vomiting
    – Decreased bicarbonate from retention of metabolites in renal failure
    – Increased bicarbonate from loss of hydrogen and chloride from vomiting
- Metabolic alkalosis with respiratory alkalosis
    – Seen with vomiting during pregnancy
    – Increased bicarbonate from loss of hydrogen and chloride from vomiting
    – Decreased CO_2 from respiratory stimulation by progesterone
- Metabolic alkalosis with respiratory acidosis
    – Seen with COPD with vomiting
    – Increased bicarbonate from loss of hydrogen and chloride with vomiting
    – Sustained elevation of CO_2 associated with COPD

PATIENTS AT RISK FOR ACID-BASE IMBALANCES

- **General information**
  - Vary in susceptibility to acid-base imbalances
  - Body's ability to compensate for imbalances affected by age- and illness-related physiologic changes
  - Infants and chronically ill patients at greatest risk

- **Infants**
  - Commonly have problems with acid-base imbalances, particularly acidosis
  - Have low residual lung volume
    – $Paco_2$ possibly changed rapidly and dramatically because of alteration in respiration
    – Change may lead to acidosis
  - Have high metabolic rates
    – Yield large amounts of metabolic wastes and acids that must be excreted by kidneys
    – Along with immature buffer system, leaves them prone to acidosis
  - Prone to airway obstruction due to more narrow airways and inability to effectively clear secretions

- **Chronically ill patients**
  - At extremely high risk because of diminished reserves
  - Any chronic diseases, such as those affecting compensatory organs of lungs and renal system, considered etiologic factors in various acid-base imbalances
  - Chronic illness: impairs body's ability to compensate for imbalances, necessitates close monitoring for these patients

Key risk factors for acid-base imbalances in infants
- Low residual lung volume
- High metabolic rates
- Prone to airway obstruction

Key risk factors for acid-base imbalances in chronically ill patients
- Diminished reserves
- Etiologic factors
- Impairment of body's ability to compensate for imbalances

TOP 10

Items to study for your next test on acid-base imbalances

1. Differences among the four types of acid-base imbalances: respiratory acidosis, respiratory alkalosis, metabolic acidosis, and metabolic alkalosis

2. Three forms of major imbalances—primary, mixed (combined), and compensated

3. Causes of the four types of acid-base imbalances

4. Drugs that impact the development of acid-base imbalances

5. Explanation of the sequence of compensation mechanisms used in correcting acid-base imbalances

6. Diagnostic results for each acid-base imbalance, including interpretation of ABG results

7. Nursing assessments for each acid-base imbalance

8. Nursing interventions used for each acid-base imbalance

9. Treatment for each acid-base imbalance, including drug management

10. Clients at risk for acid-base imbalances and the rationale for each risk factor

NCLEX CHECKS

It's never too soon to begin your NCLEX preparation. Now that you've reviewed this chapter, carefully read each of the following questions and choose the best answer. Then compare your responses to the correct answers.

1. Kussmaul's respirations are associated with which acid-base imbalance?
- ☐ **1.** Respiratory acidosis
- ☐ **2.** Respiratory alkalosis
- ☐ **3.** Metabolic acidosis
- ☐ **4.** Metabolic alkalosis

2. A client has been diagnosed with an intestinal obstruction, and has an NG tube set to low continuous suction. For which acid-base imbalance is this client at risk?
- ☐ **1.** Respiratory acidosis
- ☐ **2.** Respiratory alkalosis
- ☐ **3.** Metabolic acidosis
- ☐ **4.** Metabolic alkalosis

3. ABG results for the client above indicate that he has, indeed, developed metabolic alkalosis. Which ABG results are consistent with this finding?
- ☐ **1.** pH 7.35; $Paco_2$ 38 mm Hg; HCO_3^- 20 mEq/L
- ☐ **2.** pH 7.49; $Paco_2$ 43 mm Hg; HCO_3^- 28 mEq/L
- ☐ **3.** pH 7.30; $Paco_2$ 49 mm Hg; HCO_3^- 25 mEq/L
- ☐ **4.** pH 7.48; $Paco_2$ 32 mm Hg; HCO_3^- 23 mEq/L

4. Respiratory acidosis results from which process?
- ☐ **1.** Alveolar hyperventilation
- ☐ **2.** Hypocapnia
- ☐ **3.** Alveolar hypoventilation
- ☐ **4.** Lactic acidosis

5. A nurse has just received a client's ABG results: pH 7.31; $Paco_2$ 52 mm Hg; HCO_3^- 28 mEq/L. Which acid-base imbalance would the nurse suspect based on these results?
- ☐ **1.** Uncompensated respiratory acidosis
- ☐ **2.** Compensated respiratory acidosis
- ☐ **3.** Uncompensated metabolic acidosis
- ☐ **4.** Compensated metabolic acidosis

6. A client's ABG values show worsening respiratory acidosis. Clinically, he has rapid, shallow respirations and decreased breath sounds bilaterally. His oxygen requirement is increasing. Which intervention should be the nurse's highest priority?

☐ **1.** Prepare the client for endotracheal intubation and mechanical ventilation.

☐ **2.** Encourage the client to breathe into cupped hands.

☐ **3.** Administer diuretics as soon as possible.

☐ **4.** Administer an antibiotic for suspected pneumonia.

7. Which statement is true about oxygen therapy and clients with COPD?

☐ **1.** Clients with COPD have an increased need for oxygen to stimulate their respiratory drive.

☐ **2.** Clients with COPD typically have low CO_2 levels and, therefore, little need for oxygen therapy.

☐ **3.** Clients with COPD require 100% oxygen administration via a snug-fitting Venturi face mask.

☐ **4.** Clients with COPD should be placed on the lowest possible oxygen concentration to maintain their respiratory drive.

8. In conditions of acidosis, which electrolyte imbalance should be expected?

☐ **1.** Hyperkalemia

☐ **2.** Hypokalemia

☐ **3.** Hypercalcemia

☐ **4.** Hypermagnesemia

9. Which ABG results are consistent with compensated metabolic acidosis? Select all that apply.

☐ **1.** pH: 7.32

☐ **2.** pH: 7.49

☐ **3.** Pa_{CO_2}: 37 mm Hg

☐ **4.** Pa_{CO_2}: 31 mm Hg

☐ **5.** HCO_3^-: 21 mEq/L

☐ **6.** HCO_3^-: 28 mEq/L

10. Which acid-base imbalance should be suspected with these ABG results? pH: 7.47; Pa_{CO_2}: 30 mm Hg; HCO_3^-: 23 mEq/L

☐ **1.** Respiratory acidosis

☐ **2.** Respiratory alkalosis

☐ **3.** Metabolic acidosis

☐ **4.** Metabolic alkalosis

ANSWERS AND RATIONALES

1. CORRECT ANSWER: 3

In metabolic acidosis, acid builds up in the bloodstream. The lungs compensate with rapid, deep breathing, called *Kussmaul's respirations,* in an attempt to blow off CO_2 and increase arterial pH.

2. CORRECT ANSWER: 4
The most common cause of metabolic alkalosis is excessive acid loss from the GI tract, which can occur from vomiting or prolonged NG suctioning.

3. CORRECT ANSWER: 2
Metabolic alkalosis is characterized by a pH greater than 7.45, a normal $PaCO_2$ level, and an HCO_3^- level greater than 26 mEq/L. $PaCO_2$ level will be greater than 45 mm Hg if the respiratory system is compensating for the imbalance.

4. CORRECT ANSWER: 3
Respiratory acidosis results from alveolar hypoventilation, in which the lungs can't rid the body of adequate amounts of CO_2.

5. CORRECT ANSWER: 2
Respiratory acidosis is characterized by a pH less than 7.35 and a $PaCO_2$ greater than 45 mm Hg. An HCO_3^- level greater than 26 mEq/L indicates that the kidneys are compensating for the imbalance.

6. CORRECT ANSWER: 1
Treatment for the client's respiratory acidosis and worsening respiratory status should focus on improving ventilation. Therefore, the nurse's highest priority is to prepare the client for endotracheal intubation and mechanical ventilation. Although administering diuretics or antibiotics may also be appropriate for this client, ensuring that the client has a patent airway and is ventilating adequately takes top priority. Encouraging the client to breathe into cupped hands would be appropriate for a client with respiratory alkalosis.

7. CORRECT ANSWER: 4
Clients with COPD are accustomed to high CO_2 levels and are stimulated to breathe because of a lack of oxygen as opposed to a high CO_2 level. These clients should be placed on the lowest possible oxygen concentrations because administering too much oxygen will diminish their respiratory drive.

8. CORRECT ANSWER: 1
In conditions of acidosis, hydrogen ions move into the cells, causing potassium to move out of cells to maintain electroneutrality. This process raises serum potassium levels and causes hyperkalemia.

9. CORRECT ANSWER: 1, 4, 5
Metabolic acidosis is characterized by a pH below 7.35 and an HCO_3^- level below 22 mEq/L. Compensatory attempts by the lungs to rid the body of excess CO_2 are indicated by $PaCO_2$ levels less than 35 mm Hg.

10. CORRECT ANSWER: 2
Respiratory alkalosis is characterized by a pH above 7.45 and a $PaCO_2$ level below 35 mm Hg. Because the bicarbonate level is normal, this client's condition is uncompensated. Compensation by the metabolic system would be indicated by an HCO_3^- level below 22 mEq/L.

8

Conditions associated with imbalances

LEARNING OBJECTIVES

After studying this chapter, you should be able to:

- Identify common conditions associated with fluid, electrolyte, and acid-base imbalances.
- Describe at least two specific imbalances associated with each of these conditions.
- Discuss how the pathophysiology of these conditions leads to such imbalances.
- Describe specific nursing interventions for patients affected by fluid, electrolyte, and acid-base imbalances.

CHAPTER OVERVIEW

Various disorders can be associated with fluid, electrolyte, and acid-base imbalances. In addition, the treatments used to correct a disorder can disrupt the body's regulatory systems and result in an imbalance. To provide effective nursing care, the nurse must have knowledge of the underlying regulatory systems and the pathophysiology of the disorder. Nursing care focuses on identifying the possible imbalances and instituting measures to prevent or correct them. Patient teaching plays an important role in all aspects of care.

Common causes of balance disorders

- Disorders that disrupt the regulatory mechanism of an organ or system
- Disorders involving excessive fluid gains or losses or massive tissue destruction
- Treatments and therapy
- Dietary restrictions

Key facts about AIDS

- Progressive disorder marked by gradual destruction of CD4+ T cells
- Immunodeficiency predisposes patient to opportunistic infections, cancers, and other characteristic abnormalities

Common causes of AIDS

- Infection with the HIV retrovirus
- Contact with infected blood or body fluids; associated with identifiable high-risk behaviors

Key pathophysiologic changes in AIDS

- Results from infection with HIV, which destroys CD4+ T cells
- Immunodeficiency: results in opportunistic infections
- Fluid and electrolyte imbalances: result from underlying opportunistic infection and effects on body and from treatment measures

INTRODUCTION

- **Causes of fluid, electrolyte, and acid-base imbalances**
  - Various disorders affecting major regulatory systems
  - Various disorders that can disrupt the regulatory mechanism or action of an organ or system
  - Disorders involving excessive fluid gains or losses (such as occur in vomiting or diarrhea) or after massive tissue destruction (such as in burns and trauma)
  - Treatments instituted to correct a condition, such as diuretic therapy and nasogastric (NG) suctioning
  - Dietary restrictions
  - Electrolyte replacement therapy
  - Hormonal therapy (steroids)

ACQUIRED IMMUNODEFICIENCY SYNDROME (AIDS)

- **General information**
  - Progressive, incurable disorder marked by gradual destruction of CD4+ T cells by the human immunodeficiency virus (HIV)
  - Patient predisposed by resultant immunodeficiency to several disorders
    - Opportunistic infections
    - Unusual cancers
    - Other characteristic abnormalities

- **Causes**
  - Primary cause: infection with the HIV retrovirus
  - Transmission: occurs by contact with infected blood or body fluids; is associated with identifiable high-risk behaviors
  - Virus disproportionately represented in certain populations
    - Homosexual and bisexual men
    - I.V. drug users
    - Recipients of contaminated blood or blood products (dramatically decreased since mid-1985)
    - Heterosexual partners of persons in the former groups
    - Neonates of infected women

- **Pathophysiology**
  - Results from infection with HIV, a retrovirus that destroys the CD4+ T cells (essential regulators of normal immune response)
  - Immunodeficiency: results in opportunistic infections that eventually overwhelm immune system and invade body systems
    - Lungs
    - Bone marrow
    - Brain

Adverse reactions to commonly used HIV medications

This chart shows some of the adverse reactions to commonly used human immunodeficiency virus (HIV) medications. Many of these adverse reactions can cause or worsen fluid and electrolyte imbalances in patients infected with HIV.

MEDICATION	ADVERSE REACTIONS
Delavirdine (Rescriptor)	Rash, headache, fatigue, increased liver enzymes
Didanosine (Videx)	Upper abdominal pain, diarrhea, persistent nausea and vomiting, tingling or numbness of the extremities, difficulty breathing, headache, mental confusion
Indinavir (Crixivan)	Nephrolithiasis, hyperbilirubinemia without symptoms, hyperglycemia, anemia, elevated cholesterol and triglycerides
Lamivudine (Epivir)	Headache, fever, rash, severe abdominal pain, shortness of breath, fatigue, muscle pain, mania, psychosis, confusion, lactic acidosis, pancreatitis
Nevirapine (Viramune)	Thrombocytopenia, rash, fever, anemia, stomatitis
Ritonavir (Norvir)	Diarrhea, nausea, vomiting, anorexia, abdominal pain, body fat redistribution, hyperglycemia, hyperlipidemia
Saquinavir (Fortovase)	Diarrhea (if formulated with lactose), body fat redistribution, hyperglycemia
Stavudine (Zerit)	Numbness, pain or tingling of the extremities, neutropenia, thrombocytopenia
Zalcitabine (Hivid)	Rashes, mouth sores, upper abdominal pain, itching, numbness or tingling, confusion, seizures, fever, hyperbilirubinemia
Zidovudine (Retrovir)	Headache, fever, rash, severe abdominal pain, shortness of breath, fatigue, muscle pain, anemia, leukopenia, cardiomyopathy, cholestatic jaundice

- Fluid and electrolyte imbalances: commonly result from underlying opportunistic infection and effects on body
  - Also can result from disease treatment and patient's general disability
  - Lead to loss of appetite, decreased intake, and malnutrition (see *Adverse reactions to commonly used HIV medications*)

● **Potential imbalance: Hyponatremia**
  - Commonly develops in patients with AIDS
  - Has been associated with adrenal insufficiency and volume depletion (such as from vomiting or diarrhea)
  - Has multiple associated conditions
    - *Pneumocystis carinii* pneumonia and other pneumonias
    - Malignancies
    - Central nervous system (CNS) disease

Key facts about potential imbalances due to AIDS

Hyponatremia
- Associated with adrenal insufficiency and volume depletion
- Associated conditions: *Pneumocystis carinii* pneumonia, malignancies, and CNS disease

Key facts about potential imbalances due to AIDS

(continued)

Fluid volume deficit
- May occur through:
- Vomiting
- Diarrhea
- Fistulas
- Elevated body temperature
- Decreased fluid intake
- Weight loss associated with the wasting syndrome

Hypokalemia
- Results from GI losses of potassium
- Potassium increasingly lost by kidneys

Metabolic alkalosis
- Results from loss of gastric fluid
- Kidneys: attempt to correct pH imbalance

Hyperkalemia
- May result from trimethoprim administration
- Impairs renal excretion of potassium

Hypocalcemia
- Results from the intestinal malabsorption of vitamin D

Common assessment findings in AIDS

- Generalized lymphadenopathy
- Weight loss
- Fatigue
- Night sweats
- Fevers
- Neurologic symptoms
- Opportunistic infection or cancer

● **Potential imbalance: Isotonic fluid volume deficit**
- Large fluid losses: may occur through vomiting, diarrhea, and fistulas
- Can be caused by elevated body temperature associated with infection
  - Body's metabolism increased by fever; amount of formed metabolic wastes increased as consequence
  - Wastes: require fluid for renal excretion—causes increase in fluid loss
  - Fever: also causes hypercapnia; leads to extra water vapor loss through lungs
- Decreased fluid intake: results from extreme weakness, fatigue, or anorexia; also predisposes patient to fluid volume deficit
- Loss of body fluid also caused by weight loss associated with the wasting syndrome of AIDS

● **Potential imbalance: Hypokalemia**
- Results from the GI losses of potassium
- Caused by persistent vomiting; potassium lost in gastric fluid, increasingly lost by kidneys

● **Potential imbalance: Metabolic alkalosis**
- Occurs because of persistent vomiting and loss of gastric fluid
- Kidneys: attempt to conserve hydrogen ions to correct pH imbalance
- More potassium lost as a result

● **Potential imbalance: Hyperkalemia**
- May result when the patient receives trimethoprim (Primsol)
- Drug: impairs renal excretion of potassium

● **Potential imbalance: Hypocalcemia**
- Has been reported in patients with AIDS
- Believed to result from the intestinal malabsorption of vitamin D

● **Assessment findings**
- Persistent, generalized lymphadenopathy
- Nonspecific signs and symptoms
  - Weight loss
  - Fatigue
  - Night-sweats
  - Fevers
- Neurologic symptoms resulting from HIV encephalopathy and infection of neuroglial cells
- Opportunistic infection or cancer related to immunodeficiency

● **Diagnostic findings**
- CD4+ T-cell count of less than 200 cells/mm^3 in any HIV-infected patient
- Screening test: enzyme-linked immunosorbent assay (ELISA) and confirmatory test (Western blot) detect presence of HIV antibodies, which indicate HIV infection

- CD4$^+$ and CD8$^+$ T-lymphocyte subset counts, erythrocyte sedimentation rate, complete blood cell count, serum beta$_2$-microglobulin, p24 antigen, neopterin levels, and anergy testing: performed to support diagnosis and help evaluate severity of immunosuppression

● Treatment

- Antiretrovirals to control reproduction of HIV and slow progression of HIV-related disease
- Highly active antiretroviral therapy (commonly referred to as *HAART*) as recommended treatment for HIV; combines three or more antiretrovirals in a daily regimen
- Four classes of antiretrovirals approved by the U.S. Food and Drug Administration
  - Nonnucleoside reverse transcriptase inhibitors (such as delavirdine [Rescriptor], efavirenz [Sustiva], and nevirapine [Viramune]) to bind to and disable reverse transcriptase, a protein that HIV needs to replicate
  - Nucleoside reverse transcriptase inhibitors (such as abacavir [Ziagen], didanosine [Videx], emtricitabine [Emtriva], lamivudine [Epivir], stavudine [Zerit], tenofovir [Viread], zalcitabine [Hivid], and zidovudine [Retrovir]) to halt reproduction of the virus
  - Protease inhibitors (such as amprenavir [Agenerase], atazanavir [Reyataz], fosamprenavir [Lexiva], indinavir [Crixivan], lopinavir and ritonavir [Kaletra], nelfinavir [Viracept], ritonavir [Norvir], and saquinavir [Fortovase]) to disable protease, a protein that HIV needs to replicate
  - Fusion inhibitors (enfuvirtide [Fuzeon] is only one approved) to block HIV entry into cells
- Additional therapies
  - Immunomodulator to boost the immune system weakened by AIDS and retroviral therapy
  - Human granulocyte colony-stimulating growth factor to stimulate neutrophil production (because retroviral therapy causes anemia, patients may receive epoetin alfa [Epogen])
  - Anti-infective and antineoplastic to combat opportunistic infections and associated cancers (some prophylactically to help resist opportunistic infections)
  - Supportive therapy
    - Nutritional support
    - Fluid and electrolyte replacement therapy
    - Pain relief
    - Psychological support

● Nursing interventions

- Assess the patient carefully to determine the type and extent of fluid, electrolyte, or acid-base imbalance

---

Testing for AIDS

- CD4$^+$ T-cell count of less than 200 cells/mm^3
- ELISA and Western blot: presence of HIV antibodies

Key treatment options for AIDS

Antiretrovirals (four classes)
- Nonnucleoside reverse transcriptase inhibitors
- Nucleoside reverse transcriptase inhibitors
- Protease inhibitors
- Fusion inhibitors

Additional therapies
- Immunomodulator
- Human granulocyte colony-stimulating growth factor
- Anti-infective and antineoplastic
- Supportive therapy

Key nursing interventions for a patient with AIDS

- Assess the type and extent of imbalance.
- Maintain accurate fluid intake and output record.
- Obtain daily weight.
- Monitor vital signs.
- Monitor serum electrolyte levels.
- Monitor ECG readings.
- Administer medications, as ordered.
- Provide patient teaching as needed.

Key facts about acute renal failure

- Sudden, usually reversible disruption of normal kidney function; may progress to chronic kidney disease
- Affects nephron, which forms urine
- Kidneys: lose ability to excrete water, electrolytes, wastes, and acid-base products via urine

- Maintain an accurate fluid intake and output record; calculate insensible water losses to determine fluid balance
- Obtain daily weight and correlate results with the 24-hour intake and output record
- Monitor vital signs, including breath sounds and, when available, central venous pressure
- Monitor serum electrolyte levels for abnormalities
- Observe for signs and symptoms that may indicate electrolyte imbalance, such as tetany, paresthesia, and muscle weakness
- Monitor electrocardiogram (ECG) readings to detect changes secondary to hypokalemia, hyperkalemia, hypocalcemia, and hypercalcemia
- As necessary, restrict electrolyte intake, especially potassium and phosphorus, to prevent further imbalances
- Administer medications, as ordered, such as oral electrolyte replacements and cation exchange resins, to correct electrolyte imbalances
- Provide patient teaching as needed
    - How to calculate and record amounts (in milliliters) of fluid ingested and excreted
    - How to recognize electrolyte content in solid foods, fluids, and medications—especially over-the-counter (OTC) antacids and laxatives—to prevent excessive ingestion of electrolytes

ACUTE RENAL FAILURE

General information
- Renal system: is a major regulator of fluid, electrolyte, and acid-base balance
- Acute renal failure: involves the sudden, usually reversible disruption of normal kidney function; left untreated, may progress to chronic kidney disease (see *Understanding chronic kidney disease*)
- Affects kidneys' functional unit (*nephron*), which forms urine
- Kidneys: lose ability to excrete water, electrolytes, wastes, and acid-base products via urine; leads to imbalances
- Places patients: at risk for fluid volume, electrolyte, and metabolic acid-base imbalances
- Other problems caused by acute renal failure that alter homeostasis
    - Anemia
    - Hypertension
    - Uremia
    - Osteodystrophy

Causes
- May stem from intrarenal conditions; damage kidneys themselves
- May stem from prerenal conditions such as heart failure; causes diminished blood flow to kidneys

Understanding chronic kidney disease

Chronic kidney disease, formerly known as *chronic renal failure, chronic renal disease,* and *renal insufficiency,* affects approximately 11% of the U.S. population, and its incidence is rising. This disorder typically leads to poor outcomes, including progression to kidney failure, complications of decreasing kidney function, and cardiovascular disease. Risk factors include diabetes mellitus, hypertension, systemic lupus erythematosus, family history of the disease, and older age. Blacks also appear to be at greater risk for kidney damage than other racial groups.

The National Kidney Foundation defines chronic kidney disease as either kidney damage or decreased kidney function (decreased glomerular filtration rate [GFR]) for 3 or more months. More specifically, chronic kidney disease is present if:
- GFR is less than 60 ml/minute per 1.73 m^2, or
- GFR is ≥ 60 ml/minute per 1.73 m^2 if other evidence of kidney damage also exists.

The National Kidney Foundation has classified chronic kidney disease into five stages based on the degree of kidney damage and GFR.

STAGE 1
- Kidney damage with normal GFR: 90 ml/minute per 1.73 m^2 or above

STAGE 2
- Kidney damage with mild decrease in GFR: 60 to 89 ml/minute per 1.73 m^2

STAGE 3
- Moderate decrease in GFR: 30 to 59 ml/minute per 1.73 m^2

STAGE 4
- Severe reduction in GFR: 15 to 29 ml/minute 1.73 m^2

STAGE 5
- Kidney failure: less than 15 ml/minute 1.73 m^2

Patients with chronic kidney disease are at increased risk for fluid, electrolyte, and acid-base imbalances, especially in the later stages of disease. Specific imbalances are similar to those that occur during acute renal failure, and may include hypervolemia, hyperkalemia, metabolic acidosis, hypermagnesemia, hyperphosphatemia, and hypocalcemia. In chronic kidney disease, the patient may also develop hypernatremia as progression in the degree of kidney failure causes less sodium to be excreted.

Key facts about chronic kidney disease
- Defined as either kidney damage or decreased kidney function for 3 or more months
- Increases risk of fluid, electrolyte, and acid-base imbalances

What it causes
- Kidney failure
- Complications of decreasing kidney function
- Cardiovascular disease
- Fluid, electrolyte, and acid-base imbalances

Risk factors
- Diabetes mellitus
- Hypertension
- Systemic lupus erythematosus
- Family history of the disease
- Older age
- African-American race

Stages of chronic kidney disease
- Based on degree of kidney damage and GFR
- Stage 1: Kidney damage with normal GFR
- Stage 2: Kidney damage with mild decrease in GFR
- Stage 3: Moderate decrease in GFR
- Stage 4: Severe reduction in GFR
- Stage 5: Kidney failure

- May stem from obstructive postrenal conditions such as prostatitis; can cause backup of urine into kidneys (see *Causes of acute renal failure*, page 172)

● **Pathophysiology**
- Kidneys: can't produce urine in normal amounts or adequate concentrations
- With abnormal urine production, kidneys' ability to maintain homeostasis altered
- Proceeds in three distinct phases
  – Oliguric-anuric phase

Key pathophysiologic changes in acute renal failure

- Abnormal urine production
- Kidney's ability to maintain homeostasis altered

Three phases

- Oliguric-anuric phase: associated with a decrease in GFR
- Diuretic phase: gradual increase in daily urine output
- Recovery phase: fluid and electrolyte values start to stabilize

Common causes of acute renal failure

Prerenal

- Hypovolemia
- Peripheral vasodilation
- Severe vasoconstriction

Intrarenal

- Acute tubular necrosis
- Ischemic damage
- Trauma
- Nephrotoxins

Postrenal

- Obstruction
- Trauma

Causes of acute renal failure

The causes of acute renal failure can be divided into three categories: prerenal, intrarenal, and postrenal. Prerenal causes involve conditions that diminish blood flow to the kidneys. Intrarenal causes involve conditions that damage the kidneys themselves. Postrenal causes involve conditions that obstruct urine outflow, which causes urine to back up into the kidneys.

PRERENAL CAUSES	INTRARENAL CAUSES	POSTRENAL CAUSES
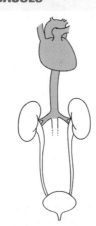	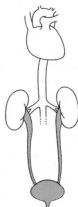	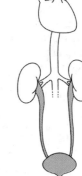

PRERENAL CAUSES
- Hypovolemia
- Peripheral vasodilation
- Renal vascular obstruction
- Serious cardiovascular disorders
- Severe vasoconstriction
- Trauma

INTRARENAL CAUSES
- Acute tubular necrosis
- Aminoglycosides or nonsteroidal anti-inflammatory drugs
- Crush injury, myopathy, sepsis, or transfusion reaction
- Eclampsia, postpartum renal failure, or uterine hemorrhage
- Heavy metals
- Ischemic damage from poorly treated renal failure
- Nephrotoxins
- Trauma

POSTRENAL CAUSES
- Bladder obstruction
- Trauma
- Ureteral obstruction
- Urethral obstruction

- Lasts 1 to 2 weeks
- Associated with a decrease in glomerular filtration rate (GFR)
- Decreased urine output first clinical sign
- Nitrogenous waste products accumulate; elevates blood urea nitrogen (BUN) and serum creatinine levels, results in uremia

– Diuretic phase
  · Lasts about 10 days
  · Starts with gradual increase in daily urine output and stabilization of the BUN level
– Recovery phase (also known as *convalescent phase*)
  · Lasts a few months
  · Begins when fluid and electrolyte values start to stabilize, indicating return to normal kidney function
  · Patient: may experience slight reduction in kidney function for the rest of his life; still at risk for fluid and electrolyte imbalances

● Potential imbalance: Hypervolemia

- Water and sodium retention during acute renal failure associated with oliguria or anuria when body can't excrete excess fluid and electrolytes
- May also occur if fluid intake exceeds urine output
- Can result in hypertension, peripheral edema, heart failure, or pulmonary edema

● Potential imbalance: Hypovolemia

- Water losses associated with the diuretic or polyuric phase of acute renal failure
- Dehydration: occurs during diuretic phase only when large volume of urine output isn't matched by adequate fluid replacement
- Can result in hypotension and circulatory collapse

● Potential imbalance: Hyperkalemia

- Usually occurs with oliguria and anuria because potassium (K) excretion is reduced as urine output is diminished
- High serum potassium levels also possibly caused by additional stressors
  – Infection
  – GI bleeding
  – Trauma
  – Surgery
- Can worsen with development of metabolic acidosis (commonly occurs in patients with acute renal failure); causes potassium to move from intracellular fluid into the ECF, further increasing serum potassium levels
- Symptoms may appear with K levels of 6 mEq/L or higher

● Potential imbalance: Hypocalcemia

- Activation of vitamin D by the kidneys decreased; results in decreased GI absorption of calcium (Ca), a potential cause of low serum calcium levels
- Afflicted patients at high risk for tetany and seizures; experience secondary hyperparathyroidism after repeated episodes of significant hypocalcemia cause parathyroid gland to hypertrophy

---

Key facts about potential imbalances due to acute renal failure

Hypervolemia
- Body can't excrete excess fluid and electrolytes
- Fluid intake exceeds urine output

Hypovolemia
- Large volume of urine output isn't matched by adequate fluid replacement

Hyperkalemia
- Potassium excretion is reduced as urine output is diminished
- Can worsen with metabolic acidosis

Hypocalcemia
- Activation of vitamin D decreased; results in decreased GI absorption of calcium
- May cause hyperphosphatemia

Hyperphosphatemia
- Kidneys lose ability to excrete phosphate
- May cause hypocalcemia

Hypermagnesemia
- Patient may retain magnesium as a result of decreased GFR or destruction of tubules
- May be due to external sources of magnesium: laxatives, antacids, I.V. solutions, or hyperalimentation solutions

Hyponatremia
- Water and sodium retention increased by decreased GFR and damaged tubules
- Dilutional hyponatremic state possibly caused by metabolic acidosis

Metabolic acidosis
- Kidneys lose ability to secrete hydrogen in urine
- Kidneys fail to hold onto bicarbonate

Key facts about potential imbalances due to acute renal failure (continued)

Metabolic alkalosis
- Rare
- Occurs only after excessive administration of bicarbonate

- Calcium mobilized from bone by overactive, enlarged parathyroid gland to replenish hypocalcemic serum
- Bone softening: known as *osteomalacia* or *renal rickets*, occurs with repeated episodes
- Serum calcium and phosphorus (P) have inverse relationship; hyperphosphatemia caused by hypocalcemia

● **Potential imbalance: Hyperphosphatemia**
- Results because the kidneys lose ability to excrete phosphate
- After developed, hypocalcemia will follow

● **Potential imbalance: Hypermagnesemia**
- Patient with acute renal failure: may retain magnesium (Mg) as a result of several factors
  - Decreased GFR
  - Destruction of tubules
- High serum magnesium level usually not recognized unless patient receives external sources of magnesium
  - Laxatives
  - Antacids
  - I.V. solutions
  - Hyperalimentation solutions
- Should be suspected if the patient demonstrates sudden changes in neurologic status

● **Potential imbalance: Hyponatremia**
- Can occur with acute renal failure; water and sodium (Na) retention increased by decreased GFR and damaged tubules
- Dilutional hyponatremic state also possibly caused by the intracellular-extracellular exchange between sodium and potassium during metabolic acidosis

● **Potential imbalance: Metabolic acidosis**
- Occurs commonly in acute renal failure
- Develops as kidneys lose ability to secrete hydrogen (H^+), an acid, in urine
- Exacerbated as kidneys fail to hold onto bicarbonate (HCO_3^-), a base

● **Potential imbalance: Metabolic alkalosis**
- Rarely occurs in acute renal failure
- Usually occurs only after excessive administration of bicarbonate in an effort to correct metabolic acidosis

● **Assessment findings**
- Early findings
  - Oliguria
  - Azotemia
  - Anuria (rare)
- GI findings
  - Anorexia

- Nausea
- Vomiting
- Diarrhea or constipation
- Stomatitis
- Bleeding
- Hematemesis
- Dry mucous membranes
- Uremic breath
- Central nervous system (CNS) findings
  - Headache
  - Drowsiness
  - Irritability
  - Confusion
  - Peripheral neuropathy
  - Seizures
  - Coma
- Integumentary findings
  - Dryness
  - Pruritus
  - Pallor
  - Purpura
  - Uremic frost (rare)
- Cardiovascular findings
  - Early in disease: hypotension
  - Later in disease: hypertension, arrhythmias, fluid overload, heart failure, systemic edema
- Respiratory findings
  - Pulmonary edema
  - Kussmaul's respirations
- Hematologic findings
  - Anemia
  - Altered clotting mechanisms

● **Diagnostic findings**
- Blood studies
  - Elevated BUN, serum creatinine, and potassium levels
  - Decreased hematocrit (HCT), bicarbonate, and hemoglobin (Hb) levels
  - Low blood pH
- Urine studies
  - Casts, cellular debris, decreased specific gravity
  - In glomerular diseases: proteinuria and urine osmolality close to serum osmolality
  - Urine Na level: less than 20 mEq/L if oliguria results from decreased perfusion, greater than 40 mEq/L if cause is intrarenal
  - Creatinine clearance: shows decreased GFR

Common assessment findings in acute renal failure

- Oliguria
- Azotemia
- Anorexia
- Nausea
- Vomiting
- Diarrhea
- Headache
- Confusion
- Seizures
- Dryness
- Pallor
- Hypertension, arrhythmias, heart failure (later in disease)
- Pulmonary edema
- Anemia

Testing for acute renal failure

Blood studies
- Elevated BUN, serum creatinine, and potassium levels
- Decreased HCT, Hb, pH, and bicarbonate levels

Urine studies
- Decreased specific gravity
- Proteinuria
- Decreased creatinine clearance

ECG
- Tall, peaked T waves
- Widening QRS complex

Key treatment options for acute renal failure

- High-calorie diet low in sodium and potassium
- Restricted protein intake
- Monitoring of electrolyte levels
- I.V. therapy
- Fluid restriction
- Diuretic therapy
- Kayexalate
- Hypertonic glucose with insulin I.V.
- Sodium bicarbonate I.V.
- Dialysis

- ECG
  - Tall, peaked T waves
  - Widening QRS complex
  - Disappearing P waves if hyperkalemia is present

● **Treatment**

- High-calorie diet low in sodium and potassium, and with restricted protein to meet metabolic needs (protein intake must be adequate enough to prevent malnourishment)
- Careful monitoring of electrolyte levels; I.V. therapy to maintain and correct fluid and electrolyte balance
- Fluid restriction to minimize edema (although fluid restoration and maintenance may be needed during the diuretic phase)
- Diuretic therapy to treat oliguric phase
- Sodium polystyrene sulfonate (Kayexalate) by mouth or enema to reverse hyperkalemia with mild hyperkalemic symptoms
  - Malaise
  - Loss of appetite
  - Muscle weakness
- Hypertonic glucose with insulin I.V. for more severe hyperkalemic symptoms
  - Numbness and tingling
  - ECG changes
- Sodium bicarbonate I.V. to treat metabolic acidosis
- Dialysis, continuous renal replacement therapy, or peritoneal dialysis to correct fluid and electrolyte imbalances

● **Nursing interventions**

- Assess the patient carefully to determine the type and extent of fluid, electrolyte, or acid-base imbalance
- Maintain an accurate fluid intake and output record; calculate insensible water losses to determine fluid balance
- Obtain daily weight and correlate results with the 24-hour intake and output record
- Monitor vital signs, including breath sounds and, when available, central venous pressure, to detect fluid abnormalities; report hypertension that may occur secondary to fluid and sodium retention
- Observe for signs and symptoms of fluid overload, such as edema, bounding pulse, jugular vein distention, crackles on lung auscultation, and shortness of breath
- Monitor serum electrolyte levels for abnormalities
- Monitor arterial blood gas (ABG) studies for pH; observe for symptomatic acidosis
- Observe for clinical signs and symptoms that may indicate an electrolyte or acid-base imbalance, such as tetany, paresthesia, muscle weakness, tachypnea, or confusion

- Monitor ECG readings to detect changes secondary to hypokalemia, hyperkalemia, hypocalcemia, hypercalcemia, hypomagnesemia, and hypermagnesemia
- As ordered, administer diuretics to patients whose kidneys can still respond to remove fluid excess; GFR should be at least 25 ml/minute
- As ordered, administer medications such as oral or I.V. electrolyte replacements and cation exchange resins to correct electrolyte imbalances, and vitamin supplements to correct nutritional deficiencies
- Know the route of excretion for medications being given; drugs excreted through the kidney or removed during dialysis will need dosage adjustments
- Expect to administer sodium bicarbonate I.V. to control acute acidosis and orally to control chronic acidosis
- Be aware of the high sodium content in a dose of sodium bicarbonate (approximately 50 mEq in one 50-ml ampule); multiple doses may result in significant hypernatremia, which could contribute to the onset of heart failure and pulmonary edema
- Maintain the patient's nutritional status: a diet high in calories and low in protein, sodium, potassium; restricted electrolyte intake, especially potassium and phosphorus, if ordered; and nutritional consultation as needed
- Be prepared to initiate dialysis for electrolyte and acid-base imbalances that don't respond to medication therapy, or when fluid removal isn't possible
- If the patient requires dialysis, check the vascular access site every 2 hours for patency and signs of clotting and feel for a bruit; check the site for bleeding after dialysis
- Don't use the extremity with the dialysis shunt or fistula for measuring blood pressure, drawing blood, or inserting I.V. catheters
- Determine the optimal "dry weight" for dialysis patients; dry weight is individualized for each patient and obtained after dialysis
- Provide emotional support to the patient and his family
- Provide patient (and family) teaching, as appropriate
  - How to calculate and record amounts (in milliliters) of fluid ingested and excreted
  - How to determine the electrolyte content in solid foods, fluids, and medications—especially OTC antacids and laxatives—to prevent ingestion of excessive electrolytes
  - How to care for the shunt, fistula, or vascular access device (patient requiring dialysis)
  - How to perform the procedure at home (patient requiring peritoneal dialysis); help in obtaining necessary supplies

Key nursing interventions for a patient with acute renal failure

- Assess type and extent of fluid, electrolyte, or acid-base imbalance.
- Accurately record fluid intake and output.
- Obtain daily weight.
- Monitor vital signs.
- Observe for signs and symptoms of fluid overload.
- Monitor serum electrolyte levels.
- Monitor ABG studies.
- Monitor ECG readings.
- Administer diuretics, as ordered.
- Administer medications to correct electrolyte imbalances.
- Be prepared to initiate dialysis.
- Provide patient (and family) teaching, as appropriate.

BURNS

● **General information**
- Involve destruction of the epidermis, dermis, or subcutaneous layers of skin
- Can be permanently disfiguring and incapacitating, both emotionally and physically, and possibly life-threatening
- Associated imbalances: result from alterations in skin integrity and internal body membranes, and from effect of heat on body water and solute losses that result from cellular destruction
- Type and severity of imbalance depend on burn type and depth, percentage of body surface area (BSA) involved, and burn phase

● **Causes**
- Thermal burns (most common): result from exposure to several sources
    - Dry heat such as flames
    - Moist heat, such as steam and hot liquids
    - Frostbite (because effects are similar to those of thermal burns)
- Mechanical burns: caused by the friction or abrasion that occurs when skin is rubbed harshly against a coarse surface
- Electrical burns: possible after contact with one of multiple causes
    - Faulty electrical wiring
    - High-voltage power lines
    - Immersion in water that has been electrified
    - Lightning strikes
- Chemical burns: result from direct contact, ingestion, inhalation, or injection of various substances
    - Acids
    - Alkali
    - Vesicants
- Radiation burns: typically associated with sunburn or radiation therapy (as for cancer treatment)

● **Pathophysiology**
- Burn phases: refer to stages that describe physiologic changes occurring after a burn
- Fluid-accumulation phase: lasts for 36 to 48 hours after a burn injury
    - Fluid: shifts from vascular compartment to interstitial space; process called *third-space shift*
    - Edema caused by shifted fluid (which typically reaches maximum extent within 8 hours after injury)
    - Circulation possibly compromised and pulses diminished from severe edema
    - Several reasons for fluid imbalances (such as hypovolemia) during this period
        • Damage to capillaries from the burn injury (alters vessel permeability)
        • Diminished kidney perfusion (decreases urine output)

Key facts about burns

- Involve destruction of the epidermis, dermis, or subcutaneous layers of skin
- Imbalances result from alterations in skin integrity and internal body membranes, and results of cellular destruction

Common causes of burns

Thermal
- Dry heat
- Moist heat
- Frostbite

Mechanical
- Friction
- Abrasion

Electrical
- Contact with faulty electrical wiring
- Contact with high-voltage power lines
- Immersion in electrified water
- Lightning strikes

Chemical
- Direct contact, ingestion, inhalation, or injection of various substances

Radiation
- Sunburn
- Radiation therapy

- Production and release of stress hormones, such as aldosterone and antidiuretic hormone (ADH), in response to burn injury (causes kidneys to retain sodium and water)
  - Respiratory problems: occur secondary to compromised, edematous airway or because circumferential burns and edema of neck or chest can restrict respirations and cause shortness of breath
  - Muscle and tissue injury: cause release of acids that can cause a drop in pH level and subsequent metabolic acidosis
  - GI problems, including Curling's ulcers (or stress ulcers): occur as result of decreased blood flow to stomach
  - Electrolyte imbalances (such as hyperkalemia, hyponatremia, hypernatremia, and hypocalcemia): common during this phase due to body's hypermetabolic needs and priority that fluid replacement takes over nutritional needs during emergency phase
- Fluid-remobilization phase: also known as the *diuresis stage*; starts about 48 hours after initial burn
  - Fluid shifted back to vascular compartment
  - Edema at burn site decreased, blood flow to the kidneys increased, (increases urine output)
  - Sodium lost through increase in diuresis; potassium either moved back into cells or lost through urine
  - Fluid and electrolyte imbalances present during initial phase after burn: can change during fluid-remobilization phase; may include hypokalemia, hypervolemia, and hyponatremia
- Convalescent phase: begins after first two phases have been resolved
  - Characterized by healing or reconstruction of burn wound
  - Major fluid shifts now resolved, but possible further fluid and electrolyte imbalances exist as result of inadequate dietary intake
  - Anemia common at this time (severe burns typically destroy red blood cells)

Potential imbalance: Hypovolemia

- Approximately 10% of plasma volume lost into tissue soon after a severe burn; result of edema caused by increased capillary permeability
- Occurs because of the third-space shift (loss of fluids from the vascular compartment); causes multiple effects
  - Decreased cardiac output
  - Tachycardia
  - Hypotension
- With burn's damage to the skin surface, decrease in skin's ability to prevent water loss; patient can lose up to 8 L of fluid per day (400 ml/hour)
- Potential for blood loss, adding to fluid volume losses

Potential imbalance: Hypervolemia

- Usually develops 3 to 5 days after a major burn injury
- Occurs during the fluid remobilization phase, as fluid shifts from the interstitial space back to the vascular compartment
- May be exacerbated by excessive administration of I.V. fluids

Key facts about potential imbalances due to burns

(continued)

Hyperkalemia
- Develops as potassium is released into ECF during fluid-accumulation phase

Hypokalemia
- Develops as potassium shifts from ECF into cells
- Occurs during fluid-remobilization phase

Hypocalcemia
- Calcium travels to damaged tissue
- Becomes immobilized at the burn site

Hyponatremia
- Results from increased loss of sodium and water from cells
- Large amounts of sodium trapped in edema fluid during fluid-accumulation phase
- Sodium also lost during fluid-remobilization phase

Hypernatremia
- Occurs as a result of aggressive use of hypertonic sodium solutions during fluid replacement therapy

Metabolic acidosis
- Fixed acids released from injured tissues accumulate

Respiratory acidosis
- Occurs secondary to inadequate ventilation, as in inhalation burns

● **Potential imbalance: Hyperkalemia**
- In burns, results from one of various causes
  - Massive cellular trauma
  - Metabolic acidosis
  - Renal failure
- Develops as potassium is released into ECF during fluid-accumulation phase

● **Potential imbalance: Hypokalemia**
- In burns, develops as potassium shifts from ECF into cells
- Usually occurs 4 to 5 days after a major burn injury, during fluid-remobilization phase

● **Potential imbalance: Hypocalcemia**
- Can develop in burns as calcium travels to damaged tissue and becomes immobilized at the burn site
- May occur 12 to 24 hours after the burn, during fluid-accumulation phase
- Also may occur due to inadequate dietary intake of calcium or inadequate supplementation during treatment

● **Potential imbalance: Hyponatremia**
- Results from increased loss of sodium and water from cells
- Large amounts of sodium trapped in edema fluid during fluid-accumulation phase
- Sodium: also lost when diuresis occurs during fluid-remobilization phase
- Sodium: contained in burn exudate, can be lost as burn exudate is secreted
- Use of aqueous silver nitrate dressings: may also contribute to this imbalance

● **Potential imbalance: Hypernatremia**
- Can occur as a result of aggressive use of hypertonic sodium solutions during fluid replacement therapy

● **Potential imbalance: Metabolic acidosis**
- Tissue perfusion: becomes ineffective because of intravascular fluid shifts and overall fluid losses
- Fixed acids released from injured tissues: accumulate, causing drop in pH

● **Potential imbalance: Respiratory acidosis**
- Can occur secondary to inadequate ventilation, as in inhalation burns
- Diminished respiratory excursion: due to circumferential chest burns, edema, or pain; also contributes to CO_2 retention

● **Assessment findings**
- Superficial partial-thickness (first-degree) burns
  - Involve superficial injury to the epidermis, marked by an uncomplicated erythematous area

Determining burn severity

The severity of a burn can be estimated by correlating its depth and size. A burn is characterized as major, moderate, or minor.

MAJOR BURNS

Major burns require care in a specialized burn facility, and include:

- second-degree burns on more than 25% of an adult's body surface area (BSA) or on more than 20% of a child's BSA
- third-degree burns on more than 10% of the BSA, regardless of body size
- burns of the hands, face, eyes, ears, feet, or genitalia
- all inhalation burns
- all electrical burns
- burns complicated by fractures or other major trauma
- all burns in high-risk patients, such as children younger than age 2, adults older than age 60, and patients who have preexisting medical conditions such as heart disease.

MODERATE BURNS

Moderate burns usually require care in either a burn care facility or a general health care facility, and include:

- third-degree burns on 2% to 10% of the BSA, regardless of body size
- second-degree burns on 15% to 25% of an adult's BSA and 10% to 20% of a child's BSA.

MINOR BURNS

Minor burns can be treated on an outpatient basis, and include:

- third-degree burns on less than 2% of the BSA, regardless of body size
- second-degree burns on less than 15% of an adult's BSA and on less than 10% of a child's BSA.

- – Localized pain
- – Skin barrier remains intact; fluid and electrolyte loss not a problem
- Partial-thickness (second-degree) burns: involve damage to the epidermis, progressing to the dermis
  - – Blisters present
  - – Mild to moderate edema and pain
  - – Possible capillary damage
  - – Possible regeneration of the epithelial layer
  - – Fluid and electrolyte imbalances associated with second-degree burns that cover significant areas of the body
- Full-thickness (third-degree) burns
  - – Involve all skin layers
  - – Regeneration impossible
  - – Skin elasticity lost, appearance altered significantly (color varies from red to black to white)
  - – No blisters present
  - – No pain if nerve endings are damaged
  - – Carry greatest risk of fluid and electrolyte imbalance (see *Determining burn severity*)

Key facts about estimating the extent of burns

For adults

- Use the Rule of Nines; divides an adult's body surface areas into percentages.
- Match the burns on your patient to the body charts
- Add the corresponding percentages
- Use the total to calculate initial fluid replacement needs.

For infants

- Infant's or child's body-section percentages differ from those of an adult
- Use the Lund-Browder classification

Estimating the extent of burns

You can quickly estimate the extent of an adult patient's burns by using the Rule of Nines. This method divides an adult's body surface areas into percentages.

To use this method, match the burns on your patient to the body charts shown below. Then add the corresponding percentages for each body section burned. Use the total—a rough estimate of burn extent—to calculate initial fluid replacement needs.

An infant or a child's body-section percentages differ from those of an adult. For instance, an infant's head accounts for a greater percentage of his total BSA when compared with an adult's. For an infant or child, use the Lund-Browder classification, as shown at right.

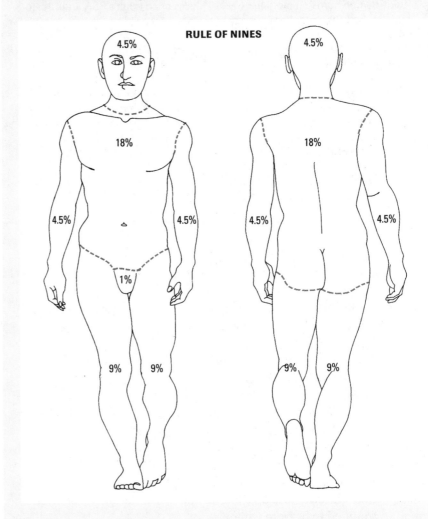

RULE OF NINES

Diagnostic findings

- Percentage of BSA involved determined by Rule of Nines or Lund-Browder classification; greater BSA involved results in greater potential for imbalances (see *Estimating the extent of burns*)

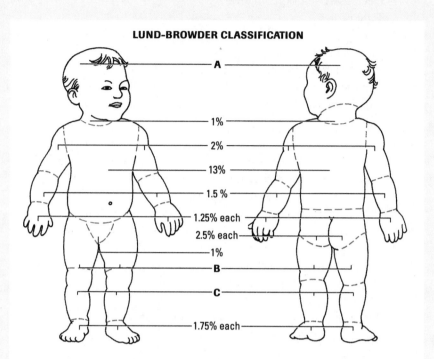

LUND-BROWDER CLASSIFICATION

A
1%
2%
13%
1.5 %
1.25% each
2.5% each
1%
B
C
1.75% each

RELATIVE PERCENTAGES OF AREAS AFFECTED BY GROWTH

	AT BIRTH	1 TO 4 YEARS	5 TO 9 YEARS	10 TO 14 YEARS	15 YEARS	ADULT
A: Half of head	9.5%	8.5%	6.5%	5.5%	4.5%	3.5%
B: Half of one thigh	2.75%	3.25%	4%	4.25	4.5%	4.75%
C: Half of one leg	2.5%	2.5%	2.75%	3%	3.25%	3.5%

- ABG levels: may be normal in early stages, may reveal hypoxemia and metabolic acidosis in later stages
- Carboxyhemoglobin level: may reveal extent of smoke inhalation due to presence of carbon monoxide

Testing for burns

Extent of burn
- Rule of Nines determines adult BSA involved
- Lund-Browder classification determines infant or child BSA involved

ABG levels
- In early stages: may be normal
- In later stages: may reveal hypoxemia and metabolic acidosis

Carboxyhemoglobin level
- May reveal extent of smoke inhalation

- Other blood studies: may reveal several findings
  - Decreased hemoglobin level
  - Total protein
  - Albumin
  - Increased HCT
  - Elevated creatine kinase and myoglobin levels
  - Leukocytosis
  - Electrolyte imbalances

● **Treatment**
- Removal of smoldering clothing (soaking first in normal saline solution if stuck to patient's skin), rings, and other constricting items
- Immersion of the burned area in cool water (55° F [12.8° C]) or application of cool compresses (minor burns)
- Pain medications as needed, or an anti-inflammatory drug
- Coverage of the area with an antimicrobial and a nonstick, bulky dressing (after debridement)
- Prophylactic tetanus injection as needed
- Prevention of hypoxia by use of several steps
  - Maintaining an open airway
  - Assessing airway, breathing, and circulation
  - Checking for smoke inhalation immediately when the patient presents
  - Assisting with endotracheal intubation
  - Administering 100% oxygen (first immediate treatment for moderate and major burns)
- Coverage of partial-thickness burns over 30% of BSA or full-thickness burns over 5% of BSA with a clean, dry, sterile bedsheet (coverage of large burns with saline-soaked dressings harmful because of drastic reduction in body temperature)
- Immediate I.V. therapy to prevent hypovolemic shock and maintain cardiac output
- Antimicrobial therapy (for all patients with major burns)
- Insertion of NG tube to decompress the stomach and avoid aspiration of stomach contents
- Irrigation of the wound with copious amounts of normal saline solution (chemical burns)
- Surgical intervention, including skin grafts and more thorough surgical cleaning (major burns)

● **Nursing interventions**
- Assess for upper airway obstruction secondary to smoke inhalation; monitor for signs and symptoms, such as tachypnea, hoarseness, wheezing, and stridor
- Provide oxygen therapy as ordered to promote optimal respiratory function; consider mechanical ventilation for a patient with inadequate ventilation for any reason, especially smoke inhalation

---

Key treatment options for burns

- Removal of smoldering clothing
- Immersion of burned area in cool water or application of cool compresses
- Pain medications
- Antimicrobial and nonstick, bulky dressing
- Prophylactic tetanus injection
- Prevention of hypoxia
- I.V. therapy
- Antimicrobial therapy
- NG tube
- Irrigation of the wound
- Surgical intervention

Using the fluid replacement formula

The Parkland formula is a commonly used formula for calculating fluid replacement in patients with burns. Always base the volume of fluid replacement on the patient's response, especially his urine output. Urine output of 30 to 50 ml/hour is a sign of adequate renal perfusion.

The Parkland formula

Over 24 hours, 4 ml of lactated Ringer's solution per kilogram of body weight per percentage of body surface area (BSA) burned.

Use this example to calculate the formula—for a person who weighs 68 kg and has 27% BSA burns: 4 ml × 68 kg × 27 = 7,344 ml over 24 hours. Give one-half of the total over the first 8 hours after the burn, and the remainder over the next 16 hours.

Key facts about Parkland formula

- Used for calculating fluid replacement in patients with burns
- Over 24 hours, 4 ml of lactated Ringer's solution per kilogram of body weight per percentage of BSA burned

- Promote respiratory airway excursion to ensure adequate gas exchange
- Assess cardiac and hemodynamic status for changes that indicate fluid imbalance, such as hypovolemia or hypervolemia
- Maintain blood pressure within the normal range to ensure adequate tissue perfusion and to prevent lactic acid production
- Assess skin for location, depth, and extent of burns
- Watch for signs of decreased tissue perfusion, increased confusion, and agitation; assess peripheral pulses for adequacy
- As ordered, administer I.V. fluid therapy to restore depleted vascular volume; lactated Ringer's solution is usually the solution of choice
  - Use Parkland formula or another fluid resuscitation formula to calculate amount of fluid replacement, as ordered by the physician (see *Using the fluid replacement formula*)
  - Maintain I.V. fluid replacement; base on daily assessment of fluid, electrolyte, acid-base, nutritional needs
- Don't administer colloid solutions in the immediate postburn period; colloids will increase osmotic pressure in the interstitial space, which may exacerbate burn edema and increase the risk of vascular collapse
- Administer I.V. electrolyte replacement therapy as ordered during the initial postburn period; monitor for signs and symptoms of hypokalemia, hyponatremia, and hypocalcemia
- Watch for signs and symptoms of pulmonary edema, which can result from fluid replacement therapy and the shift of fluid back to the vascular compartment
- Observe the pattern of third-space shifting, which causes generalized edema, ascites, and pulmonary or intracranial edema
- If bowel sounds are present, provide a diet high in potassium, protein, vitamins, fats, nitrogen, and calories to maintain the patient's preburn weight

Key nursing interventions for a patient with burns

- Assess for upper airway obstruction.
- Provide oxygen therapy as ordered.
- Assess cardiac and hemodynamic status.
- Assess skin for location, depth, and extent of burns.
- Administer I.V. fluid therapy, as ordered.
- Assess for signs and symptoms of metabolic acidosis.
- Monitor ECG readings.
- Assess fluid and hydration status.
- Monitor ABG values and serum electrolyte levels.
- Perform burn care.
- Observe for signs and symptoms of infection.
- Provide patient teaching as appropriate.

- If necessary, feed the patient enterally until he can tolerate oral feedings; if he can't tolerate oral or enteral feedings, administer total parenteral nutrition (TPN); TPN may also be necessary to meet the patient's increased metabolic needs
- Assess for signs and symptoms of metabolic acidosis, such as headache, disorientation, drowsiness, nausea, vomiting, and rapid, shallow breathing
- Monitor ECG readings for changes pointing to fluid and electrolyte imbalances, especially potassium imbalances
- Assess fluid and hydration status, including skin turgor, daily weight, and hourly urine output, for significant changes
- Monitor ABG values and serum electrolyte levels to detect any significant changes
- Monitor the patient for temperature changes because skin impairment leads to body alterations and chills as well as infection
- Maintain core body temperature by covering the patient with a sterile blanket and exposing only small areas of his body at a time
- Insert an NG tube, if ordered, to decompress the stomach; avoid aspiration of stomach contents during the procedure
- Perform burn care as ordered; monitor the patient's response
- Observe the patient for signs and symptoms of infection, such as fever, tachycardia, and purulent wound drainage; the patient has an increased risk of infection exacerbated by destruction of the skin barrier and nutrient losses
- Provide patient teaching as appropriate
  - Explanation of individualized treatment plan
  - Teaching management of burn wound (give complete instructions for home care)
  - Importance of taking pain medication as needed, especially before dressing changes
  - Role of good nutrition in wound healing

CIRRHOSIS

Key facts about cirrhosis

- Widespread destruction and fibrotic regeneration of hepatic cells
- Liver structure and normal vasculature altered

Common causes of cirrhosis

- Various types of hepatitis
- Toxic exposures
- Alcoholism

● **General information**
- Chronic hepatic disorder
- Characterized by widespread destruction and fibrotic regeneration of hepatic cells
- As progresses, liver structure and normal vasculature altered
  - Impaired blood and lymph flow
  - Ultimate hepatic insufficiency

● **Causes**
- Various types of hepatitis (such as nonviral hepatitis or viral types A, B, C, or D)
- Toxic exposures
- Alcoholism

What happens in portal hypertension

Portal hypertension (elevated pressure in the portal vein) occurs when blood flow meets increased resistance. This common result of cirrhosis may also stem from mechanical obstruction and occlusion of the hepatic veins (Budd-Chiari syndrome).

As the pressure in the portal vein rises, blood backs up into the spleen and flows through collateral channels to the venous system, bypassing the liver. Thus, portal hypertension causes:
- splenomegaly with thrombocytopenia
- dilated collateral veins (esophageal varices, hemorrhoids, or prominent abdominal veins)
- ascites.

In many patients, the first sign of portal hypertension is bleeding esophageal varices (dilated tortuous veins in the submucosa of the lower esophagus).

Esophageal varices commonly cause massive hematemesis, requiring emergency care to control hemorrhage and prevent hypovolemic shock.

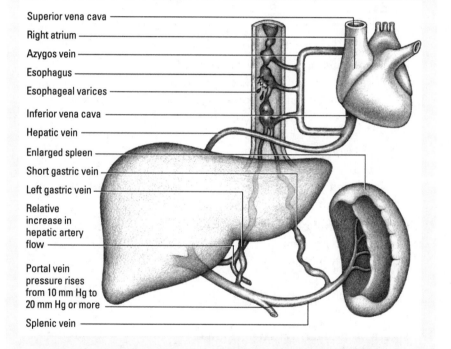

Superior vena cava
Right atrium
Azygos vein
Esophagus
Esophageal varices
Inferior vena cava
Hepatic vein
Enlarged spleen
Short gastric vein
Left gastric vein
Relative increase in hepatic artery flow
Portal vein pressure rises from 10 mm Hg to 20 mm Hg or more
Splenic vein

- Sarcoidosis
- Chronic inflammatory bowel disease

Pathophysiology
- Fibrotic tissue in the liver: increases hepatic pressure, reduces liver's capacity to do its job
- Ascites: accumulates as venous outflow impeded through fibrotic liver, seeping from the liver's surface into the peritoneal cavity (see *What happens in portal hypertension*)

Key facts about portal hypertension
- Occurs when blood flow meets increased resistance
- May also stem from mechanical obstruction and occlusion of the hepatic veins
- As pressure in the portal vein rises, blood backs up into the spleen and flows through collateral channels to the venous system, bypassing the liver
- Causes splenomegaly with thrombocytopenia, dilated collateral veins, and ascites

Key pathophysiologic changes in cirrhosis
- Fibrotic tissue in the liver: increases hepatic pressure, reduces liver's capacity to do its job
- Ascites: occurs as fluid; seeps from the liver's surface into the peritoneal cavity
- Additional fluid pulled from surfaces of intestines
- Arterial volume decreases
- Edema also occurs

Key facts about potential imbalances due to cirrhosis

Fluid volume excess
- Excess of total body fluid produced by ascites and edema
- Kidneys: retain sodium and water

Hyponatremia
- Results from body's inability to excrete wastes
- May result from persistent release of ADH

Hypokalemia
- Causes: may include low dietary intake and renal losses of potassium by hyperaldosteronism and diuretics

Hyperkalemia
- Commonly associated with use of potassium-sparing diuretics and potassium supplements

Hypomagnesemia
- May result from magnesium loss through vomiting

Hypocalcemia
- Results from inadequate storage of vitamin D by the liver

Respiratory alkalosis
- Increasing ammonia levels stimulate hyperventilation

Respiratory acidosis
- Severe ascites interferes with diaphragmatic excursion
- Results in hypoventilation and CO_2 retention

Metabolic alkalosis
- Associated with use of potassium-sparing diuretics
- Possibly caused by vomiting and NG suctioning

- Fluid high in protein; as a result, additional fluid pulled from surfaces of intestines
- Arterial volume decreases
  - Total ECF volume normal or expanded
  - Kidneys: respond as if underperfused
  - Sodium retained
  - Urine concentrated
- Edema: also results with ascites
  - Increased pressure in vena cava (from the ascitic fluid and enlarged liver)
  - Interference with venous drainage from lower extremities
  - Hypoalbuminemia: lowers plasma oncotic pressure; promotes shift of fluid from the intravascular to interstitial spaces

● **Potential imbalance: Fluid volume excess**
- Excess of total body fluid produced by ascites and edema
- Kidneys: attempt to increase intravascular volume by retaining sodium and water
- Plasma aldosterone levels commonly above normal because of increased adrenal secretion and liver's inability to deactivate it

● **Potential imbalance: Hyponatremia**
- Common in patients with advanced cirrhosis
  - Usually results from body's inability to excrete wastes
  - May result from persistent release of ADH
- Occurs in addition to fluid volume excess
  - Abnormal retention of sodium and water
  - However, relatively greater degree of water retention
- Also caused by sodium losses due to frequent paracenteses, excessive diuretic use, or excessive sodium restriction

● **Potential imbalance: Hypokalemia**
- Common in patients with chronic liver disease
- Causes: may include low dietary intake and renal losses of potassium by hyperaldosteronism and diuretics
- Possibly contributed to by losses from the GI tract, such as through vomiting

● **Potential imbalance: Hyperkalemia**
- Occasionally seen
- Commonly associated with use of potassium-sparing diuretics and with potassium supplements

● **Potential imbalance: Hypomagnesemia**
- May result from magnesium loss through vomiting
- Also may result from poor dietary intake and renal wasting of magnesium in patients with cirrhosis due to alcoholism

● **Potential imbalance: Hypocalcemia**
  • Believed to result from inadequate storage of vitamin D by the liver
  • Also associated with hypoalbuminemia

● **Potential imbalance: Respiratory alkalosis**
  • Most common acid-base imbalance associated with cirrhosis
  • Increasing ammonia levels thought to stimulate hyperventilation, resulting in respiratory alkalosis
  • Elevated progesterone levels (normally degraded by the liver) also thought to play a role as a respiratory stimulant

● **Potential imbalance: Respiratory acidosis**
  • May occur if ascites is severe enough to interfere with diaphragmatic excursion
  • Results in hypoventilation and CO_2 retention

● **Potential imbalance: Metabolic alkalosis**
  • Usually associated with use of potassium-sparing diuretics
  • Also possibly caused by vomiting and NG suctioning, or sources such as antacids or citrate from blood transfusion

● **Assessment findings**
  • Early stages
    – Anorexia
    – Constipation
    – Diarrhea
    – Dull abdominal ache
    – Indigestion
    – Nausea and vomiting
  • Late stages
    – Respiratory system
      · Pleural effusion and limited thoracic expansion
      · Interference with efficient gas exchange
    – CNS
      · Lethargy
      · Mental changes
      · Slurred speech
      · Asterixis (flapping tremor)
      · Peripheral neuritis
      · Paranoia
      · Hallucinations
      · Coma
    – Endocrine system
      · Testicular atrophy
      · Menstrual irregularities
      · Gynecomastia
      · Loss of chest and axillary hair

Common assessment findings in cirrhosis

Early stages
● Anorexia
● Diarrhea
● Nausea and vomiting

Late stages
● Pleural effusion and limited thoracic expansion
● Lethargy
● Asterixis (flapping tremor)
● Coma
● Bleeding tendencies
● Jaundice
● Hepatomegaly
● Ascites
● Severe pruritus
● Pain in right upper abdominal quadrant
● Bleeding from esophageal varices

– Hematologic system
  · Bleeding tendencies (nosebleeds, easy bruising, and bleeding gums)
  · Anemia
– Hepatic system
  · Jaundice
  · Hepatomegaly
  · Ascites
– Skin
  · Severe pruritus
  · Extreme dryness
  · Poor tissue turgor
  · Abnormal pigmentation
  · Spider angiomas
– Miscellaneous
  · Musty breath
  · Enlarged superficial abdominal veins
  · Muscle atrophy
  · Pain in right upper abdominal quadrant that worsens when patient sits up or leans forward
  · Palpable liver or spleen
  · Temperature of 101° to 103° F (38.3° to 39.4° C)
  · Bleeding from esophageal varices that results from portal hypertension

● **Diagnostic findings**
  • Liver biopsy: reveals tissue destruction and fibrosis
  • Abdominal X-ray
    – Enlarged liver
    – Cysts
    – Gas within the biliary tract or liver
    – Liver calcification
    – Massive fluid accumulation (ascites)
  • Computed tomography (CT) and liver scans
    – Increased liver size
    – Abnormal masses
    – Impaired hepatic blood flow and obstruction
  • Esophagogastroduodenoscopy
    – Bleeding esophageal varices
    – Stomach irritation or ulceration
    – Duodenal bleeding and irritation
  • Blood studies
    – Elevated levels of liver enzymes, total serum bilirubin, and indirect bilirubin
    – Decreased levels of total serum albumin, protein, hemoglobin, and electrolytes
    – Prolonged prothrombin time

Testing for cirrhosis

- Liver biopsy: tissue destruction and fibrosis
- Abdominal X-ray: enlarged liver and ascites
- CT and liver scans: impaired hepatic blood flow and obstruction
- Esophagogastroduodenoscopy: bleeding esophageal varices, duodenal bleeding and irritation
- Elevated liver enzyme and bilirubin levels
- Decreased total serum albumin levels
- Prolonged prothrombin time

- Decreased HCT
- Deficiency of vitamins A, C, and K
- Urine studies: show increased bilirubin and urobilirubinogen levels
- Fecal studies: show decreased fecal urobilirubinogen level

Treatment

- Vitamins and nutritional supplements to help heal damaged liver cells and improve nutritional status
- Antacid to reduce gastric distress and decrease the potential for GI bleeding
- Potassium-sparing diuretic to reduce fluid accumulation
- Vasopressin to treat esophageal varices
- Esophagogastric intubation with multilumen tubes to control bleeding from esophageal varices or other hemorrhage sites by using balloons to exert pressure on the bleeding site
- Gastric lavage until contents are clear; with an antacid and histamine antagonist if the bleeding is secondary to a gastric ulcer
- Paracentesis to relieve abdominal pressure and remove ascitic fluid
- Surgical shunt placement to divert ascites into venous circulation, leading to weight loss, decreased abdominal girth, increased sodium excretion from kidneys, and improved urine output
- Sclerosing agent injected into oozing vessels to cause clotting and sclerosis
- Transjugular intrahepatic portosystemic shunt (radiologic procedure) to reduce pressure in the varices, preventing them from bleeding
- Insertion of portosystemic shunts to control bleeding from esophageal varices and decrease portal hypertension (diverts a portion of the portal vein blood flow away from the liver; seldom performed)

Nursing interventions

- Assess the patient carefully to determine the type and extent of fluid, electrolyte, or acid-base imbalance; observe for signs and symptoms that may indicate electrolyte imbalance, such as tetany, paresthesia, and muscle weakness
- Maintain an accurate fluid intake and output record; calculate insensible water losses to determine fluid balance
- Obtain daily weight and correlate results with the 24-hour intake and output record
- Monitor vital signs, including breath sounds and, when available, central venous pressure, to detect fluid abnormalities
- Observe signs and symptoms of fluid overload, such as edema, bounding pulse, and shortness of breath
- Measure abdominal girth at least once every 12 hours
  - Mark abdomen: to ensure consistent and accurate measurements
  - Notify physician: of any increases or decreases
- Monitor serum electrolyte levels for abnormalities

Key treatment options for cirrhosis

- Vitamins and nutritional supplements
- Vasopressin
- Paracentesis
- Surgical shunt placement
- Sclerosing agent injected into oozing vessels
- Transjugular intrahepatic portosystemic shunt

Key nursing interventions for a patient with cirrhosis

- Assess type and extent of fluid, electrolyte, or acid-base imbalance.
- Maintain an accurate fluid intake and output record.
- Obtain daily weight.
- Monitor vital signs.
- Monitor abdominal girth.
- Monitor serum electrolyte levels.
- Monitor ECG readings.
- Monitor ABG studies.
- Administer medications as ordered.
- Monitor LOC.
- Provide patient teaching as appropriate.

- Monitor ECG readings to detect changes secondary to hypokalemia, hyperkalemia, hypocalcemia, hypercalcemia, and hypomagnesemia
- Monitor ABG studies for pH
- As ordered, administer diuretics to patients whose kidneys can still respond to remove fluid excess; GFR should be at least 125 ml/minute
- Administer medications as ordered, such as diuretics, potassium, and protein and vitamin supplements, and restrict fluid and sodium intake
- Monitor the patient's level of consciousness (LOC) for changes; institute safety precautions to prevent injury
- Provide patient teaching as appropriate
  - Importance of rest and good nutrition to conserve energy and decrease metabolic demands on the liver; urge small, frequent meals
  - How to calculate and record amounts (in milliliters) of fluid ingested and excreted
  - How to determine electrolyte content in solid foods, fluids, and medications, especially OTC antacids and laxatives, to prevent ingestion of excessive electrolytes

DIABETES INSIPIDUS

General information
- Metabolic disorder
- Caused by deficiency of ADH (vasopressin)
- Disorder of water metabolism; characterized by excessive fluid intake and hypotonic polyuria

Causes
- Acquired, familial, idiopathic, neurogenic, or nephrogenic
- Most common cause: failure of ADH secretion in response to normal stimuli
- Less common cause: kidneys' failure to respond to ADH
- Associated with stroke, hypothalamic or pituitary tumors, and cranial trauma or surgery
- Certain drugs, such as lithium (Eskalith) and phenytoin (Dilantin), or alcohol
- X-linked recessive trait or end-stage renal failure

Pathophysiology
- Normally, ADH synthesized in the hypothalamus and stored by the posterior pituitary gland
- ADH released into general circulation, acts on distal and collecting tubules of kidney; permeability to water increased, water reabsorbed
- ADH absence: allows filtered water to be excreted in urine instead of being reabsorbed
- Large quantities of dilute fluid passed throughout body; consequent plasma hyperosmolarity develops
- Dehydration: develops rapidly if fluids aren't replaced

Key facts about diabetes insipidus
- Metabolic disorder
- Characterized by excessive fluid intake and hypotonic polyuria

Common causes of diabetes insipidus
- Failure of ADH secretion in response to normal stimuli
- Kidneys' failure to respond to ADH

Key pathophysiologic changes in diabetes insipidus
- ADH absence: allows filtered water to be excreted in urine instead of being reabsorbed
- Large quantities of dilute fluid passed throughout body; consequent plasma hyperosmolarity develops

- **Potential imbalance: Hypernatremia**
  - Water diuresis: leads to large volume of water excretion and resultant sodium loss
  - Serum sodium level: will remain within normal limits if patient experiences thirst and drinks sufficient fluid to replace the lost volume,

- **Potential imbalance: Intracellular fluid (ICF) volume deficit**
  - Results from disproportionately high loss of water in relation to sodium in ECF
  - ECF left hypertonic from excessive water loss; draws water from ICF to ECF
  - Most likely to occur if patient has impaired or absent thirst mechanism

- **Assessment findings**
  - Polydipsia (cardinal sign): fluid intake of 5 to 20 qt (5 to 20 L)/day
  - Polyuria (cardinal sign): urine output of 2 to 20 L/24-hour period of dilute urine
  - Nocturia
  - Changes in LOC
  - Hypotension and tachycardia
  - Headache and vision disturbance
  - Abdominal fullness, anorexia, and weight loss

- **Diagnostic findings**
  - Almost colorless urine of low osmolarity (50 to 200 mOsm/L [less than that of plasma]) and low specific gravity (less than 1.005)
  - Water deprivation test to identify vasopressin deficiency: shows renal inability to concentrate urine

- **Treatment**
  - Vasopressin (Pitressin) to control fluid balance and prevent dehydration
  - Hydrochlorothiazide (Microzide) with potassium supplement to reduce urine volume by creating mild sodium depletion
  - Desmopressin acetate (DDAVP), a synthetic vasopressin analogue administered intranasally, to enhance reabsorption of water in the kidneys
  - Lypressin (Diapid), a synthetic vasopressin replacement administered intranasally, to prevent or control frequent urination, increased thirst, and loss of water
  - Chlorpropamide (Diabinese) to decrease thirst sensation in patients with continued hypernatremia

- **Nursing interventions**
  - Monitor the patient's fluid intake and output hourly, vital signs and urine specific gravity as ordered, and weight daily
  - Assess the patient for changes in LOC
  - Institute safety precautions to prevent injury

Key facts about potential imbalances due to diabetes insipidus

Hypernatremia
- Large volume of water excretion and resultant sodium loss

ICF volume deficit
- Disproportionately high loss of water in relation to sodium in ECF

Common assessment findings in diabetes insipidus
- Polydipsia
- Polyuria
- Changes in LOC
- Hypotension and tachycardia

Testing for diabetes insipidus
- Colorless urine of low osmolarity and low specific gravity
- Water deprivation test to identify vasopressin deficiency: renal inability to concentrate urine

Key treatment options for diabetes insipidus
- Vasopressin
- Desmopressin acetate

Key nursing interventions for a patient with diabetes insipidus

- Monitor intake and output.
- Assess for changes in LOC.
- Institute safety precautions.
- Administer vasopressin.
- Begin fluid replacement therapy.
- Monitor serum electrolyte levels.
- Provide patient teaching as appropriate.

Key facts about DKA

- Acute condition resulting from insulin deficiency in a patient with type 1 diabetes
- Characterized by hyperglycemia, ketonuria, hyperosmolality, ketonemia, and acidosis

Common causes of DKA

- Illness
- Insufficient or absent insulin

Key pathophysiologic changes in DKA

- Insufficient insulin: results in an inability to metabolize glucose
- Fats then burned for energy; results in ketosis
- Ketone bodies accumulated in ECF, hydrogen ions exchanged for potassium
- Lungs: attempt to eliminate excess acids through deep and rapid respirations
- Kidneys: attempt to increase acid excretion in urine

- Administer vasopressin cautiously to a patient with coronary artery disease because the drug may cause vasoconstriction
- Assess the patient receiving vasopressin for signs and symptoms of water intoxication, including drowsiness, light-headedness, headache, seizures and, possibly, coma
- Begin fluid replacement therapy using hypotonic solutions as ordered; expect to administer 1 ml of fluid for every 1 ml of urine output
- Keep in mind that hypernatremia must be corrected slowly to avoid rapid fluid shifts in the brain, which could lead to cerebral edema, seizures, or permanent neurologic damage
- Monitor serum electrolyte levels, especially sodium, BUN levels, and serum osmolality for changes
- Provide patient teaching as appropriate
  - Adequate fluid intake during the day to prevent severe dehydration but limit fluids in the evening to prevent nocturia
  - Need for long-term hormone replacement therapy; emphasize that the medication must not be discontinued abruptly without the physician's advice, and instruct patient on all aspects of medication regimen

DIABETIC KETOACIDOSIS (DKA)

● **General information**
- Is an acute condition resulting from insulin deficiency in a patient with type 1 diabetes
- Insufficient insulin available to metabolize glucose; condition may result from patient's failure to take prescribed insulin dose or from additional stressors
  - Infection
  - Trauma
  - Surgery
- Characterized by hyperglycemia, ketonuria, hyperosmolality, ketonemia, and acidosis
- Imbalances primarily a result of hyperglycemia

● **Causes**
- Infection
- Illness
- Surgery
- Stress
- Insufficient or absent insulin

● **Pathophysiology**
- Insufficient insulin: results in an inability to metabolize glucose; reflected by elevated serum glucose levels (exceeding 200 mg/dl)
- Fats then burned for energy; results in ketosis (*ketones* are strong metabolic body acids)

- Ketone bodies accumulated in ECF, hydrogen ions exchanged for potassium
- Elevated serum osmolality created by large volumes of glucose in the serum
- Elevated glucose levels in the renal tubules: precipitate osmotic diuresis, with losses of water, sodium, chloride, and potassium
- Inadequate volume replacement followed by significant dehydration and electrolyte deficits (see *Understanding DKA*, pages 196 and 197)
- Pulmonary and renal compensatory mechanisms triggered by these deficits
- Lungs: attempt to eliminate excess acids through deep and rapid respirations (Kussmaul's respirations) to compensate for increase in ketones
- Kidneys: attempt to increase acid excretion in urine (ketonuria)

Potential imbalance: Hypovolemia
- ECF volume deficit caused by massive fluid loss from osmotic diuresis
- Excessive water lost as kidneys attempt to rid body of excess acids

Potential imbalance: Hypokalemia
- In DKA, results from osmotic diuresis
- Aldosterone secretion: increased by ECF volume deficit; in turn, leads to potassium loss
- Can be exacerbated by intracellular movement of potassium in response to ketone accumulation and metabolic acidosis

Potential imbalance: Hyponatremia
- Elevated blood glucose levels: result in osmotic diuresis
- Sodium lost along with water and other electrolytes

Potential imbalance: Hypophosphatemia
- Osmotic diuresis: results in increased phosphorus loss in urine
- Insulin therapy: causes phosphorus to reenter intracellular space, thereby decreasing serum levels

Potential imbalance: Metabolic acidosis
- In DKA, fats broken down for energy into ketones
- Ketones: accumulate in blood, increasing amount of fixed acids and, thus, lowering pH (results in this imbalance)

Assessment findings
- Rapid onset of drowsiness, stupor, and coma
- Severe dehydration
- Kussmaul's respirations
- Fruity breath odor
- Polyuria, polydipsia, and polyphagia
- Weight loss
- Muscle wasting
- Vision changes
- Recurrent infections

Key facts about potential imbalances due to DKA

Hypovolemia
- Massive fluid loss from osmotic diuresis

Hypokalemia
- Results from osmotic diuresis

Hyponatremia
- Results from osmotic diuresis

Hypophosphatemia
- Results from osmotic diuresis
- Insulin therapy: causes phosphorus to reenter intracellular space, thereby decreasing serum levels

Metabolic acidosis
- Ketones: accumulate in blood

Common assessment findings in DKA

- Drowsiness, stupor, and coma
- Severe dehydration
- Kussmaul's respirations
- Fruity breath odor
- Polyuria, polydipsia, and polyphagia
- Nausea and vomiting

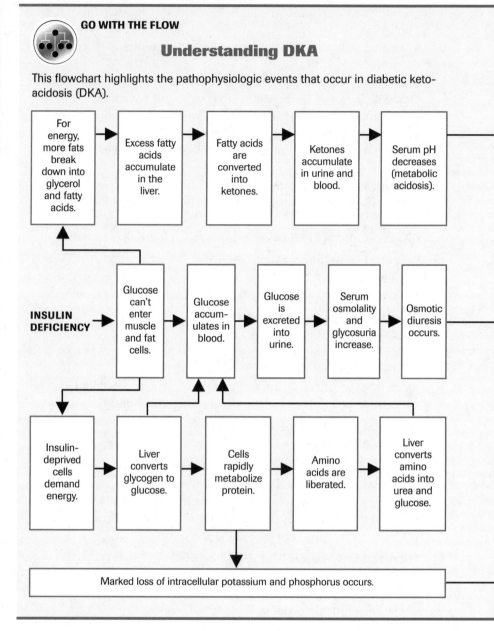

GO WITH THE FLOW

Understanding DKA

This flowchart highlights the pathophysiologic events that occur in diabetic keto-acidosis (DKA).

For energy, more fats break down into glycerol and fatty acids. → Excess fatty acids accumulate in the liver. → Fatty acids are converted into ketones. → Ketones accumulate in urine and blood. → Serum pH decreases (metabolic acidosis).

INSULIN DEFICIENCY → Glucose can't enter muscle and fat cells. → Glucose accumulates in blood. → Glucose is excreted into urine. → Serum osmolality and glycosuria increase. → Osmotic diuresis occurs.

Insulin-deprived cells demand energy. → Liver converts glycogen to glucose. → Cells rapidly metabolize protein. → Amino acids are liberated. → Liver converts amino acids into urea and glucose.

Marked loss of intracellular potassium and phosphorus occurs.

Testing for DKA

- Elevated serum glucose level
- Increased serum ketone level
- Positive urine acetone
- ABG analysis: metabolic acidosis

- Abdominal cramps
- Nausea and vomiting
- Leg cramps

● **Diagnostic findings**

- Elevated serum glucose (200 to 800 mg/dl)
- Increased serum ketone level
- Positive urine acetone
- ABG analysis that reveals metabolic acidosis

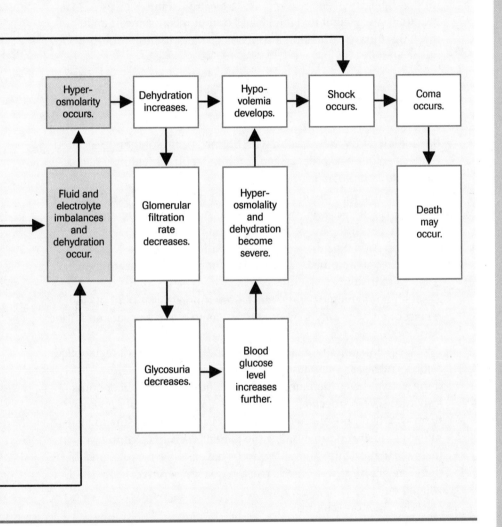

- Initially, normal potassium or hyperkalemia, depending on the level of acidosis, and then hypokalemia
- ECG changes related to hyperkalemia (tall, tented T waves and widened QRS complex); later, with hypokalemia, flattened T wave and presence of U wave
- Elevated serum osmolality

● **Treatment**
- Airway support and mechanical ventilation if patient is comatose
- I.V. fluids to rehydrate and restore electrolyte and acid-base balance

- Insulin therapy to control glucose levels
- **Nursing interventions**
  - Carefully monitor serum glucose and electrolyte levels, serum osmolality, and ABG results
  - Monitor vital signs frequently; institute cardiac monitoring to evaluate for possible arrhythmias secondary to electrolyte imbalances
  - Monitor daily weight and intake and output records; insert an indwelling urinary catheter in a comatose patient to monitor urine output accurately
  - Administer insulin (Humulin), as ordered, correlating dosage with serum glucose levels; remember that blood glucose levels must be reduced gradually to prevent cerebral fluid shifting and subsequent cerebral edema
  - Provide initial I.V. rehydration with normal saline solution or lactated Ringer's solution as ordered; rapid volume replacement may necessitate a rate as rapid as 1 L/hour
  - When the patient's blood glucose level approaches 250 mg/dl, anticipate the addition of dextrose to the fluid replacement regimen; dextrose is necessary to prevent hypoglycemia while also allowing for continued use of insulin to correct the patient's acidosis
  - Be prepared to administer bicarbonate for severe acidosis that doesn't respond to insulin
  - Assess hemodynamic parameters to determine the amount of volume replacement necessary to maintain adequate blood pressure and urine output
  - Replace potassium gradually with I.V. fluids; correction of metabolic acidosis releases potassium from cells
  - If the patient has experienced prolonged acidosis or if phosphorus levels are severely decreased, anticipate phosphorus replacement therapy; when phosphorus replacement is required, be sure to institute it gradually and to monitor the patient's serum calcium levels (remember that calcium and phosphorus have an inverse relationship; therefore, if phosphorus levels rise too quickly, serum calcium levels will fall quickly)
  - Provide patient teaching as appropriate
    - Review of prescribed diabetic regimen (monitor patient's compliance)
    - Emphasis on importance of strictly complying with prescribed therapy; discuss diet, medications, exercise, monitoring techniques, hygiene and foot care, sick-day rules, and how to prevent and recognize hypoglycemia and hyperglycemia
    - Reinforcement of teaching: how blood glucose control affects long-term health

---

Key nursing interventions for a patient with DKA

- Monitor serum glucose and electrolyte levels, serum osmolality, and ABG results.
- Monitor vital signs.
- Monitor intake and output.
- Administer insulin as ordered.
- Provide I.V. rehydration.
- Administer electrolyte supplements as ordered.
- Provide patient teaching as appropriate.

HEART FAILURE

● General information

- Heart can't pump sufficient blood volume to meet body's metabolic demands
- Typically, left side first to fail
- Multiple steps in left-sided heart failure
  - Left ventricle: can't propel blood volume forward into aorta
  - Blood: backs up in pulmonary vascular bed, increases pulmonary capillary pressure; results in pulmonary venous congestion (see *How left-sided heart failure develops*)
  - Pulmonary circulation: engorged; rising capillary pressure pushes sodium and water into interstitial space, causes pulmonary edema
  - Right ventricle: stressed from pumping against greater pulmonary vascular resistance and left ventricular pressure
  - Commonly leads to, and is main cause of, right-sided heart failure
- Multiple steps in right-sided heart failure
  - Right ventricle: begins failure, symptoms worsen
  - Right ventricle: has difficulty propelling blood forward into pulmonary circulation; blood pooled in right ventricle and right atrium
  - Backed-up blood: causes pressure and congestion in venae cavae and systemic circulation (see *How right-sided heart failure develops*, page 200)

How left-sided heart failure develops

This illustration shows what happens when left-sided heart failure develops. The left side of the heart normally receives oxygenated blood returning from the lungs, and then pumps it through the aorta to all tissues. Left-sided heart failure causes blood to back up in the lungs, which results in such respiratory symptoms as tachypnea and shortness of breath.

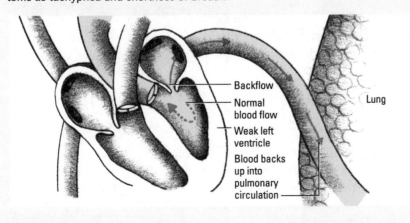

Backflow

Normal blood flow

Weak left ventricle

Blood backs up into pulmonary circulation

Lung

Key facts about heart failure

- Heart can't pump sufficient blood volume to meet body's metabolic demands

Left-sided

- Left ventricle: can't propel blood volume forward
- Pulmonary circulation: engorged; rising capillary pressure pushes sodium and water into interstitial space
- Commonly leads to right-sided heart failure

Right-sided

- Right ventricle: has difficulty propelling blood forward into pulmonary circulation
- Backed-up blood: causes pressure and congestion in venae cavae and systemic circulation
- Rising capillary pressure: forces excess fluid from capillaries into interstitial space; causes tissue edema

How right-sided heart failure develops

This illustration shows what happens when right-sided heart failure develops. The right side of the heart normally receives deoxygenated blood returning from the tissues and then pumps that blood through the pulmonary artery into the lungs. Right-sided heart failure causes blood to back up past the vena cava and into the systemic circulation. This, in turn, causes enlargement of the abdominal organs and tissue edema.

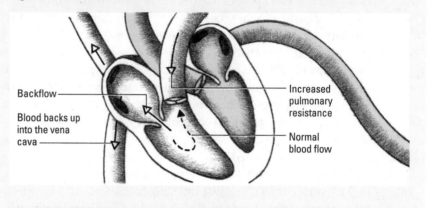

Backflow

Blood backs up into the vena cava

Increased pulmonary resistance

Normal blood flow

- Blood: distends visceral veins, especially hepatic vein; as liver and spleen become engorged, function is impaired
- Rising capillary pressure: forces excess fluid from capillaries into interstitial space; causes tissue edema, especially in lower extremities and abdomen
- Afflicted patients at risk for fluid-volume, electrolyte, and metabolic acid-base imbalances
- Imbalances: may result from heart's failure to pump and adequately perfuse tissues; from stimulation of renin-angiotensin-aldosterone mechanism; or from treatments such as diuretic administration

● **Causes**
- Conditions that directly damage the heart
  - Myocardial infarction (MI)
  - Myocarditis
  - Myocardial fibrosis
  - Ventricular aneurysm
- Conditions that cause ventricular overload
  - Aortic insufficiency
  - Ventricular septal defect
  - Systemic or pulmonary hypertension
  - Elevation in pressure against which the heart must pump
- Conditions that cause restricted ventricular diastolic filling
  - Constrictive pericarditis or cardiomyopathy
  - Tachyarrhythmias

Common causes of heart failure

- Conditions that directly damage the heart
- Conditions that cause ventricular overload
- Conditions that cause restricted ventricular diastolic filling
- Conditions that result in inadequate venous return
- Circulatory overload

– Cardiac tamponade
– Mitral or aortic stenosis
- Conditions that result in inadequate venous return
    – Chronic obstructive pulmonary disease (COPD)
    – Pulmonary hypertension
- Circulatory overload, such as in excessive vascular volume expansion

Pathophysiology

- Failing heart: can't generate enough energy to propel ventricular blood volume forward
- Blood backed up in system
- Fallen cardiac output and hydrostatic pressure in the vascular space; reflected in blood pressure drop
- Renin-angiotensin-aldosterone mechanism triggered by kidneys (sensitive to renal hypoperfusion state resulting from decreased cardiac output)
- Angiotensin II: produced from the conversion of renin and angiotensin I, acts directly on vessels to produce massive peripheral vasoconstriction; also stimulates release of aldosterone, which enhances sodium reabsorption at the nephron level
- Cardiac muscle: pumps against a vasoconstricted vessel, results in increased workload (increased afterload) and exacerbated failure
- Sodium reabsorption accompanied by water reabsorption; together cause increased vascular volume, compounding existing cardiac compromise

Potential imbalance: Hypervolemia

- Is the most common fluid imbalance associated with heart failure
- Results from the heart's failure to propel blood forward, consequent vascular pooling, and sodium and water reabsorption triggered by renin-angiotensin-aldosterone mechanism
- Commonly causes peripheral edema

Potential imbalance: Hypovolemia

- Is usually associated with overaggressive diuretic therapy
- Can be especially dangerous in elderly patients; causes confusion and hypotension

Potential imbalance: Hypokalemia

- Caused by prolonged diuretic use without adequate potassium replacement
- In patients taking digoxin (Lanoxin), potentiates digoxin toxicity
- Can lead to life-threatening arrhythmias

Potential imbalance: Hyperkalemia

- May be caused by use of potassium-sparing diuretic to treat heart failure
- Can also lead to life-threatening arrhythmias

Key pathophysiologic changes in heart failure

- Failing heart: can't propel ventricular blood volume forward
- Cardiac output falls and blood pressure drops
- Renin-angiotensin-aldosterone mechanism triggered by kidneys
- Cardiac muscle: pumps against a vasoconstricted vessel; results in increased workload and exacerbated failure
- Sodium reabsorption accompanied by water reabsorption: cause increased vascular volume

Key facts about potential imbalances due to heart failure

Hypervolemia
- Results from the heart's failure to propel blood forward, consequent vascular pooling, and sodium and water reabsorption triggered by renin-angiotensin-aldosterone mechanism

Hypovolemia
- Usually associated with overaggressive diuretic therapy

Hypokalemia
- Caused by prolonged diuretic use without adequate potassium replacement

Hyperkalemia
- Caused by use of potassium-sparing diuretic to treat heart failure

Hyponatremia
- May result from sodium loss because of diuretic abuse

Hypernatremia
- May occur if diuretic use produces more water loss than sodium loss

Hypochloremia
- May result from diuretic therapy

Hypomagnesemia
- May result from diuretic therapy

Metabolic acidosis
- Results from decreased cardiac output and poor systemic perfusion

Metabolic alkalosis
- May result from excessive diuretic use, leading to bicarbonate retention
- May also result from reduction in circulating blood volume

Respiratory acidosis
- Caused by CO_2 accumulation
- Impairs gas exchange

Common assessment findings in heart failure

Left-sided
- Fatigue
- Tachypnea
- Tachycardia
- Third and fourth heart sounds
- Crackles

Right-sided
- Jugular vein distention
- Edema and weight gain
- Enlarged and slightly tender liver

Potential imbalance: Hyponatremia
- May result from sodium loss because of diuretic abuse
- In some cases, may result from a dilutional effect that occurs when there's more water reabsorption than sodium reabsorption

Potential imbalance: Hypernatremia
- May occur if diuretic use produces more water loss than sodium loss
- Also may be linked to overactive renin mechanism that causes excessive sodium reabsorption

Potential imbalance: Hypochloremia
- May result from diuretic therapy
- Increased excretion of chloride in urine caused by loop and thiazide diuretics

Potential imbalance: Hypomagnesemia
- May accompany hypokalemia, particularly if patient is receiving a diuretic (many diuretics cause kidneys to excrete magnesium)
- May also result from diuretic therapy; loop and thiazide diuretics increase excretion of magnesium

Potential imbalance: Metabolic acidosis
- Results from decreased cardiac output and poor systemic perfusion
- Linked to excessive lactic acid production and renal failure from poorly perfused kidneys

Potential imbalance: Metabolic alkalosis
- May result from excessive diuretic use, leading to bicarbonate retention
- Also may result from reduction in effective circulating blood volume due to edema, which decreases kidney perfusion; in turn leads to enhanced hydrogen ion secretion and bicarbonate retention

Potential imbalance: Respiratory acidosis
- Progressed heart failure: further impairs gas exchange
- Caused by resulting carbon dioxide (CO_2) accumulation

Assessment findings
- Left-sided heart failure
  - Fatigue, weakness, orthopnea, and exertional dyspnea
  - Paroxysmal nocturnal dyspnea requiring two to three pillows to elevate head while sleeping
  - Tachypnea
  - Coughing; may produce pink, frothy sputum if pulmonary edema is present
  - Tachycardia
  - Third and fourth heart sounds possibly heard on auscultation
  - Restlessness, confusion, and progressive decrease in LOC
  - Crackles heard on auscultation (later stages)
  - Oliguria (later stages)

- Right-sided heart failure
  - Jugular vein distention
  - Edema and weight gain
  - Cyanotic nail beds
  - Anorexia, abdominal fullness, and nausea
  - Nocturia
  - Enlarged and slightly tender liver
  - Ascites
  - Jaundice

● **Diagnostic findings**
- Elevated serum levels of brain natriuretic peptide (strongly indicative of heart failure along with clinical signs such as edema)
- ECG
  - Arrhythmias
  - MI
  - Presence of coronary artery disease
- Chest X-rays
  - Cardiomegaly
  - Alveolar edema
  - Pleural effusion
  - Pulmonary edema
- Echocardiograms
  - Enlarged heart chambers
  - Changes in ventricular function
  - Presence of valvular disease
- Hemodynamic pressure readings
  - Increased central venous pressure
  - Increased pulmonary artery wedge pressure

● **Treatment**
- Treatment of underlying cause, if known
- Angiotensin-converting enzyme (ACE) inhibitor to reduce production of angiotensin II
- Digoxin to increase myocardial contractility, improve cardiac output, reduce the volume of the ventricle, and decrease ventricular stretch
- Diuretics to reduce fluid volume overload and venous return
- Beta-adrenergic blockers to promote peripheral vasodilation, thereby decreasing systemic pressure directly and cardiac workload indirectly
- Diuretics, nitrates, morphine (Duramorph), and oxygen to treat pulmonary edema
- Coronary artery bypass graft surgery or angioplasty for patients with heart failure due to coronary artery disease
- Heart transplantation in patients receiving aggressive medical treatment but still experiencing limitations or repeated hospitalizations
- Other surgery or invasive procedures
  - Cardiomyoplasty

Testing for heart failure

- Elevated serum levels of brain natriuretic peptide
- Arrhythmias
- Alveolar edema
- Pulmonary edema
- Enlarged heart chambers
- Increased central venous pressure
- Increased pulmonary artery wedge pressure

Key treatment options for heart failure

- Treatment of underlying cause
- ACE inhibitor
- Digoxin
- Diuretics
- Beta-adrenergic blockers
- Surgery or invasive procedure
- Lifestyle modifications

- Insertion of an intra-aortic balloon pump
- Partial left ventriculectomy
- Use of a mechanical ventricular assist device
- Implantation of an implantable cardioverter-defibrillator or a biventricular pacemaker
• Lifestyle modifications to reduce symptoms of heart failure
  - Weight loss (if obese)
  - Limited sodium (3 g/day) and alcohol intake
  - Reduced fat intake
  - Smoking cessation
  - Stress reduction
  - Development of an exercise program

Nursing interventions

• Monitor vital signs, including blood pressure, pulse, respirations, and breath sounds, for abnormalities that might indicate a fluid excess or deficit; report any changes immediately
• Maintain continuous cardiac monitoring during acute and advanced stages of disease to identify arrhythmias promptly
• Assess for signs and symptoms of impending cardiac failure, such as fatigue, restlessness, hypotension, rapid and thready pulse, decreased heart sounds, murmurs, gallop rhythms, rapid respirations, dyspnea, coughing, decreased urine output, and rapid liver enlargement
• Check weight and fluid intake and output daily for significant changes to detect fluid overload; if the patient gains 2 or more pounds over 24 hours, additional diuretic therapy may be needed
• Assess for the presence, amount, and location of edema; note the presence and degree of any pitting
• Assess the patient's mental status and report changes immediately
• Monitor serum electrolyte levels, especially sodium and potassium, for changes that may indicate an imbalance; remember that hypokalemia can lead to digoxin toxicity
• Monitor ABG results to assess the adequacy of ventilation
• Monitor sodium and fluid intake as ordered, because hyponatremia and fluid-volume deficit can stimulate the renin-angiotensin-aldosterone mechanism and exacerbate heart failure; usually, a mild sodium restriction—such as "no added salt"—with no water restriction is implemented
• Administer medications as ordered, such as digoxin, diuretics, ACE inhibitors, and potassium supplements, to support cardiac function and minimize symptoms
• Administer oral potassium supplements in orange juice or with meals to promote absorption and prevent gastric irritation
• Place the patient in Fowler's position and give supplemental oxygen as ordered to help him breathe more easily
• Encourage the patient to perform activities of daily living independently, as tolerated (bed rest may be required for some patients)

Key nursing interventions for a patient with heart failure

- Monitor vital signs.
- Provide continuous cardiac monitoring.
- Check weight and fluid intake and output daily.
- Assess for edema.
- Assess mental status.
- Monitor serum electrolyte levels.
- Monitor ABG results.
- Monitor sodium and fluid intake.
- Administer medications as ordered.
- Place the patient in Fowler's position.
- Give supplemental oxygen as ordered.
- Provide patient teaching as appropriate.

TIME-OUT FOR TEACHING

Patient teaching: Heart failure

When teaching a patient with heart failure, be sure to cover this information, and then evaluate the patient's learning:

- Teach the patient and his family about heart failure, including its causes and associated risks.
- Instruct the patient and his family to notify the staff of any changes in the patient's condition, such as increased shortness of breath, chest pain, or dizziness.
- Advise the patient to avoid foods high in sodium, such as canned or commercially prepared foods and dairy products, to curb fluid overload.
- Teach a patient taking a potassium-wasting diuretic to watch for and report symptoms of hypokalemia, such as weakness and excessive urine output.
- Explain to the patient that the potassium he loses through diuretic therapy may need to be replaced by taking a prescribed potassium supplement and eating foods high in potassium, such as bananas and apricots.
- Stress the importance of taking digoxin (Lanoxin) exactly as prescribed. Tell the patient to watch for and immediately report signs of toxicity, such as anorexia, vomiting, and yellow vision.
- Instruct the patient to call the physician if his pulse rate is irregular, if it measures fewer than 60 beats/minute, or if he experiences dizziness, blurred vision, shortness of breath, a persistent dry cough, palpitations, increased fatigue, nocturnal dyspnea that comes and goes, swollen ankles, or decreased urine output.

- Reposition the patient every 1 to 2 hours as needed (edematous skin is prone to breakdown)
- Provide patient teaching as appropriate (see *Patient teaching: Heart failure*)

HYPEROSMOLAR HYPERGLYCEMIC NONKETOTIC SYNDROME (HHNS)

General information
- Characterized by insulin deficiency in a patient with diabetes
- Is an acute condition
- Some insulin present, but not enough to metabolize glucose
- Characterized by hyperglycemia, hyperosmolarity, and osmotic diuresis; no ketosis and ketonuria present (see *Distinguishing between DKA and HHNS,* page 206)
- Associated imbalances: include fluid-volume and electrolyte imbalances that result primarily from osmotic diuresis

Causes
- Typically occurs in patients with type 2 diabetes; may also occur in other types of patients

Distinguishing between DKA and HHNS

Diabetic ketoacidosis (DKA) and hyperosmolar hyperglycemic nonketotic syndrome (HHNS) are two acute complications of diabetes. Use this decision tree to help distinguish between these two complications when assessing your patient.

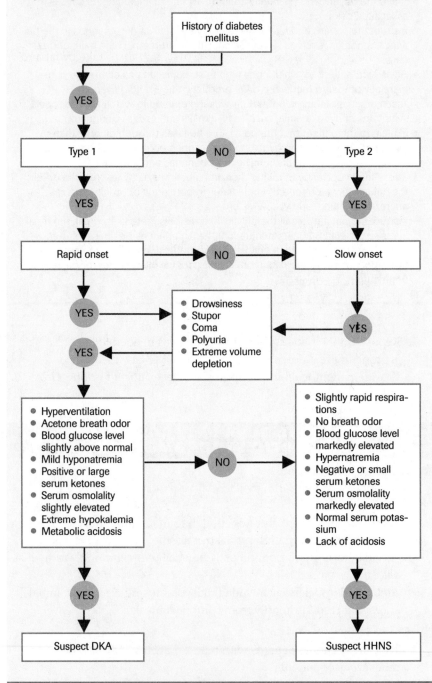

– Anyone whose insulin tolerance is strained (such as from illness, infection, or stress)
– Patients who have undergone certain therapeutic procedures
  · Peritoneal dialysis
  · Hemodialysis
  · Tube feedings
  · TPN

● **Pathophysiology**
  • Insulin present in sufficient amounts to prevent ketosis but in insufficient amounts to prevent hyperglycemia; glucose uptake by fat and muscle cells hindered by inadequate insulin
  • Liver: responds to demands of energy-starved cells by converting glycogen to glucose, releasing glucose into blood; further increases blood glucose level
  • Hyperglycemia: when exceeds renal threshold, excess glucose excreted in urine
  • Insulin-deprived cells: can't utilize glucose, respond by rapidly metabolizing protein
    – Results in loss of intracellular potassium and phosphorus
    – Also results in excessive liberation of amino acids
    – Liver: converts these amino acids into urea and glucose
  • Hyperglycemia: results from these processes, causes hyperosmolarity and osmotic diuresis
  • Massive fluid loss from osmotic diuresis: causes fluid and electrolyte imbalances and dehydration
  • Water loss: exceeds electrolyte loss, contributes to hyperosmolarity; in turn, perpetuates dehydration, decreases GFR, reduces amount of glucose excreted in urine

● **Potential imbalance: Hypovolemia**
  • Is related to osmotic diuresis
  • Electrolyte loss exceeded by water loss, resulting in hyperosmolarity

● **Potential imbalance: Hypokalemia**
  • Results from osmotic diuresis
  • May decrease further as fluid resuscitation initiates (dilutes serum concentrations) and insulin therapy starts (glucose pulls potassium into cells, further lowering serum levels)

● **Potential imbalance: Hypernatremia**
  • Results from proportionately greater water loss than sodium loss, causing hemoconcentration
  • Indicates severe fluid loss and dehydration

● **Assessment findings**
  • Severe dehydration
  • Hypotension and tachycardia
  • Diaphoresis
  • Tachypnea

Key pathophysiologic changes in HHNS

• Insulin present in sufficient amounts to prevent ketosis but in insufficient amounts to prevent hyperglycemia
• Liver: converts glycogen to glucose
• Insulin-deprived cells: can't utilize glucose, respond by rapidly metabolizing protein
• Hyperglycemia: causes hyperosmolarity and osmotic diuresis
• Massive fluid loss: causes fluid and electrolyte imbalances and dehydration

Key facts about potential imbalances due to HHNS

Hypovolemia
• Related to osmotic diuresis

Hypokalemia
• Results from osmotic diuresis
• Fluid resuscitation and insulin therapy: may decrease potassium levels

Hypernatremia
• Results from proportionately greater water loss than sodium loss, causing hemoconcentration

Common assessment findings in HHNS

• Severe dehydration
• Hypotension and tachycardia
• Tachypnea
• Polyuria, polydipsia, and polyphagia
• Rapid onset of lethargy

- Polyuria, polydipsia, and polyphagia
- Vision changes
- Rapid onset of lethargy
- Stupor and coma
- Neurologic changes

● **Diagnostic findings**
- Elevated serum glucose (may be as high as 800 to 2,000 mg/dl)
- Negative urine and serum ketone results (ketones are absent)
- Positive urine glucose levels
- Increased serum osmolality
- Elevated serum sodium level and normal serum potassium level
- Normal ABG results; no evidence of acidosis

● **Treatment**
- Isotonic or half-normal saline I.V. fluid administration to correct dehydration
- I.V. insulin to lower hyperglycemia
- Electrolyte replacement therapy to correct electrolyte imbalances

● **Nursing interventions**
- Assess the patient's LOC; most patients with HHNS experience some type of altered mental status, and about one-half of patients are comatose
- Monitor vital signs frequently; assess hemodynamic status and institute continuous cardiac monitoring to evaluate for possible arrhythmias secondary to electrolyte imbalances
- Assess hydration status for changes indicating imbalances by monitoring intake and output, daily weight, and skin turgor
- Monitor serum glucose and electrolyte levels, and serum osmolality for changes
- Administer I.V. fluid replacement therapy with isotonic or half-normal saline solution, typically giving one-half of the replacement (determined by the extent of fluid deficit) during the first 12 hours
  - Give the remainder of the replacement amount over the next 24 hours
  - Anticipate addition of dextrose to fluid replacement regimen when patient's blood glucose levels approach 250 mg/dl (to prevent hypoglycemia)
- Administer insulin as ordered, adjusting the dosage according to serum glucose levels; remember that blood glucose levels must be reduced gradually to prevent cerebral fluid shifting and subsequent cerebral edema
  - Less insulin usually needed to reduce the glucose level when compared with that required for DKA because the patient typically secretes some insulin and may be extremely sensitive to additional doses

---

Testing for HHNS
- Elevated serum glucose level
- Negative urine and serum ketone results
- Increased serum osmolality
- Normal ABG results

Key treatment options for HHNS
- I.V. fluid administration
- I.V. insulin
- Electrolyte replacement therapy

Key nursing interventions for a patient with HHNS
- Assess LOC.
- Monitor vital signs.
- Monitor serum glucose and electrolyte levels, and serum osmolality.
- Administer I.V. fluid replacement therapy.
- Administer insulin as ordered.
- Administer electrolyte replacement therapy as ordered.
- Provide patient teaching as appropriate.

- Evaluate renal function before administering potassium replacement; potassium can be added to the I.V. fluid or given as an oral supplement
- Be aware that severe hypophosphatemia may be treated with potassium phosphate; carefully monitor patients receiving potassium phosphate for hyperphosphatemia, especially a patient with diminished renal function
- Provide patient teaching as appropriate
  - Review of prescribed diabetic regimen; monitor patient compliance
  - Emphasis on importance of strict compliance with prescribed therapy; discuss diet, medications, exercise, monitoring techniques, hygiene and foot care, sick-day rules, and how to prevent and recognize hypoglycemia and hyperglycemia
  - Reinforcement of teaching: how blood glucose control affects long-term health

INTESTINAL OBSTRUCTION

- **General information**
  - Involves interference with the normal peristaltic movement of intestinal contents
  - May result from a physical barrier or from impairment of bowel innervation, resulting in inability to move digested food forward
  - Associated imbalances: fluid-volume and metabolic acid-base imbalances

- **Causes**
  - Small-bowel obstruction typically caused by adhesions and strangulated hernias; large-bowel obstruction typically caused by carcinomas
  - Mechanical intestinal obstruction resulting from foreign bodies (fruit pits, gallstones, or worms), or compression of bowel wall caused by one of several disorders
    - Stenosis
    - Intussusception
    - Volvulus of the sigmoid or cecum
    - Tumors
    - Atresia
  - Nonmechanical obstruction resulting from physiologic disturbances
    - Paralytic ileus
    - Electrolyte imbalances
    - Toxicity (uremia or generalized infection)
    - Neurogenic abnormalities (spinal cord lesions)
    - Thrombosis or embolism of mesenteric vessels

Key facts about intestinal obstruction

- Interference with the normal peristaltic movement of intestinal contents
- May result from a physical barrier or from impairment of bowel innervation

Common causes of intestinal obstruction

- Adhesions and strangulated hernias
- Carcinomas
- Mechanical obstruction resulting from foreign bodies
- Compression of bowel wall
- Nonmechanical obstruction resulting from physiologic disturbances

Key pathophysiologic changes in intestinal obstruction

- Partial or complete blockage of the lumen of the intestine
- Fluid, air, and gas collect near site
- Peristalsis temporarily increased
- Intestinal mucosa is injured
- Distention occurs
- Bowel secretes water, sodium, and potassium into fluid pooled in lumen

Key facts about potential imbalances due to intestinal obstruction

Hypovolemia
- Results from trapped fluid in the intestines, prolonged vomiting, excessive GI suctioning, or third space shifting

Metabolic acidosis
- Results from vomiting larger amounts of alkaline intestinal fluids than acidic gastric fluids

Metabolic alkalosis
- Upper intestine obstruction; may cause excessive vomiting of large amounts of gastric fluid

Respiratory acidosis
- Linked to marked abdominal distention; impairs respiratory excursion

Common assessment findings in intestinal obstruction

- Colicky pain
- Nausea and vomiting
- Constipation
- Abdominal distention
- Abdominal tenderness or pain

Pathophysiology
- Can be a partial or complete blockage of the lumen in the small or large bowel
- When occurs, fluid, air, and gas collect near site
- Peristalsis temporarily increased as bowel attempts to force contents through obstruction
  - Injures intestinal mucosa, causes distention at and above the obstruction site
  - Distention: blocks flow of venous blood and halts normal absorptive processes
  - Results: bowel secretes water, sodium, and potassium into fluid pooled in lumen; causes several disorders
    · Hypovolemia
    · Hyponatremia
    · Hypokalemia
    · Distention
    · Retention of enormous amounts of fluid in the gut
- Ultimately may lead to ischemia, necrosis, and death

Potential imbalance: Hypovolemia
- Results from trapped fluid in the intestines, prolonged vomiting, excessive GI suctioning, or third space shifting
- Volume loss: may be 5 L or more

Potential imbalance: Metabolic acidosis
- May result from vomiting larger amounts of alkaline intestinal fluids than acidic gastric fluids
- Vomiting: usually occurs from obstruction in the distal small intestines

Potential imbalance: Metabolic alkalosis
- Rare occurrence
- Upper intestine obstruction: may cause excessive vomiting of large amounts of gastric fluid
- Can result from consequent dehydration and loss of gastric hydrochloric acid

Potential imbalance: Respiratory acidosis
- Is usually linked to marked abdominal distention
- Distention: increases pressure on diaphragm and impairs respiratory excursion

Assessment findings
- Colicky pain
- Nausea and vomiting
- Constipation
- Abdominal distention (may be severe in large-bowel obstruction)
- Abdominal tenderness

- Leakage of liquid stools around the obstruction (common in partial obstruction)
- Fecal vomiting and continuous pain (complete obstruction)

● **Diagnostic findings**

- Abdominal films (small-bowel obstruction): show typical "stepladder pattern," with alternating fluid and gas levels apparent in 3 to 4 hours
- Barium enema (large-bowel obstruction): reveals distended, air-filled colon or closed loop of sigmoid with extreme distention (in sigmoid volvulus)
- Decreased sodium, chloride, and potassium levels (due to vomiting)
- Slightly elevated white blood cell (WBC) count (with necrosis, peritonitis, or strangulation)
- Increased serum amylase level (possibly from irritation of pancreas by bowel loop)

● **Treatment**

- Preoperative therapy
  - Correction of fluid and electrolyte imbalances
  - Decompression of the bowel to relieve vomiting and distention
  - Treatment of shock and peritonitis
- Blood replacement and I.V. fluid administration usually needed for strangulated obstruction
- Passage of NG tube, followed by use of longer and weighted Miller-Abbott or Cantor tube; usually accomplishes decompression, especially in small-bowel obstruction
- Close monitoring of patient's condition to determine duration of treatment; surgery necessary if patient fails to improve or if his condition deteriorates
- Large-bowel obstruction: decompression with an NG tube commonly followed by surgical resection with anastomosis, colostomy, or ileostomy
- TPN for patient with protein deficit from chronic obstruction, surgery, paralytic ileus, or infection
- Drug therapy, including an analgesic, sedative, and antibiotic for peritonitis due to bowel strangulation or infarction

● **Nursing interventions**

- Administer I.V. isotonic or hypotonic solutions (usually lactated Ringer's solution or dextrose 5% in water) to replace fluid losses; administer at the prescribed rate to prevent overload
- Remember that isotonic normal saline solution may be used if gastric fluid loss is excessive
- Administer sodium, potassium, and chloride replacements based on the patient's serum electrolyte levels; monitor these levels closely to prevent imbalances

Testing for intestinal obstruction

- Abdominal films: typical "stepladder pattern"
- Barium enema: distended, air-filled colon

Key treatment options for intestinal obstruction

- Correction of fluid and electrolyte imbalances
- Decompression of the bowel
- Surgical resection
- TPN
- Drug therapy

Key nursing interventions for a patient with intestinal obstruction

- Administer I.V. solutions and electrolyte replacements.
- Monitor intake and output and daily weight.
- Monitor vital signs.
- Assess bowel sounds and stool quantity and character.
- Prepare for possible surgical intervention.

- Provide patient teaching as appropriate.

- Assess hydration status by monitoring intake and output, daily weight, and skin turgor
- Monitor vital signs, especially pulse rate and blood pressure, to detect changes indicating fluid imbalance
- Evaluate the need for TPN or alternate feeding methods to maintain or restore nutritional status
- Assess the presence and character of bowel sounds and stool quantity and character to detect resolution of the obstruction
- Monitor GI suction for amount and character of drainage
- Keep the patient in semi-Fowler's position as much as possible to promote pulmonary ventilation and ease respiratory distress from abdominal distention
- Prepare the patient for possible surgical intervention
- Provide patient teaching as appropriate
  - Encourage ambulation, activity to help promote return of peristalsis (during recovery period and postoperatively)
  - Arrange patient consult with enterostomal therapist (for patients requiring surgery and ostomy)

PANCREATITIS

● **General information**
- Nonbacterial inflammation of the pancreas
- Occurs in acute and chronic disease forms; may result in edema, necrosis, or hemorrhage

● **Causes**
- Abnormal organ structure
- Alcoholism
- Biliary tract disease
- Blunt trauma or surgical trauma
- Drugs
  - Glucocorticoids
  - Sulfonamides
  - Thiazides
  - Hormonal contraceptives
  - Nonsteroidal anti-inflammatory drugs (NSAIDs)
- Endoscopic examination of the bile ducts and pancreas
- Kidney failure or transplantation
- Metabolic or endocrine disorders
  - High cholesterol levels
  - Overactive thyroid
- Pancreatic cysts or tumors
- Penetrating peptic ulcers

● **Pathophysiology**
- Pancreatitis: involves autodigestion

Key facts about pancreatitis

- Nonbacterial inflammation of the pancreas
- Acute and chronic disease forms

Common causes of pancreatitis

- Alcoholism
- Biliary tract disease
- Trauma
- Drugs
- Pancreatic cysts or tumors

- Pancreatic tissue digested by enzymes normally excreted by the pancreas; leads to peripancreatic edema and fluid loss from blood into retroperitoneal tissue
- Digestive enzymes released from inflamed pancreas: can cause a peritoneal burn that, when severe, can equal a burn covering up to one-half of the body's surface; this causes fluid to shift from the ECF

Potential imbalance: Hypovolemia
- Occurs because fluid shifts from ECF to retroperitoneal space and peritoneal cavity
- Also contributed to by fluid loss from vomiting or NG suctioning

Potential imbalance: Hypocalcemia
- May be related to hypoalbuminemia associated with protein-rich fluid leaking into peritoneal cavity
- Ionized calcium decreased, but exact cause unknown

Potential imbalance: Hypomagnesemia
- Has been attributed to deposition of magnesium ions in the inflamed tissue
- Thought to be related to hypoalbuminemia
- Magnesium: also directly lost by vomiting, gastric suctioning, diarrhea, and diuretic use

Potential imbalance: Hypophosphatemia
- May occur in patients experiencing respiratory alkalosis
- Other possible causes
  - Increased catecholamine production
  - Alteration in circulating insulin or glucose
  - I.V. administration of glucose

Potential imbalance: Metabolic alkalosis
- May result from frequent vomiting
- Development contributed to by gastric suctioning used to rest the pancreas

Potential imbalance: Metabolic acidosis
- May occur from poor tissue perfusion
- Also may result from complications of acute renal failure

Potential imbalance: Respiratory acidosis
- May occur from respiratory complications associated with pancreatitis
- Severe pain: may interfere with patient's ability to breathe deeply and expand lungs adequately
- Pancreatic enzymes: released into circulation, damage pulmonary vessels; stimulate inflammation; cause alveolocapillary leakage—results in intrapulmonary shunting, hypoxemia and, possibly, pleural effusion

Potential imbalance: Respiratory alkalosis
- May occur from respiratory complications associated with pancreatitis
- May be caused by severe pain may that stimulates ventilation

---

Key pathophysiologic changes in pancreatitis

- Pancreatic tissue digested by enzymes normally excreted by the pancreas
- Digestive enzymes released from inflamed pancreas: can cause a peritoneal burn, causing fluid to shift from the ECF

Key facts about potential imbalances due to pancreatitis

Hypovolemia
- Fluid shifts from ECF to retroperitoneal space and peritoneal cavity
- May also result from excessive vomiting or NG suctioning

Hypocalcemia
- Related to hypoalbuminemia associated with protein-rich fluid leaking into peritoneal cavity

Hypomagnesemia
- Attributed to deposition of magnesium ions in the inflamed tissue

Hypophosphatemia
- May result from respiratory alkalosis

Metabolic alkalosis
- May result from frequent vomiting or gastric suctioning

Metabolic acidosis
- May occur from poor tissue perfusion

Respiratory acidosis
- Pancreatic enzymes cause alveolocapillary leakage that results in intrapulmonary shunting, hypoxemia and, possibly, pleural effusion

Respiratory alkalosis
- May occur from respiratory complications associated with pancreatitis

Common assessment findings in pancreatitis

- Midepigastric pain
- Tachycardia
- Restlessness
- Persistent vomiting

Testing for pancreatitis

- Serum amylase and lipase levels elevated
- CT scan and abdominal ultrasound: enlarged pancreas with cysts and pseudocysts

Key treatment options for pancreatitis

- I.V. replacement of fluids, protein, and electrolytes
- Withholding of food and oral fluids
- NG tube suctioning
- Antiemetics and analgesics
- Insulin
- Surgical drainage
- Laparotomy

Assessment findings

- Midepigastric pain, which can radiate to the back
- Mottled skin
- Tachycardia
- Low-grade fever
- Cold, sweaty extremities
- Restlessness
- Extreme malaise
- Several findings in severe attacks
  - Persistent vomiting
  - Abdominal distention
  - Diminished bowel activity
  - Crackles at lung bases
  - Left pleural effusion

Diagnostic findings

- Serum amylase and lipase levels elevated; confirm diagnosis
- Blood and urine glucose tests: reveal transient glucose in urine and hyperglycemia
- WBC count elevated
- Serum bilirubin level elevated
- Serum calcium level: may be decreased
- Stool analysis: shows elevated lipid and trypsin levels
- Abdominal and chest X-rays: detect pleural effusions and differentiate pancreatitis from diseases that cause similar symptoms; may detect pancreatic calculi
- CT scanning and abdominal ultrasonography: show enlarged pancreas with cysts and pseudocysts
- Endoscopic retrograde cholangiopancreatography: identifies ductal system abnormalities, such as calcification or strictures; helps to differentiate pancreatitis from other disorders, such as pancreatic cancer

Treatment

- I.V. replacement of fluids, protein, and electrolytes to treat shock
- Fluid-volume replacement to help correct metabolic acidosis
- Blood transfusions to replace blood loss from hemorrhage
- Withholding of food and oral fluids to rest the pancreas and reduce pancreatic enzyme secretion
- NG tube suctioning to decrease stomach distention and suppress pancreatic secretions
- Antiemetic to alleviate nausea and vomiting
- Morphine to relieve abdominal pain
- Antacid to neutralize gastric secretions
- Histamine antagonist to decrease hydrochloric acid production
- Antibiotic to fight bacterial infections
- Anticholinergic to reduce vagal stimulation, decrease GI motility, and inhibit pancreatic enzyme secretion

- Insulin to correct hyperglycemia
- Surgical drainage to treat a pancreatic abscess or pseudocyst or to reestablish drainage of the pancreas
- Laparotomy (if biliary tract obstruction causes acute pancreatitis) to remove obstruction

● **Nursing interventions**
- Assess the patient's level of pain and administer analgesics as ordered
- Assess pulmonary status frequently to detect signs of respiratory complications early
- Monitor intake and output, daily weight, and laboratory studies
- Evaluate the patient's metabolic and nutritional status, and monitor for signs of electrolyte imbalances
- Maintain an NG tube for drainage or suction
- Keep airway and suction apparatus available in case hypocalcemia develops
- Place the patient in a comfortable position that allows for maximal chest expansion
- If allowed, encourage the patient to drink plenty of fluids; administer I.V. fluids as ordered
- Be alert for signs and symptoms of fluid overload; patients with acute pancreatitis commonly receive large amounts of fluid replacement therapy
- When allowed, provide a diet high in carbohydrates, low in proteins, and low in fat
- Provide patient teaching as appropriate
  - Explain disorder, signs and symptoms, possible treatments
  - Stress need to avoid factors that precipitate acute pancreatitis, especially alcohol use

RESPIRATORY FAILURE

● **General information**
- Lungs: major regulator of fluid, electrolyte, acid-base balance; can't maintain adequate gas exchange in respiratory failure
- Patients with respiratory insufficiency at risk for fluid volume, electrolyte, and acid-base imbalances
- Imbalances: result from ventilatory impairment (leads to excessive CO_2 retention or elimination, or to excessive fluid loss through lungs)

● **Causes**
- Hypoxemia secondary to increased pulmonary capillary pressure or permeability
  - Left-sided heart failure
  - Pneumonia
- Conditions impairing normal CO_2 elimination
  - COPD

Key nursing interventions for a patient with pancreatitis

- Assess level of pain; administer analgesics.
- Assess pulmonary status.
- Monitor intake and output, daily weight, and laboratory studies.
- Maintain an NG tube.
- Administer I.V. fluids as ordered.
- Provide patient teaching as appropriate.

Key facts about respiratory failure

- Lungs can't maintain adequate gas exchange in respiratory failure
- Leads to excessive CO_2 retention or elimination, or to excessive fluid loss through lungs

Common causes of respiratory failure

Brain
- Anesthesia
- Drug overdose
- Head trauma

Lungs
- Acute respiratory distress syndrome
- COPD
- Massive bilateral pneumonia
- Obstruction

Muscles and nerves
- Amyotrophic lateral sclerosis
- Multiple sclerosis
- Spinal cord trauma

Pulmonary circulation
- Heart failure
- Pulmonary edema
- Pulmonary embolism

Key pathophysiologic changes in respiratory failure

Gas exchange diminished by any combination of three factors:
- Alveolar hypoventilation
- $\dot{V}/\dot{Q}$ mismatch
- Intrapulmonary shunting

Causes of respiratory failure

Problems with the brain, lungs, muscles, and nerves, or problems with pulmonary circulation can impair gas exchange and cause respiratory failure. This chart lists conditions that can cause respiratory failure.

BRAIN
- Anesthesia
- Cerebral hemorrhage
- Cerebral tumor
- Drug overdose
- Head trauma
- Skull fracture

LUNGS
- Acute respiratory distress syndrome
- Asthma
- Chronic obstructive pulmonary disease
- Cystic fibrosis
- Flail chest
- Massive bilateral pneumonia
- Sleep apnea
- Tracheal obstruction

MUSCLES AND NERVES
- Amyotrophic lateral sclerosis
- Guillain-Barré syndrome
- Multiple sclerosis
- Muscular dystrophy
- Myasthenia gravis
- Polio
- Spinal cord trauma

PULMONARY CIRCULATION
- Heart failure
- Pulmonary edema
- Pulmonary embolism

  - Asthmatic crisis
- Neuromuscular impairment of the respiratory drive; can result from various causes
  - Drug overdoses
  - Spinal cord injury
  - Multiple sclerosis
  - Myasthenia gravis (see *Causes of respiratory failure*)

● **Pathophysiology**
- In patients with respiratory failure, gas exchange diminished by any combination of three factors
  - Alveolar hypoventilation
  - Ventilation-perfusion ($\dot{V}/\dot{Q}$) mismatch
  - Intrapulmonary shunting (see *How acute respiratory failure develops*)
- Inadequate oxygenation: results in hypoxemia, leading to hypocapnia and an increased respiratory rate
- Increased respiratory rate: leads to increased insensible fluid loss through lungs and excessive elimination of CO_2
- Insufficient respiratory center stimulation: results in hypercapnia, leading to hypoxemia
- Airway obstruction: results in CO_2 retention and hypercapnia, limiting amount of CO_2 eliminated by the lungs; respiratory rate may be normal or increased

How acute respiratory failure develops

Three major malfunctions account for impaired gas exchange and subsequent acute respiratory failure: alveolar hypoventilation, ventilation-perfusion ($\dot{V}/\dot{Q}$) mismatch, and intrapulmonary (right-to-left) shunting.

ALVEOLAR HYPOVENTILATION

In alveolar hypoventilation, shown here as the result of airway obstruction, the amount of oxygen brought to the alveoli is diminished, causing a drop in the partial pressure of arterial oxygen and an increase in alveolar carbon dioxide (CO_2). The accumulation of CO_2 in the alveoli prevents diffusion of adequate amounts of CO_2 from the capillaries, which increases the partial pressure of arterial carbon dioxide.

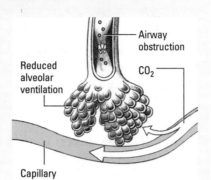

$\dot{V}/\dot{Q}$ MISMATCH

$\dot{V}/\dot{Q}$ mismatch, the leading cause of hypoxemia, occurs when insufficient ventilation exists with a normal flow of blood, or when, as shown, normal ventilation exists with an insufficient flow of blood.

INTRAPULMONARY SHUNTING

Intrapulmonary shunting occurs when blood passes from the right side of the heart to the left side without being oxygenated, as shown. Shunting can result from untreated ventilation or perfusion mismatches.

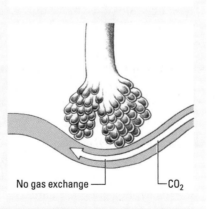

Development of acute respiratory failure

From alveolar hypoventilation
- Oxygen to alveoli diminished
- Partial pressure of arterial oxygen dropped and alveolar CO_2 increased
- CO_2: accumulates in alveoli, prevents diffusion of CO_2 from capillaries

From $\dot{V}/\dot{Q}$ mismatch
- Occurs when insufficient ventilation exists with normal blood flow, or when normal ventilation exists with insufficient blood flow

From intrapulmonary shunting
- Blood: passes from right to left side of heart without oxygen
- Can result from untreated $\dot{V}/\dot{Q}$ mismatches

● **Potential imbalance: Respiratory acidosis**
  - Due to hypoventilation; results from the lungs' inability to eliminate adequate amounts of CO_2
  - Excessive CO_2: combines with water (H_2O) to form carbonic acid (H_2CO_3)

Key facts about potential imbalances due to respiratory failure

Respiratory acidosis
- Results from the lungs' inability to eliminate adequate amounts of CO_2

Respiratory alkalosis
- Results from too-rapid respirations or from hyperventilation, causing excessive CO_2 elimination

Metabolic acidosis
- Hypoxia induces cells to use anaerobic metabolism

Hypervolemia
- Excessive fluid absorption possibly caused by increased pulmonary capillary pressure or permeability

Hypovolemia
- Excessive water loss caused by fever or any condition that increases metabolic rate and, thus, respiratory rate

Hyperkalemia
- Potassium ions: move out of cells and into blood to balance positive charges between the two fluid compartments

Hypokalemia
- Results from hyperventilation

Common assessment findings in respiratory failure

- Cyanosis
- Tachypnea and tachycardia
- Cold, clammy, ashen skin
- Diminished breath sounds
- Agitation

- Increased carbonic acid levels: result in decreased pH, contribute to imbalance

● **Potential imbalance: Respiratory alkalosis**
- Results from too-rapid respirations or from hyperventilation, causing excessive CO_2 elimination
- CO_2 loss: decreases serum's acid-forming potential, results in imbalance

● **Potential imbalance: Metabolic acidosis**
- Hypoxia caused by various conditions; induces cells to use anaerobic metabolism
- Increased lactic acid production caused by anaerobic metabolism; can lead to imbalance

● **Potential imbalance: Hypervolemia**
- Prolonged respiratory treatment (as with nebulizers): can lead to inhalation of water vapor and its absorption through lung tissue
- Excessive fluid absorption possibly caused by increased pulmonary capillary pressure or permeability
- Pulmonary edema possibly precipitated by this excessive fluid absorption

● **Potential imbalance: Hypovolemia**
- Water as vapor normally eliminated from lungs during respiration
- Excessive water loss caused by fever or any condition that increases metabolic rate and, thus, respiratory rate

● **Potential imbalance: Hyperkalemia**
- Excess hydrogen ions: move into cells during acidosis
- Potassium ions: move out of cells and into blood to balance positive charges between the two fluid compartments; this imbalance may result

● **Potential imbalance: Hypokalemia**
- Alkalosis possibly results from patient hyperventilation
- Hydrogen: moves out of cells and potassium ions move from blood into cells; shift can cause this imbalance

● **Assessment findings**
- Nasal flaring and use of accessory muscles of respiration to breathe
- Cyanosis of the oral mucosa, lips, and nail beds
- Tachypnea and tachycardia
- Strong and rapid pulse initially, progressing to thready and irregular in later stages
- Cold, clammy, ashen skin and frank diaphoresis, especially around the forehead and face
- Diminished breath sounds on auscultation; adventitious breath sounds (such as wheezes, rhonchi, or crackles) may be heard
- Agitation that may progress to confusion and disorientation

Diagnostic findings
- ABG analysis: indicates respiratory failure
- Chest X-rays: identify an underlying pulmonary disease or condition
- ECG changes: may show arrhythmias
- Pulse oximetry: reveals decreasing arterial oxygen saturation
- Blood cultures: may aid in identifying pathogens
- Serum potassium level: may be high or low depending on acid-base balance

Treatment
- Oxygen therapy to promote oxygenation and raise partial pressure of arterial oxygen level
- Bidirectional positive-pressure airway mask over the oronasal region, or mechanical ventilation with an endotracheal or a tracheostomy tube if needed, to provide adequate oxygenation and reverse acidosis
- High-frequency ventilation, if patient doesn't respond to treatment, to force airways open, promoting oxygenation and preventing alveoli collapse
- Antibiotic to treat infection
- Bronchodilator to maintain airway patency
- Corticosteroid to decrease inflammation
- Fluid restrictions to reduce volume and cardiac workload
- Diuretic to reduce edema and fluid overload
- Deep breathing with pursed lips, if patient isn't intubated, to help keep airway patent
- Incentive spirometry to increase lung volume

Nursing interventions
- Monitor ABG levels to assess oxygenation and pH status
- Assess lung status; monitor rate, depth, and character of respirations, being sure to check breath sounds for abnormalities
- Monitor vital signs frequently; evaluate ECG results for arrhythmias; monitor oxygen saturation values with a pulse oximeter
- Monitor the patient's neurologic status; it may become depressed as respiratory failure worsens
- Perform ongoing respiratory assessment by monitoring accessory muscle use, changes in breath sounds, ABG analysis, secretion production and clearance, and respiratory rate, depth, and pattern; notify the physician if interventions don't improve the patient's condition
- Monitor fluid status by maintaining accurate fluid intake and output records; obtain daily weights
- Evaluate serum electrolyte levels for abnormalities that can occur with acid-base imbalances
- Intervene to correct the underlying respiratory problem and associated alterations in acid-base status, as needed
- Keep a handheld resuscitation bag at the patient's bedside

Testing for respiratory failure
- ABG analysis: respiratory failure
- Chest X-rays: pulmonary disease or condition
- ECG changes: possible arrhythmias
- Pulse oximetry: decreasing arterial oxygen saturation

Key treatment options for respiratory failure
- Oxygen therapy
- Bronchodilator
- Fluid restrictions
- Diuretics, antibiotics, or corticosteroids

Key nursing interventions for a patient with respiratory failure

- Monitor ABG levels.
- Assess lung status.
- Monitor vital signs.
- Monitor neurologic status.
- Monitor fluid status.
- Monitor electrolyte levels.
- Administer oxygen.
- Perform chest physiotherapy and postural drainage.
- Provide patient teaching as appropriate.

- Maintain patent I.V. access as ordered for medication and I.V. fluid administration
- Administer oxygen as ordered to help maintain adequate oxygenation and restore the normal respiratory rate
- Administer oxygen to the patient with COPD cautiously because adequate serum oxygen levels depress the stimulus for breathing
- Perform chest physiotherapy and postural drainage as needed to promote adequate ventilation
- Encourage slow, deep breaths with pursed lips if the patient is retaining CO_2; urge him to cough up secretions; if he can't mobilize secretions, suction him when necessary
- Increase the patient's fluid intake to 2 qt (2 L)/day to help liquefy secretions (unless he's retaining fluid or has heart failure)
- Position the patient for optimum lung expansion; as tolerated, sit the conscious patient upright in a supported, forward-leaning position to promote diaphragm movement, and supply an overbed table and pillows for support
- If the patient isn't on a ventilator, avoid giving him an opioid analgesic or another CNS depressant because either may further suppress respirations
- Limit carbohydrate intake and increase protein intake, because carbohydrate metabolism causes more CO_2 production than protein metabolism
- Calm and reassure the patient while providing care, because anxiety can increase oxygen demands
- Pace care activities to maximize the patient's energy level and provide needed rest; limit his need to respond verbally because talking may cause shortness of breath
- Implement safety measures as needed to protect the patient; reorient him if he's confused
- Provide patient (and family) teaching as appropriate
  - How to recognize signs and symptoms of overexertion, fluid retention, and heart failure
    - Weight gain of 2 to 3 lb [0.9 to 1.4 kg]/day
    - Edema of the feet or ankles
    - Nausea
    - Loss of appetite
    - Shortness of breath
    - Abdominal tenderness
  - Developing knowledge and skills needed to perform pulmonary hygiene
  - Need for adequate hydration to thin secretions, while watching for and reporting signs of fluid retention or heart failure

SYNDROME OF INAPPROPRIATE ANTIDIURETIC HORMONE (SIADH)

General information
- Characterized by inappropriate secretion of ADH triggered by stimuli other than increased ECF osmolality and decreased ECF volume
- May result from various disorders
  - Head trauma (including neurosurgery)
  - Cancers
  - CNS disorders
  - Pulmonary disorders
  - Endocrine disorders
  - Use of certain medications, such as osmotic diuretics
- Associated imbalances: fluid-volume and electrolyte imbalances

Causes
- Most common: oat cell carcinoma of the lung
- Other neoplastic diseases
  - Pancreatic and prostate cancer
  - Hodgkin's disease
  - Thymoma (tumor on the thymus)
  - Renal carcinoma
- CNS disorders
  - Brain tumor or abscess
  - Stroke
  - Head injury
  - Guillain-Barré syndrome
- Drugs that either increase ADH production or potentiate ADH action
  - Antidepressants
  - NSAIDs
  - Chlorpropamide
  - Vincristine (Oncovin)
  - Cyclophosphamide (Cytoxan)
  - Carbamazepine (Tegretol)
  - Clofibrate (Atromid-S)
  - Metoclopramide (Reglan)
  - Morphine
- Pulmonary disorders
  - Pneumonia
  - Tuberculosis
  - Lung abscess
  - Aspergillosis
  - Bronchiectasis
  - Positive-pressure ventilation
- Miscellaneous conditions
  - Psychosis
  - Myxedema

Key facts about SIADH
- Characterized by inappropriate secretion of ADH triggered by stimuli other than increased ECF osmolality and decreased ECF volume
- May result from various disorders

Common causes of SIADH
- Oat cell carcinoma of the lung
- Neoplastic diseases
- CNS disorders
- Drugs
- Pulmonary disorders
- Miscellaneous conditions

Key pathophysiologic changes in SIADH

- Prolonged ADH secretion: results in water retention, which leads to serum hypo-osmolality
- Water reabsorption in tubules increased, resulting in increased intravascular fluid volume
- Intravascular fluid volume increased, inhibits release of renin and aldosterone; results in further urine sodium losses

Key facts about potential imbalances due to SIADH

Hypervolemia
- Tubular reabsorption of water increased because of continued ADH secretion

Hyponatremia
- Occurs as a result of excessive water retention and aldosterone inhibition

Common assessment findings in SIADH

- Thirst, anorexia, fatigue, and lethargy
- Weight gain, edema, water retention, and decreased urine output
- Neurologic signs and symptoms

Testing for SIADH

- Serum osmolality less than 280 mOsm/kg of water
- Hyponatremia
- Elevated urinary Na level and osmolality
- Elevated serum ADH level

- AIDS
- Physiologic stress
- Pain

● **Pathophysiology**
- ADH secretion continuous and inappropriate
- Prolonged ADH secretion: results in water retention, which leads to serum hypo-osmolality
- Urine osmolality greater than serum osmolality
- Water reabsorption in tubules increased, resulting in increased intravascular fluid volume
- GFR increased, inhibiting reabsorption of sodium and water
- Intravascular fluid volume increased, inhibits release of renin and aldosterone; results in further urine sodium losses (see *What happens in SIADH*)

● **Potential imbalance: Hypervolemia**
- Tubular reabsorption of water increased because of continued ADH secretion
- Water retained, leading to increased intravascular fluid volume

● **Potential imbalance: Hyponatremia**
- Occurs as a result of excessive water retention and aldosterone inhibition
- Decreased aldosterone secretion: results in further urine sodium losses

● **Assessment findings**
- Thirst, anorexia, fatigue, and lethargy (earliest signs and symptoms), followed by vomiting and intestinal cramping
- Weight gain, edema, water retention, and decreased urine output
- Neurologic signs and symptoms
  - Restlessness
  - Confusion
  - Headache
  - Irritability
  - Decreasing reflexes
  - Seizures
  - Coma

● **Diagnostic findings**
- Serum osmolality less than 280 mOsm/kg of water
- Hyponatremia (serum Na level less than 135 mEq/L); lower values indicate worsening condition
- Elevated urinary Na level (more than 20 mEq/L) and increased osmolarity (greater than 150 mOsm/L)
- Elevated serum ADH level
- Normal BUN level
- Urine osmolality elevated

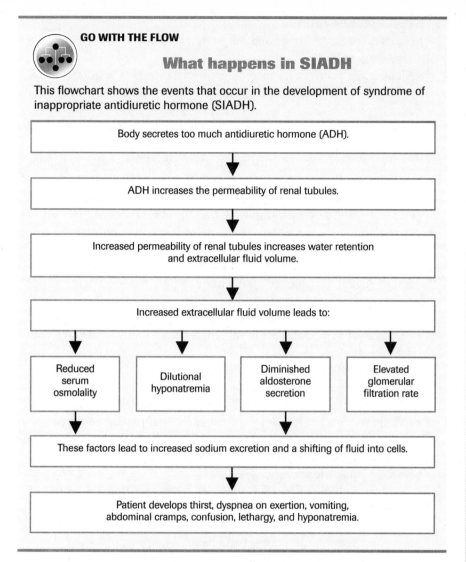

GO WITH THE FLOW

What happens in SIADH

This flowchart shows the events that occur in the development of syndrome of inappropriate antidiuretic hormone (SIADH).

Body secretes too much antidiuretic hormone (ADH).

↓

ADH increases the permeability of renal tubules.

↓

Increased permeability of renal tubules increases water retention and extracellular fluid volume.

↓

Increased extracellular fluid volume leads to:

| Reduced serum osmolality | Dilutional hyponatremia | Diminished aldosterone secretion | Elevated glomerular filtration rate |

↓

These factors lead to increased sodium excretion and a shifting of fluid into cells.

↓

Patient develops thirst, dyspnea on exertion, vomiting, abdominal cramps, confusion, lethargy, and hyponatremia.

● Treatment
- Restricted water intake (16 to 32 oz [480 to 960 ml]/day) as symptomatic treatment
- Administration of 200 to 300 ml of 3% saline solution to slowly and steadily increase serum sodium level (severe water intoxication); if too rapid a rise, cerebral edema may result
- Correction of underlying cause of SIADH, when possible
- Surgical resection, irradiation, or chemotherapy to alleviate water retention for SIADH resulting from cancer
- Demeclocycline (Declomycin) to block renal response to ADH (if fluid restriction is ineffective)
- Furosemide (Lasix) with normal or hypertonic saline to maintain urine output and block ADH secretion

Key treatment options for SIADH

- Restricted water intake
- Administration of 3% saline solution
- Correction of underlying cause

Key nursing interventions for a patient with SIADH

- Maintain accurate intake and output records.
- Monitor daily weight.
- Monitor serum sodium levels.
- Administer I.V. hypertonic saline solution.
- Restrict fluids as ordered
- Provide patient teaching as appropriate.

● **Nursing interventions**

- Maintain accurate intake and output records; monitor for fluid intake exceeding output
- Monitor daily weight for increases; correlate weights with fluid gains or losses; a 1-lb (0.5-kg) weight gain is equal to 500 ml of fluid
- Monitor serum sodium levels for abnormalities, and assess for signs and symptoms of hyponatremia; monitor serum and urine osmolarity for changes
   - Severe hyponatremia: expect to administer I.V. hypertonic saline solution to replace sodium
   - Use a volume-control device (to prevent overload)
- Expect to administer a diuretic (usually Lasix or mannitol [Osmitrol]) concomitantly with I.V. hypertonic saline solution to promote water excretion
- Depending on urine output, restrict daily fluid intake to approximately 500 to 700 ml; consider all intake routes when imposing fluid restrictions
- Intervene as appropriate to treat the underlying cause of SIADH
- Institute safety precautions to minimize risk of injury in patients with sensory changes
- Be aware that the doctor may order lithium or Dilantin as possible therapy; keep in mind that demeclocycline also may be used to decrease the renal response to ADH, thereby promoting fluid excretion
- Elevate the head of the bed approximately 10 to 20 degrees to promote venous return; remember that decreased venous return is a stimulus for ADH release
- Provide patient teaching as appropriate
   - Need for fluid restrictions (ways to decrease patient's discomfort from thirst)
   - Self-monitoring techniques for fluid retention, including measurement of intake and output and daily weight
   - Signs and symptoms that require immediate medical intervention

NCLEX CHECKS

It's never too soon to begin your NCLEX preparation. Now that you've reviewed this chapter, carefully read each of the following questions and choose the best answer. Then compare your responses to the correct answers.

1. A client with chronic kidney disease who is in kidney failure (stage 5) would have a GFR of:
   ☐ **1.** less than 15 ml/minute.
   ☐ **2.** 15 to 29 ml/minute.
   ☐ **3.** 30 to 59 ml/minute.
   ☐ **4.** 60 to 89 ml/minute.

2. A client with kidney failure has developed hypocalcemia. For which other electrolyte imbalance should the nurse monitor the client because of its association with hypocalcemia?

□ **1.** Hypermagnesemia
□ **2.** Hyponatremia
□ **3.** Hyperphosphatemia
□ **4.** Hypophosphatemia

3. In respiratory failure, the client's lungs can't eliminate sufficient quantities of CO_2, placing the client at risk for developing which acid-base imbalance?

□ **1.** Metabolic acidosis
□ **2.** Metabolic alkalosis
□ **3.** Respiratory acidosis
□ **4.** Respiratory alkalosis

4. During the fluid-accumulation phase of a burn injury, which condition can the nurse expect?

□ **1.** Hypovolemia
□ **2.** Hypervolemia
□ **3.** Hypokalemia
□ **4.** Increased urine output

5. Using the Parkland formula for determining fluid replacement in clients with burns, calculate the 24-hour fluid replacement volume for a client who weighs 56 kg and has 30% BSA burns. How many milliliters of fluid should be given over 24 hours? _____

6. What's the most common fluid imbalance associated with heart failure?

□ **1.** Hypovolemia
□ **2.** Hypervolemia
□ **3.** Third-space fluid shift
□ **4.** Osmotic diuresis

7. What type of breathing should be encouraged for a client with CO_2 retention?

□ **1.** Slow, deep breathing with pursed lips
□ **2.** Breathing into cupped hands
□ **3.** Rapid, shallow breathing
□ **4.** Breathing into a paper bag

8. Which drug may be administered to treat conditions of acidosis?

□ **1.** Mannitol
□ **2.** Lasix
□ **3.** Epinephrine
□ **4.** Sodium bicarbonate

TOP 10

Items to study for your next test on conditions associated with imbalances

1. Pathophysiology and regulatory systems for each imbalance condition

2. Nursing assessments and treatments for each condition

3. Correlation of phases of acute renal failure to specific diagnostic results

4. Comparing and contrasting acute renal failure and chronic kidney disease to various imbalances

5. Correlation of heart failure to fluid, electrolyte, and acid-base imbalances

6. Treatment for each imbalance correlated to heart failure

7. Correlation of respiratory failure to each type of imbalance

8. Each phase of burn management in relation to fluid, electrolyte, and acid-base imbalances and their related treatments

9. Relationship of AIDS, cirrhosis, diabetes insipidus, DKA, HHNS, intestinal obstruction, pancreatitis, and SIADH to different types of imbalances

10. Drugs used to restore balances in fluid, electrolyte, and acid-base imbalances

9. Which clinical finding is characteristic of diabetes insipidus?
- ☐ **1.** Increased urine output with highly concentrated urine
- ☐ **2.** Decreased urine output with highly dilute urine
- ☐ **3.** Increased urine output with highly dilute urine
- ☐ **4.** Plasma hypo-osmolality

10. Which electrolyte imbalance is the most common adverse effect of diuretic use?
- ☐ **1.** Hyperkalemia
- ☐ **2.** Hypokalemia
- ☐ **3.** Hypernatremia
- ☐ **4.** Hyponatremia

ANSWERS AND RATIONALES

1. CORRECT ANSWER: 1
A client with chronic renal failure and a GFR less than 10 ml/minute is in the stage known as *end-stage renal disease.*

2. CORRECT ANSWER: 3
Because calcium and phosphorus have an inverse relationship, the client with hypocalcemia may also have developed hyperphosphatemia.

3. CORRECT ANSWER: 3
When the pulmonary system can't rid the body of adequate amounts of CO_2, serum levels of CO_2 will increase and pH will decrease, resulting in respiratory acidosis.

4. CORRECT ANSWER: 1
During the fluid-accumulation phase, fluid shifts from the vascular compartment to the interstitial space, causing hypovolemia. Hypervolemia, hypokalemia, and increased urine output are associated with the fluid-remobilization phase.

5. CORRECT ANSWER: 6720
The client should receive 4 ml of lactated Ringer's solution per kilogram of body weight per percentage of BSA burned over a period of 24 hours. As it applies to this particular client: 4 ml $\times$ 56 kg $\times$ 30 = 6,720 ml of fluid over 24 hours.

6. CORRECT ANSWER: 2
Hypervolemia results from the heart's failure to propel blood forward, which causes vascular pooling. Hypervolemia commonly causes the peripheral edema associated with a third-space fluid shift.

7. CORRECT ANSWER: 1
To promote ventilation and aid in the elimination of CO_2, the client should be encouraged to take slow, deep breaths.

8. CORRECT ANSWER: 4

Sodium bicarbonate, an alkalinizing agent, is used to manage conditions of acidosis by neutralizing the hydrogen ion concentration and raising blood pH.

9. CORRECT ANSWER: 3

In diabetes insipidus, the absence of ADH allows for large quantities of dilute fluids to be excreted in the urine. This process leaves behind hyperosmolar plasma.

10. CORRECT ANSWER: 2

Hypokalemia is the most common, and most serious, electrolyte imbalance associated with the use of diuretics.

9

Fluid and electrolyte replacement therapy

LEARNING OBJECTIVES

After studying this chapter, you should be able to:

● Identify administration routes used for fluid and electrolyte replacement therapies.

● List examples of isotonic, hypotonic, and hypertonic I.V. solutions.

● Discuss nursing interventions for patients receiving nasogastric tube feedings, I.V. fluid replacement therapy, and blood and blood products.

CHAPTER OVERVIEW

Fluid and electrolyte replacement therapy aims to restore and maintain homeostasis. It may be administered via the oral, nasogastric, or I.V. route. Depending on the type of imbalance, therapy may include the use of water, crystalloids, enteral and parenteral nutrition supplements, colloids, and blood and blood products. Nursing care focuses on measures to correct the fluid or electrolyte losses, meet the patient's daily fluid and electrolyte needs, prevent new imbalances from occurring, and preserve renal function.

I.V. delivery methods

The choice of I.V. delivery methods is based on the purpose of the therapy and its duration; the patient's diagnosis, age, and health history; and the condition of the patient's veins. I.V. solutions can be delivered through a peripheral or a central vein.

PERIPHERAL LINES

Peripheral I.V. therapy is administered for short-term or intermittent therapy through a vein in the arm, hand, leg, or foot. Potential I.V. sites include the metacarpal, cephalic, basilic, median cubital, and greater saphenous veins. Using veins in the leg or foot is unusual because of the risk of thrombophlebitis. However, veins in the foot are commonly used in neonates and infants.

CENTRAL LINES

Central venous therapy involves administering solutions through a catheter placed in a central vein, typically the subclavian or internal jugular vein; less commonly, the femoral vein. This type of I.V. therapy is used for patients who have inadequate peripheral veins, need long-term I.V. access, need access for blood sampling, require a large volume of fluid, need a hypertonic solution or caustic medication, or need a high-calorie nutritional supplement.

INTRODUCTION

- **Description**
  - Aimed at restoring and maintaining homeostasis
  - Methods: include oral and gastric feedings, and parenteral therapy
  - Choice of therapy affected by several factors
    - Type and severity of imbalance
    - Patient's overall health status and age, renal and cardiovascular status
    - Usual maintenance requirements

- **Administration routes**
  - Oral route: oral ingestion of fluids and electrolytes as liquids or solids administered directly into GI tract
  - Nasogastric (NG) route: instillation of fluids and electrolytes through feeding tubes, such as NG, gastrostomy, and jejunostomy tubes
  - I.V. route: administration of fluids and electrolytes directly into bloodstream using continuous infusion, bolus, or I.V. push injection through peripheral or central venous site (see *I.V. delivery methods*)

- **Categories of replacement fluids**
  - Categorized by concentration (tonicity)
  - Usually prepared in isotonic, hypotonic, and hypertonic concentrations (see *Comparing fluid tonicity,* page 230)
  - Isotonic solutions
    - Same osmolality as plasma (approximately 275 to 295 mOsm/kg)

Key facts about fluid and electrolyte replacement therapy

- Aimed at restoring and maintaining homeostasis
- Includes oral and gastric feedings, and parenteral therapy

Administration routes for fluid and electrolyte replacement therapy

- Oral route: ingestion of fluids and electrolytes directly into GI tract
- NG route: instillation of fluids and electrolytes through feeding tubes
- I.V. route: administration of fluids and electrolytes directly into bloodstream

Categories of replacement fluids

Isotonic solutions
- Same osmolality as plasma
- Examples: D_5W, normal saline solution, Ringer's solution, lactated Ringer's solution

Hypotonic solutions
- Lower osmolality than plasma
- Examples: 0.45% NaCl, 0.33% NaCl

Hypertonic solutions
- Higher osmolality than plasma
- Examples: whole blood, albumin, TPN, concentrated dextrose solution (10% and greater), fat emulsions, elemental oral diets, tube feedings

These illustrations show the effects of different types of I.V. fluids on fluid movement and cell size.

ISOTONIC

Isotonic fluids, such as normal saline solution, have a concentration of dissolved particles, or tonicity, equal to that of intracellular fluid (ICF). Therefore, osmotic pressure is the same inside and outside the cells, so they neither shrink nor swell with fluid movement.

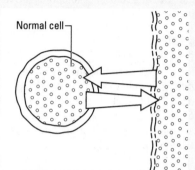

Normal cell

Key facts about fluid tonicity

Isotonic
- Concentration of dissolved particles equal to that of ICF
- Cells neither shrink nor swell with fluid movement

Hypertonic
- Has a tonicity greater than that of ICF
- Draws water out of the cells and into the more highly concentrated ECF

Hypotonic
- Has a tonicity less than that of ICF
- Osmotic pressure draws water into the cells from the ECF

HYPERTONIC

Hypertonic fluid has a tonicity greater than that of ICF, so osmotic pressure is unequal inside and outside the cells. Dehydration or rapidly infused hypertonic fluids, such as 3% saline or 50% dextrose, draws water out of the cells and into the more highly concentrated extracellular fluid (ECF).

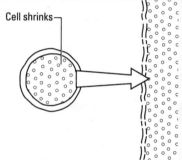

Cell shrinks

HYPOTONIC

Hypotonic fluids, such as half-normal saline solution, have a tonicity less than that of ICF, so osmotic pressure draws water into the cells from the ECF. Severe electrolyte losses or inappropriate use of I.V. fluids can make body fluids hypotonic.

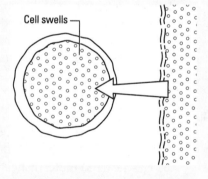

Cell swells

- Vascular space osmolality not altered by infusion
- Expand intracellular and extracellular spaces equally; degree of expansion correlates with amount of fluid infused
- No solution-related shifting between intracellular fluid (ICF) and extracellular fluid (ECF) spaces
- Examples: dextrose 5% in water (D_5W), normal saline solution, Ringer's solution, lactated Ringer's solution
- Hypotonic solutions

- Lower osmolality than plasma (usually less than 275 mOsm/kg)
- Hypo-osmolality possible with infusion because solutions have a lower concentration of electrolytes than plasma does
- Transcend all membranes from vascular space to tissue to cell
- Examples: 0.45% sodium chloride (NaCl), 0.33% NaCl
- Hypertonic solutions
  - Higher osmolality than plasma (usually greater than 295 mOsm/kg)
  - Infusion: can significantly raise plasma osmolality
  - Can cause vascular volume expansion and ICF deficit
  - Complications possible with excessive administration
    - Excessive vascular volume
    - Potential for pulmonary edema and heart failure
  - Examples: whole blood, albumin, total parenteral nutrition (TPN), concentrated dextrose solution (10% and greater), fat emulsions, elemental oral diets, tube feedings

● **Nursing interventions: oral fluid and electrolyte replacement therapy**
- Work with the physician to calculate the patient's daily fluid requirements
- Use a standard chart to calculate the patient's total body surface area (BSA) and accurately determine fluid needs
- Administer 1,500 ml of water for each square meter of BSA to meet the patient's daily fluid needs
- Increase the amount of fluid replacement to 2,400 ml/m^2 of BSA for moderate fluid losses, and to 3,000 ml/m^2 for severe fluid losses
- Position the patient in semi-Fowler's or high Fowler's position to ensure safe ingestion of fluids and to avoid aspiration
- Prepare foods and fluids as necessary, such as mixing replacement fluid with table foods, and provide portions compatible with the patient's appetite
- Check the temperature of oral fluids before administration to prevent oral mucosa burns and to promote ingestion
- Provide a relaxed, pleasant environment to enhance the patient's appetite and promote compliance with therapy
- Maintain accurate fluid intake and output records
- Obtain the patient's daily weight, and correlate any weight gain or loss with the 24-hour total on the fluid intake and output record
- Assess the effectiveness of fluid replacement therapy by monitoring urine output, serum sodium levels, blood urea nitrogen (BUN) levels, and serum osmolality
- Provide patient teaching as appropriate
  - Guidelines with goals for total daily fluid volumes the patient should try to meet
  - Instructions for monitoring intake and output

Key nursing interventions for a patient receiving oral replacement therapy
- Administer fluid replacement.
- Position the patient in semi-Fowler's or high Fowler's position to avoid aspiration.
- Maintain accurate fluid intake and output records.
- Obtain daily weight.
- Monitor serum sodium levels, BUN levels, and serum osmolality.
- Provide patient teaching as appropriate.

Key tube feeding problems

- Aspiration of gastric secretions
- Tube obstruction
- Oral, nasal, or pharyngeal irritation or necrosis
- Vomiting, bloating, diarrhea, or cramps
- Constipation
- Electrolyte imbalance
- Hyperglycemia

Managing tube feeding problems

COMPLICATION	NURSING INTERVENTIONS
Aspiration of gastric secretions	• Discontinue feeding immediately. • Perform tracheal suction of aspirated contents if possible. • Notify the physician; prophylactic antibiotics and chest physiotherapy may be ordered. • Check tube placement before feeding to prevent complication.
Tube obstruction	• Flush the tube with warm water; if necessary, replace the tube. • Flush the tube with 50 ml of water after each feeding to remove excess sticky formula, which could occlude the tube.
Oral, nasal, or pharyngeal irritation or necrosis	• Provide frequent oral hygiene using mouthwash or sponge-tipped mouth swabs; use petroleum jelly on cracked lips. • Change the tube's position; if necessary, replace the tube.
Vomiting, bloating, diarrhea, or cramps	• Reduce the flow rate. • Administer metoclopramide (Reglan) to increase GI motility. • Warm the formula to prevent GI distress. • For 30 minutes after feeding, position the patient on his right side with his head elevated to facilitate gastric emptying. • Notify the physician; he may want to reduce the amount of formula being given during each feeding.
Constipation	• Provide additional fluids if the patient can tolerate them. • Administer a bulk-forming laxative. • Increase fruit, vegetable, or sugar content of the feeding.
Electrolyte imbalance	• Monitor serum electrolyte levels; administer supplements. • Notify the physician; he may want to adjust the formula content to correct the deficiency.
Hyperglycemia	• Monitor blood glucose levels and notify the physician of elevated levels; he may adjust the sugar content of the formula. • Administer insulin if ordered.

Key nursing interventions for a patient receiving NG tube feedings

- Position the patient in semi-Fowler's or high Fowler's position to prevent aspiration.
- Check NG tube placement.
- Check for retention of formula.
- Administer adequate amounts of water.
- Provide patient teaching as appropriate.

● Nursing interventions: NG tube feedings

- Constitute tube feedings as ordered, or use preconstituted liquid tube feedings to prevent administration of hypertonic fluids
- Position the patient in semi-Fowler's or high Fowler's position to prevent aspiration by gastroesophageal reflux, and to promote digestion
- For intubated patients, inflate the endotracheal tube cuff during feedings
- Check NG tube placement, according to institutional policy, before administering feedings
  – No tube feeding until proper placement of NG tube verified in patient's stomach; administering feeding through misplaced tube can cause formula to enter lungs
  – Safest way to verify placement: with X-ray or by checking pH of aspirated gastric fluid (should be 4 or less)
  – Verifying tube placement not necessary for gastric and jejunostomy tubes (surgically positioned)
- Check for retention of formula by withdrawing aspirant

TIME-OUT FOR TEACHING

Patient teaching: Enteral tube feedings

When teaching a patient about enteral tube feedings, be sure to cover this information; then evaluate your patient's learning.

- Inform the patient that he'll receive nourishment through tube feedings. Tell him why the tube feedings are necessary and explain the tube-insertion procedure.
- Teach the patient about the type of formula he'll be receiving. If intermittent feedings are ordered, provide the patient with a schedule of feeding times.
- Tell the patient about signs and symptoms of adverse reactions and which ones to report, including vomiting, abdominal cramping or distention, diarrhea, and constipation.
- If the patient will need to administer enteral tube feedings at home, cover the following teaching topics with the patient and a family member:
  - How and where to obtain needed equipment
  - How to insert the tube and verify tube placement
  - How to prepare and store formula
  - How to administer formula through the tube
  - How to recognize and report adverse reactions such as vomiting, abdominal cramping or distention, diarrhea, and constipation
  - How to care for all supplies
  - How to troubleshoot problems with the tube or feeding equipment.

Key patient teaching topics for enteral tube feedings

- Nourishment through tube feedings
- Types of formula
- Schedule of feeding times
- Signs and symptoms of adverse reactions
- Administering enteral tube feedings at home

  - Retention indicated by volume greater than 160 ml
  - Aspiration not recommended for patient with temporary feeding tube (such as a Flexiflo tube); may cause tube to collapse
- Make sure feedings are at room temperature to prevent abdominal cramping on administration (see *Managing tube feeding problems*)
- Wean the patient gradually onto hypertonic tube feeding; start with small, diluted amounts (approximately 50 to 60 ml per feeding) in an effort to prevent diarrhea; isotonic tube feedings may be started at full strength
- Stop the feeding immediately if the patient becomes nauseated or vomits; vomiting may occur if the stomach becomes distended from overfeeding or delayed gastric emptying
- After administering the feeding, leave the patient in semi-Fowler's or high Fowler's position for at least 30 minutes to prevent aspiration
- Administer adequate amounts of water via the feeding tube or parenteral route when necessary to meet total fluid needs
- Consider using a mechanical feeding pump for continuous infusion to prevent possible fluid overload
- Always use clean equipment and technique; this is especially important for gastrostomy and jejunostomy tubes, which carry a high infection risk because they enter the peritoneum
- Provide patient teaching as appropriate (see *Patient teaching: Enteral tube feedings*)

Key nursing interventions for a patient receiving parenteral replacement therapy

- Follow standard precautions.
- Label and time-tape the bottle or bag.
- Calculate and adjust the flow rate as ordered.
- Measure intake and output.
- Assess the compatibility of all medications with the type of fluid being administered.
- Provide patient teaching.

● **Nursing interventions: parenteral fluid and electrolyte replacement therapy**

- Assess veins, degree of limb mobility, and type of fluid ordered for infusion to determine the optimal site for parenteral line placement
- Follow standard precautions and use appropriate equipment for each specific purpose; for example, a butterfly needle for temporary infusions and an I.V. catheter for long-term therapy or for infusing irritating solutions or medications
- Label and time-tape the bottle or bag to ensure that the proper administration rate is used
- Apply a dressing at the insertion site after stabilizing the needle with tape to prevent infection
- Calculate and adjust the flow rate as ordered to prevent fluid overload
- Monitor daily weights to document fluid retention or loss; a 2.2 lb (1 kg) change corresponds to 1 qt (1 L) of fluid gained or lost
- Measure intake and output carefully at scheduled intervals
- Change dressings and I.V. tubing according to institutional protocol; assess the insertion site for redness, tenderness, and swelling (see *Complications of I.V. therapy*)
- Use caution when infusing hypotonic solutions because they cause fluid to move from the extracellular space into cells, causing the cells to swell; this fluid shift can cause cardiovascular collapse from vascular fluid depletion, and increased intracranial pressure from fluid shifting into brain cells
- Use caution when infusing hypertonic solutions because rapid infusion can precipitate heart failure (use of an infusion pump is recommended)
- Administer protein infusions after 3 to 4 days of carbohydrate infusion; the daily protein requirement is 1 g/kg of body weight for adults, and 1 to 2 g/kg of body weight for children
- Assess the compatibility of all medications with the type of fluid being administered to prevent complications; for example, phenytoin (Dilantin) is incompatible with dextrose 5% in water (D_5W)
- Note the pH of the I.V. solutions, which can alter the effect and stability of medications mixed in the I.V. bag; consult the manufacturer's package insert, a drug handbook or formulary, or a pharmacist if you have questions
- Consider vitamin administration after 3 days of parenteral therapy to prevent possible vitamin deficiencies
- Provide patient teaching, especially if he'll be discharged home on parenteral therapy
    - What to expect before, during, and after the I.V. insertion procedure
    - Signs and symptoms of complications and when to report them
    - Any activity or diet restrictions
    - Proper care of the I.V. line

(Text continues on page 240.)

Complications of I.V. therapy

COMPLICATIONS	SIGNS AND SYMPTOMS	POSSIBLE CAUSES	INTERVENTIONS
Local complications			
Phlebitis	• Tenderness at the tip of and above the venipuncture device • Redness at the tip of the catheter and along the vein • Puffy area over the vein • Vein hard on palpation • Possible fever	• Poor blood flow around the venipuncture device • Tip of the catheter located next to the vessel wall • Friction from movement of the catheter in the vein • Venipuncture device left in the vein too long • Clotting at the catheter tip (thrombophlebitis) • Drug or solution with a high or low pH, or high osmolarity	• Remove the venipuncture device. • Apply warm soaks. Elevate the extremity if edema is present. • Notify the physician; document the patient's condition and your interventions. ***Prevention*** • Restart the infusion, preferably in the other arm, using a larger vein for an irritating solution, or restart with a smaller-gauge device to ensure adequate blood flow. • Tape the device securely to prevent motion.
Extravasation	• Swelling at and above the I.V. site (may extend along the entire limb) • Discomfort, burning, or pain at the site (but may be painless) • Tight feeling at the site • Decreased skin temperature around the site • Blanching at the site • Continuing fluid infusion even when the vein is occluded (although the rate may decrease)	• Venipuncture device dislodged from the vein or perforated vein • Vesicant in the tissue	• Remove the venipuncture device; notify the physician and follow facility policy. • Monitor the patient's pulse and capillary refill time. • Restart the infusion in another limb. • Document the patient's condition and your interventions. ***Prevention*** • Check the site often. • Don't obscure the area above the site with tape. • Teach the patient to observe the I.V. site and advise him to report pain or swelling.
Catheter dislodgment	• Catheter partially backed out of the vein • Solution infiltrating the tissue	• Loosened tape or tubing snagged in the bed linens, resulting in partial retraction of the catheter • Catheter pulled out by a confused patient	• Remove the I.V. catheter. ***Prevention*** • Tape the venipuncture device securely on insertion. *(continued)*

Key complications of I.V. therapy

Local
• Phlebitis
• Extravasation
• Catheter dislodgment
• Occlusion
• Vein irritation or pain at the I.V. site
• Severed catheter
• Hematoma
• Venous spasm
• Vasovagal reaction
• Thrombosis
• Thrombophlebitis
• Nerve, tendon, or ligament damage

Complications of I.V. therapy *(continued)*

COMPLICATIONS	SIGNS AND SYMPTOMS	POSSIBLE CAUSES	INTERVENTIONS
Local complications *(continued)*			
Occlusion	• I.V. fluid that doesn't flow	• I.V. flow interrupted • Saline lock not flushed • Backflow of blood in the line when the patient walks • Line clamped too long	• Use a mild flush injection; don't force it (if you're unsuccessful, reinsert the I.V. line). ***Prevention*** • Maintain the I.V. flow rate. • Flush the line soon after intermittent piggyback administration. • Have the patient walk with his arm folded to his chest to reduce the risk of blood backflow.
Vein irritation or pain at the I.V. site	• Pain during infusion • Possible blanching if vasospasm occurs • Red skin over the vein during infusion • Rapidly developing signs of phlebitis	• Solution with a high or low pH, or high osmolarity, such as 40 mEq/L of potassium chloride (KCl), phenytoin (Dilantin), and some antibiotics (erythromycin [Erythrocin], nafcillin, and vancomycin [Vancocin])	• Decrease the flow rate. • Try using an electronic flow device to achieve a steady flow. • Change the I.V. site. ***Prevention*** • Dilute the solutions before administration; for example, give antibiotics in a 250-ml solution rather than a 100-ml solution. • If long-term therapy with an irritating drug is planned, ask the physician to use a central I.V. line.
Severed catheter	• Leakage from the catheter shaft	• Catheter inadvertently cut by scissors • Reinsertion of the needle into the catheter	• If a broken part is visible, attempt to retrieve it (if you're unsuccessful, notify the physician). • If a portion of the catheter enters the bloodstream, place a tourniquet above the I.V. site to prevent progression of the broken part. Immediately notify the physician and the radiology department. • Document the patient's condition and your interventions. ***Prevention*** • Don't use scissors around the I.V. site. • Never reinsert a needle into the catheter. • Remove an unsuccessfully inserted catheter and needle together.

Complications of I.V. therapy *(continued)*

COMPLICATIONS	SIGNS AND SYMPTOMS	POSSIBLE CAUSES	INTERVENTIONS
Local complications *(continued)*			
Hematoma	• Tenderness at the venipuncture site • Bruised area around the site	• Vein punctured through the opposite wall at the time of insertion • Leakage of blood into the tissue	• Remove the venipuncture device and restart the infusion in the opposite limb. • Apply pressure and cold compresses to the affected area. • Recheck the site for bleeding. • Document the patient's condition and your interventions. ***Prevention*** • Choose a vein that can accommodate the size of the venipuncture device. • Release the tourniquet as soon as a successful insertion is achieved.
Venous spasm	• Pain along the vein • Sluggish flow rate when the clamp is completely open • Blanched skin over the vein	• Severe vein irritation as a result of irritating drugs or fluids • Administration of cold fluids or blood products • Very rapid flow rate (with fluids at room temperature)	• Apply warm soaks over the vein and surrounding area. • Decrease the flow rate. ***Prevention*** • Use a blood warmer for blood or packed red blood cells.
Vasovagal reaction	• Sudden collapse of the vein during venipuncture • Sudden pallor, sweating, faintness, dizziness, and nausea • Decreased blood pressure	• Vasospasm as a result of anxiety or pain	• Lower the head of the bed. • Have the patient take deep breaths. • Check the patient's vital signs. ***Prevention*** • To relieve the patient's anxiety, prepare him for the procedure. • Use a local anesthetic to prevent pain.
Thrombosis	• Painful, reddened, and swollen vein • Sluggish or stopped I.V. flow	• Injury to the endothelial cells of the vein wall, allowing platelets to adhere and thrombi to form	• Remove the venipuncture device, then restart the infusion in the opposite limb, if possible; notify the physician. • Apply warm soaks. • Watch for an I.V. therapy–related infection. ***Prevention*** • Use proper venipuncture techniques to reduce injury to the vein.

(continued)

Key complications of I.V. therapy

Systemic
- Circulatory overload
- Systemic infection (septicemia or bacteremia)
- Speed shock
- Air embolism
- Allergic reaction

Complications of I.V. therapy *(continued)*

COMPLICATIONS	SIGNS AND SYMPTOMS	POSSIBLE CAUSES	INTERVENTIONS
Local complications *(continued)*			
Thrombophlebitis	• Severe discomfort at the site • Reddened, swollen, and hardened vein	• Thrombosis and inflammation	• Follow the interventions for thrombosis; notify the physician. ***Prevention*** • Check the site frequently; remove the venipuncture device at the first sign of redness and tenderness.
Nerve, tendon, or ligament damage	• Extreme pain (similar to electric shock when the nerve is punctured), numbness, and muscle contraction • Delayed effects, including paralysis, numbness, and deformity	• Improper venipuncture technique, resulting in injury to the surrounding nerves, tendons, or ligaments • Tight taping or improper splinting with an arm board	• Stop the procedure. ***Prevention*** • Don't repeatedly penetrate tissues with the venipuncture device. • Don't apply excessive pressure when taping. Don't encircle the limb with tape. • Pad the arm boards and the tape securing the arm boards, if possible.
Systemic complications			
Circulatory overload	• Discomfort • Jugular vein distention • Respiratory distress • Increased blood pressure • Crackles • Increased difference between fluid intake and output	• Roller clamp loosened to allow run-on infusion • Flow rate too rapid • Miscalculation of fluid requirements	• Raise the head of the bed. • Administer oxygen if needed. • Reduce the infusion rate to a keep-vein-open rate and notify the physician. • Give drugs as ordered. ***Prevention*** • Use a pump, controller, or rate-minder for an elderly or compromised patient. • Recheck calculations of the patient's fluid requirements. • Monitor the infusion frequently.

Complications of I.V. therapy *(continued)*

COMPLICATIONS	SIGNS AND SYMPTOMS	POSSIBLE CAUSES	INTERVENTIONS
Systemic complications *(continued)*			
Systemic infection (septicemia or bacteremia)	• Fever, chills, and malaise for no apparent reason • Contaminated I.V. site, usually with no visible signs of infection at the site	• Failure to maintain sterile technique during insertion or site care • Severe phlebitis, causing organism growth • Poor taping that permits the venipuncture device to move, introducing organisms into the bloodstream • Prolonged indwelling time • Compromised immune system	• Notify the physician. • Administer medications, as prescribed. • Culture the site and the device. • Monitor the patient's vital signs. ***Prevention*** • Use scrupulous sterile technique when handling solutions and tubing, inserting a venipuncture device, and discontinuing the infusion. • Secure all connections. • Change the I.V. solutions, tubing, and venipuncture device at the recommended times.
Speed shock	• Flushed face, headache • Tightness in the chest • Irregular pulse • Syncope • Rapid hypertension • Shock • Cardiac arrest	• Too rapid injection of drug, causing plasma levels to become toxic • Improper administration of a bolus infusion (especially additives)	• Discontinue the infusion. • Begin an infusion of dextrose 5% in water at a keep-vein-open rate. • Notify the physician. ***Prevention*** • Check the infusion guidelines before giving a drug. • Dilute the drug with a compatible solution.
Air embolism	• Respiratory distress • Unequal breath sounds • Chest pain, dyspnea • Anxiety • Weak, rapid pulse • Increased central venous pressure • Decreased blood pressure • Altered consciousness	• Solution container empty • Tubing disconnected	• Discontinue the infusion. • Place the patient in left lateral Trendelenburg's position to allow air to enter the right atrium and disperse through the pulmonary artery. • Administer oxygen. • Notify the physician. • Document the patient's condition and your interventions. ***Prevention*** • Purge the tubing of air completely before starting an infusion. • Use the air-detection device on the pump or an air-eliminating filter proximal to the I.V. site. • Secure all connections.

(continued)

Key facts about water

- Most ingested directly orally
- Ingested indirectly through consumption of fruits, vegetables, and meats

Key uses of water

- Replace pure water losses
- Increase intravascular fluid volume

Administration routes for water

- Oral
- NG

Key nursing interventions for a patient receiving water

- Monitor intake and output.
- Follow the same nursing interventions as for NG tube feedings.

Complications of I.V. therapy *(continued)*

COMPLICATIONS	SIGNS AND SYMPTOMS	POSSIBLE CAUSES	INTERVENTIONS
Systemic complications *(continued)*			
Allergic reaction	• Itching • Watery eyes and nose • Broncho-spasm • Wheezing • Urticarial rash • Anaphylactic reaction, which may occur within minutes (flushing, chills, anxiety, agitation, itching, palpitations, paresthesia, throbbing in the ears, wheezing, coughing, seizures, cardiac arrest)	• Allergens such as medications	• If a reaction occurs, stop the infusion immediately. • Maintain a patent airway. • Notify the physician. • Administer an antihistaminic corticosteroid and antipyretic as ordered. • Give 0.2 to 0.5 ml of 1:1,000 aqueous epinephrine (Adrenalin) subcutaneously as ordered; repeat at 3-minute intervals and as needed. ***Prevention*** • Obtain the patient's allergy history; look for cross-allergies. • Assist with test dosing. • Monitor the patient carefully during the first 15 minutes of administering of a new drug.

WATER

General information
- Most ingested orally and directly
- Also can be ingested indirectly through consumption of fruits, vegetables, and meats
- NG replacement sometimes used if the patient is unable to consume fluids or foods orally

Uses
- To replace pure water losses
- To increase intravascular fluid volume

Administration routes
- Oral
- NG

Nursing interventions
- Keep in mind that nursing interventions are similar to those for oral fluid and electrolyte replacement therapy and NG tube feedings
- Be aware that many fluid imbalances have an iatrogenic origin; carefully record all water intake to accurately monitor intake and output

ENTERAL NUTRITIONAL SUPPLEMENTATION

- **General information**
  - Administered to restore or maintain nutritional status
  - Contains essential nutrients
    - Amino acids
    - Calories
    - Electrolytes
    - Vitamins

- **Composition**
  - Elemental diets
    - Combination of water and a powdered mixture
    - Mixture: contains essential and nonessential amino acids, fatty acids, glucose, electrolytes, and minerals
  - Tube feedings
    - Liquid mixture of water, protein, carbohydrates, fats, minerals, and vitamins
    - Mixture: can be commercially prepared or made from liquefied whole foods

- **Types**
  - Hyperosmolar elemental diets, such as Vivonex
  - Hyperosmolar tube feedings, such as Ensure and Sustacal
  - Iso-osmolar tube feedings, such as Osmolite and Isocal

- **Uses**
  - Provide a caloric supplement
  - Restore and maintain nutritional status
  - Provide an additional energy source

- **Administration routes**
  - Oral
  - NG
  - Gastric (through gastrostomy or jejunostomy tube, or gastrostomy button)

- **Nursing interventions**
  - Keep in mind that nursing interventions are similar to those for oral and NG tube feedings
  - Be aware of risks and complications of enteral nutritional supplementation
    - Dehydration due to inadequate dilution or water supplementation, especially in geriatric patients
    - Aspiration of tube feedings

Key facts about enteral nutritional supplementation

- Administered to restore or maintain nutritional status
- Contains essential nutrients

Composition of enteral nutritional supplementation

- Elemental diets
- Tube feedings

Common types of enteral nutritional supplementation

- Hyperosmolar elemental diets
- Hyperosmolar tube feedings
- Iso-osmolar tube feedings

Key uses of enteral nutritional supplementation

- Caloric supplement
- Restoration and maintenance of nutritional status
- Additional energy source

Administration routes for enteral nutritional supplementation

- Oral
- NG
- Gastric

Key nursing interventions for a patient receiving enteral nutritional supplementation

- Follow the same nursing interventions as for oral and NG tube feedings.
- Be aware of risks and complications.

CRYSTALLOIDS

● **General information**
  - Used primarily for hydration and replacement therapy
  - Composed mainly of water with dissolved electrolytes or dextrose
  - Can be isotonic, hypertonic, or hypotonic (see *Comparing I.V. solutions*)
  - Isotonic: include D_5W, normal saline solution, and lactated Ringer's solution
  - Hypertonic: include dextrose 10% in water ($D_{10}W$) and dextrose 50% in water
  - Hypotonic: include half-normal saline solution and 0.25% NaCl solution

● **Composition**
  - Water included in crystalloid solutions
  - Carbohydrate solutions: contain dextrose in 5% to 50% concentrations
  - Electrolyte solutions: can include sodium, potassium (K), chloride, and other electrolytes
  - Acid-base components: include acetate, lactate, or ammonium chloride

● **Types**
  - D_5W (dextrose 5% in water)
  - Normal saline solution (water, 154 mEq/L of Na, and 154 mEq/L of Cl)
  - Dextrose 5% and half-normal saline solution (water, dextrose, 77 mEq/L of Na, and 77 mEq/L of Cl)
  - Dextrose 5% and 0.25% NaCl solution (water, dextrose, 34 mEq/L of Na, and 34 mEq/L of Cl)
  - Ringer's solution (water and a range of electrolytes, including 130 mEq/L of Na, 109 mEq/L of Cl, 4 mEq/L of K, and 3 mEq/L of calcium [Ca])
  - Lactated Ringer's solution (water and all the electrolytes listed for Ringer's solution, plus 28 mEq/L of lactate)

● **Uses**
  - Provide hydration
  - Provide calories
  - Provide electrolyte replacement
  - Protect protein from being used as a source of energy (when solutions containing dextrose are used)
  - Replace ECF losses (normal saline solution)
  - Correct acidosis (lactated Ringer's solution)

● **Administration routes**
  - Peripheral or central I.V.

Comparing I.V. solutions

This chart shows examples of some commonly used I.V. fluid solutions and includes some of the uses and special considerations associated with them.

I.V. SOLUTION	USES	SPECIAL CONSIDERATIONS
Hypertonic		
Dextrose 5% in half-normal saline solution	• Diabetic ketoacidosis (DKA) after initial treatment with normal saline solution and half-normal saline solution—prevents hypoglycemia and cerebral edema (occurs when serum osmolality is reduced too rapidly)	• In patients with DKA, use the solution only when glucose falls under 250 mg/dl.
Dextrose 5% in normal saline solution	• Addisonian crisis • Hypotonic dehydration • Syndrome of inappropriate antidiuretic hormone (or use 3% NaCl) • Temporary treatment of circulatory insufficiency and shock if plasma expanders aren't available	• Don't use this in patients with cardiac or renal disorders because of risk of heart failure and pulmonary edema.
Dextrose 10% in water	• Conditions in which some nutrition with glucose is required • Water replacement	• Monitor serum glucose levels.
Hypotonic		
0.45% NaCl (half-normal saline solution)	• DKA after initial normal saline solution and before dextrose infusion • Gastric fluid loss from nasogastric suctioning or vomiting • Hypertonic dehydration • Sodium and chloride depletion • Water replacement	• Use this cautiously; it may cause cardiovascular collapse or increased intracranial pressure. • Don't use this in patients with liver disease, trauma, or burns.
Isotonic		
Dextrose 5% in water	• Fluid loss and dehydration • Hypernatremia	• The solution is isotonic initially and becomes hypotonic when dextrose is metabolized. • Don't use this for resuscitation; it can cause hyperglycemia. • Use this cautiously in patients with renal or cardiac disease; it can cause fluid overload. • It doesn't provide enough daily calories for prolonged use and may cause eventual protein breakdown.

(continued)

Key uses of I.V. solutions

Hypertonic
• DKA
• Addisonian crisis
• Hypotonic dehydration
• SIADH
• Circulatory insufficiency and shock
• Conditions requiring glucose
• Water replacement

Hypotonic
• DKA after initial normal saline and before dextrose infusion
• Gastric fluid loss
• Hypertonic dehydration
• Water replacement

Isotonic
• Fluid loss and dehydration
• Hypernatremia
• Resuscitation
• Shock
• Acute blood loss
• Burns
• Metabolic alkalosis or acidosis
• Lower GI tract fluid loss

Administration routes for crystalloids

- Peripheral I.V.
- Central I.V.

Key nursing interventions for a patient receiving crystalloids

- Follow the same nursing interventions as for parenteral fluid replacement therapy.
- Never administer hypertonic solutions to a patient at risk for cellular dehydration.

Key facts about colloids

- Administered during an acute situation
- Indicated for patients with a protein deficit

Comparing I.V. solutions (continued)

I.V. SOLUTION	USES	SPECIAL CONSIDERATIONS
Isotonic *(continued)*		
0.9% NaCl (normal saline solution)	• Blood transfusions • Fluid challenges • Fluid replacement in patients with DKA • Hypercalcemia • Hyponatremia • Metabolic alkalosis • Resuscitation • Shock	• Because it replaces extracellular fluid, don't use this in patients with heart failure, edema, or hypernatremia; it can lead to overload.
Lactated Ringer's solution	• Acute blood loss • Burns • Dehydration • Hypovolemia due to third-space shifting • Lower GI tract fluid loss • Mild metabolic acidosis • Salicylate overdose	• Electrolyte content is similar to that of serum but doesn't contain magnesium. • This contains potassium; don't use it in patients with renal failure because it can cause hyperkalemia. • Don't use this in patients with liver disease because they can't metabolize lactate (a functional liver converts it to bicarbonate); don't give it if a patient's pH is more than 7.5.

Nursing interventions
- Keep in mind that nursing interventions are similar to those for parenteral fluid replacement therapy
- Administer normal saline solution to correct sodium or chloride deficits
- Never administer hypertonic solutions to patients at risk for cellular dehydration, such as those with diabetic ketoacidosis, because hypertonic solutions draw fluids from cells

COLLOIDS

General information
- Administered during an acute situation, such as hypovolemia, to expand intravascular volume and maintain blood pressure
- Indicated for patients with a protein deficit, which can come from multiple sources
  - Starvation
  - Liver disease
  - Alcohol abuse

- Pull fluid into the bloodstream; effects last several days if lining of capillaries is normal
- **Composition**
  - Plasma: composed of water, protein, and small amounts of carbohydrates and lipids
  - Serum protein and albumin: composed of albumin and globulins
- **Types**
  - Fresh frozen plasma
  - Albumin (Albuminar)
  - Plasma protein fraction (Plasmanate)
- **Uses**
  - Restore serum protein levels
  - Restore albumin levels
  - Expand intravascular volume
  - Correct hypotensive episodes
- **Administration routes**
  - Peripheral or central I.V.
- **Nursing interventions**
  - Keep in mind that nursing interventions are similar to those for parenteral fluid replacement therapy
  - Be aware that colloid administration can greatly expand intravascular volume, putting the patient at risk for heart failure and pulmonary edema
  - Closely monitor the patient during a colloid infusion for increased blood pressure, dyspnea, and bounding pulse, which are all signs of hypervolemia
  - Monitor serum protein and albumin levels for deficits during colloid administration

PARENTERAL NUTRITIONAL SUPPLEMENTATION

- **General information**
  - Administered to restore or maintain nutritional status
  - Contains essential nutrients
    - Amino acids
    - Caloric sources
    - Electrolytes
    - Vitamins
  - TPN: provides concentrated source of calories (approximately 1,000 calories/L) and total nutrient requirements; administered through central I.V. line; peripheral parenteral nutrition may be infused through peripheral I.V. line

Composition of colloids
- Plasma
- Serum protein and albumin

Common types of colloids
- Fresh frozen plasma
- Albumin
- Plasma protein fraction

Key uses of colloids
- Restoration of serum protein levels
- Restoration of albumin levels
- Expanding intravascular volume

Administration routes for colloids
- Peripheral I.V.
- Central I.V.

Key nursing interventions for a patient receiving colloids
- Follow the same nursing interventions as for parenteral fluid replacement therapy.
- Monitor serum protein and albumin levels.

Key facts about parenteral nutritional supplementation
- Administered to restore or maintain nutritional status
- Contains essential nutrients

Composition of parenteral nutritional supplementation

- Carbohydrate parenteral nutrients
- Protein parenteral solutions
- Fat emulsions
- TPN
- Alcohol solutions
- Vitamins

Common types of parenteral nutritional supplementation

- Crystalline amino acids
- Fat emulsions
- Ethyl alcohol solutions
- Vitamins

Key uses of parenteral nutritional supplementation

- Providing calories
- Restoring and maintaining nutritional status

Administration routes for parenteral nutritional supplementation

- Peripheral I.V
- Central I.V.

- Lipid emulsions: provide calories and assist in wound healing, red blood cell (RBC) production, prostaglandin synthesis
- Caloric requirements
  - Approximately 400 calories/day: must be administered to prevent protein from being used as a source of energy
  - 1,600 calories/day required to meet daily adult energy needs
- Protein requirements
  - Adults: average 1 g/kg of body weight daily
  - Children: 1 to 2 g/kg of body weight daily
- Ethyl alcohol: provides rich source of calories, with 1 gram yielding approximately 7 calories

● **Composition**
- Carbohydrate parenteral nutrients: carbohydrates available as dextrose solutions in concentrations of 5% to 50%
- Protein parenteral solutions: crystalline amino acids or colloidal elements
- Fat emulsions: lipids in 10% and 20% concentrations
- TPN: dextrose (25% to 50%), amino acids, and selected amounts of multiple elements
  - Potassium
  - Sodium
  - Calcium
  - Phosphorus
  - Magnesium
  - Possibly, water and fat-soluble vitamins (see *Common TPN additives*)
- Alcohol solutions: contain ethyl alcohol (rich source of calories)
- Vitamins: may include both fat-soluble and water-soluble vitamins

● **Types**
- Crystalline amino acids or albumin-type products
- Fat emulsions
- Ethyl alcohol solutions
- Vitamin C, vitamin B-complex, or fat-soluble vitamins

● **Uses**
- Provide calories
- Restore and maintain nutritional status
- Prevent protein breakdown (if 400 calories/day administered)
- Provide additional energy source

● **Administration routes**
- Peripheral or central I.V.

Common TPN additives

Common components of total parenteral nutrition (TPN) solutions—such as dextrose 10% in water ($D_{10}W$), amino acids, and other additives—are used for specific purposes. For instance, $D_{10}W$ provides calories for metabolism. This list contains other common additives and the purposes each serve. Lipids may be infused separately.

ELECTROLYTES
- Calcium promotes development of bones and teeth, and aids in blood clotting.
- Chloride regulates acid-base balance and maintains osmotic pressure.
- Magnesium helps the body absorb carbohydrates and protein.
- Phosphorus is essential for cell energy and calcium balance.
- Potassium is needed for cellular activity and cardiac function.
- Sodium helps control water distribution and maintains normal fluid balance.

VITAMINS
- Folic acid is needed for deoxyribose nucleic acid formation and promotes growth and development.
- Vitamin B complex aids in the final absorption of carbohydrates and protein.
- Vitamin C helps in wound healing.
- Vitamin D is essential for bone metabolism and maintenance of serum calcium levels.
- Vitamin K helps prevent bleeding disorders.

OTHER ADDITIVES
- Acetate prevents metabolic acidosis.
- Amino acids provide the proteins necessary for tissue repair.
- Micronutrients, such as zinc, cobalt, and manganese, help in wound healing and red blood cell synthesis.

● **Nursing interventions**
- Keep in mind that nursing interventions are similar to those for parenteral fluid replacement therapy
- Use a mechanical infusion pump for TPN administration to reduce the risk of hyperosmolality with rapid infusion
- Infuse TPN through a central line only due to its higher dextrose concentrations
- Never add medications to a TPN solution container
- Use a 0.22-micron filter for TPN infusion; this size inhibits passage of *Pseudomonas* bacteria and decreases the risk of contamination
- Return the bag to the pharmacy if you see particulate matter, cloudiness, or an oily layer in the bag when preparing to hang a TPN solution; the solution should be clear or pale yellow if multivitamins are added
- Use meticulous sterile technique when changing TPN central-line tubing and dressings; patients are at high risk for infection because of the solution's concentrated glucose content

Key nursing interventions for a patient receiving parenteral nutritional supplementation

- Follow the same nursing interventions as for parenteral fluid replacement therapy.
- Use a mechanical infusion pump.
- Infuse TPN through a central line.
- Never add medications.
- Use sterile technique when changing TPN central-line tubing and dressings.
- Assess laboratory studies.
- Monitor fingerstick blood glucose levels.

– Change I.V. administration set according to institutional policy (usually every 24 hours for TPN); don't allow TPN solutions to hang for more than 24 hours

– Site care and dressing changes per institutional policy, or whenever dressing becomes wet, soiled, or nonocclusive

• Assess the patient every 15 minutes during the first hour of TPN therapy to determine tolerance, then every 30 minutes for 1 hour (or according to institutional policy) thereafter

• Be aware that starting TPN in a severely malnourished patient may cause refeeding syndrome, which includes a rapid drop in potassium, magnesium, and phosphorus levels; to avoid compromising cardiac function, initiate feeding slowly and monitor the patient's electrolyte levels closely until they stabilize

• Assess laboratory studies, such as serum BUN, creatinine, and electrolyte levels, every 12 to 24 hours (or whenever the patient's condition changes) for indications of an imbalance

• Be aware that the common imbalances associated with TPN infusion include hyperkalemia, azotemia, hypophosphatemia, metabolic acidosis, hyperglycemia, and hyperosmolar nonketotic syndrome

• Assess liver function with liver function tests and bilirubin, triglyceride, and cholesterol levels; abnormal values may indicate intolerance

• Monitor fingerstick blood glucose levels as ordered, and monitor for signs and symptoms of hyperglycemia (thirst and polyuria); consider the need for insulin if hyperglycemia occurs

• When discontinuing TPN, decrease the infusion slowly, depending on current glucose intake; this minimizes the risk of hyperinsulinemia and resulting hypoglycemia

• While a filter must always be used when administering TPN, remember that the fat emulsion infusion line doesn't need one

• Remember that fat emulsions are contraindicated in patients with conditions that disrupt normal fat metabolism (for example, pancreatitis, pathologic hyperlipidemia, and lipid nephrosis)

• When administering fat emulsions, assess for adverse reactions such as vomiting, headache, dyspnea, allergic reaction, hyperlipidemia, temperature elevation, flushing, sweating, hepatomegaly, fat-overload syndrome, and shock; also continue to monitor for delayed reactions

BLOOD AND BLOOD PRODUCTS

● **General information**
• Normal adult blood volume: averages about 75 ml/kg of body weight; 15% to 20% plasma volume deficit associated with hypovolemic shock
• Transfusions performed to restore blood volume, correct deficiencies in blood's oxygen-carrying capacity and coagulation components

Identifying compatible blood types

A blood transfusion will most likely be safe if the donor and recipient have compatible blood types. Use this chart as a guide to blood-type compatibility.

RECIPIENT'S BLOOD TYPE	COMPATIBLE DONOR TYPES
A	A, O
B	B, O
AB	A, B, AB, O
O	O

- Donor-recipient blood compatibility: must be established before transfusion; degree affected by various antigens in blood (ABO blood group, rhesus [Rh] factor, human leukocyte antigen [HLA] blood group)
  - ABO blood group
    - ABO blood typing used to identify two antigens (A and B) in RBCs; person can have both (type AB), only one (type A or type B), or neither (type O)
    - Person with A antigens: has anti-B antibodies in plasma
    - Person with B antigens: has anti-A antibodies in plasma
    - Transfusion reaction: may occur if patient receives blood type for which he has antibodies (see *Identifying compatible blood types*)
    - People with type AB: called *universal recipients*; don't have antibodies; can receive blood types O, A, B, or AB without having an ABO reaction
    - People with type O: called *universal donors,* may donate blood for transfusion into person with any blood type; may receive only type O blood safely because they have both anti-A and anti-B antibodies
    - In emergency (when inadvisable to wait for crossmatch): patient possibly given plasma-volume expanders, or blood from a universal donor
  - Rh factor
    - Rh antigen found on membrane of RBCs
    - Rh antigen present in about 85% of U.S. population (known as *Rh-positive*); remainder don't have Rh antigen (known as *Rh-negative*)
    - No natural antibodies to Rh antigens, but may develop in Rh-negative people exposed to Rh-positive blood; sensitization usually caused by first exposure, fatal hemolytic reaction (such as can occur during transfusions or pregnancy) may be caused by second

· If Rh-negative patient exposed to Rh-positive blood, problem possibly corrected with injection of Rh_o(D) immune globulin (RhoGAM) given within 72 hours of exposure to inhibit antibody formation

– HLA blood group
  · HLA located on surface of circulating platelets, white blood cells, and most tissue cells
  · Responsible for febrile reactions in patients receiving blood transfusion containing platelets from several donors
    - Antigen-antibody reaction: causes platelet destruction; patient now less responsive to platelet transfusions
    - Risk of antigen-antibody reactions: greatly reduced by giving HLA-matched platelets
  · Patients receiving multiple transfusions over long time period, or frequent transfusions during short-term illness, generally benefitted by HLA tests

Composition of blood and blood products

- Whole blood: contains erythrocytes and all coagulation factors except VIII and V; lacks platelets
- Packed RBC volume: contains erythrocytes and 100 ml plasma
- Fresh frozen plasma: contains multiple components; lacks platelets
- Platelets: contain only platelets
- Cryoprecipitate: contains factor VIII and fibrinogen
- Albumin: contains human albumin

● **Composition**
• Whole blood
  – Available volume: 500 ml bags
  – Contains erythrocytes and all coagulation factors except VIII and V
  – Lacks platelets
• Packed RBC volume
  – Available volume: 250 to 300 ml bags
  – Contains erythrocytes and 100 ml plasma
• Fresh frozen plasma
  – Available volume: 200 to 250 ml bags
  – Contains multiple components
    · Plasma
    · Water
    · Fibrinogen
    · Some clotting factors
    · Electrolytes
    · Sugar
    · Vitamins
    · Minerals
    · Hormones
    · Antibodies
  – Lacks platelets (a colloid)
• Platelets
  – Available volume: 50 ml bags
  – Contain only platelets
• Cryoprecipitate
  – Available volume: 10 to 25 ml
  – Contains factor VIII and fibrinogen

- Albumin
  - Available volume: 50 (25%) to 250 (5%) ml
  - Contains human albumin
  - Carries virtually no risk of hepatitis or human immunodeficiency virus (because of heat treatment process used during manufacturing)

● **Types**
- Whole blood
  - Rarely used unless patient has lost more than 25% of total blood volume
  - Used to treat hemorrhage, trauma, or major burns
  - Should be avoided if fluid overload is a concern
  - Stored whole blood high in potassium
  - ABO compatibility and Rh matching required before administration
- Packed RBCs
  - Prepared by removing about 90% of plasma surrounding cells and adding anticoagulant preservative
  - Has several uses
    · Helps restore or maintain oxygen-carrying capacity of blood in patients with anemic conditions
    · Corrects blood losses during or after surgery
  - About 70% of leukocytes in packed cells removed before transfusion; reduces risk of febrile, nonhemolytic reactions
  - ABO compatibility and Rh matching required
- Fresh frozen plasma
  - Prepared by separating plasma from RBCs and freezing it within 6 hours of collection
  - Has several uses
    · Treats hemorrhage
    · Expands plasma volume
    · Corrects undetermined coagulation factor deficiencies
    · Replaces specific clotting factors
    · Corrects factor deficiencies resulting from liver disease
  - Large-volume transfusions: may require correction for hypocalcemia; citric acid in transfusion binds with and depletes patient's own serum calcium
  - ABO compatibility testing unnecessary; Rh matching preferred
- Platelets
  - Prepared by pooling platelet components separated from whole blood or through plateletpheresis
  - Used for patients with one of several disorders or conditions
    · Platelet dysfunctions or thrombocytopenia
    · Multiple transfusions of stored blood
    · Acute leukemia or bone marrow abnormalities
  - ABO compatibility testing not required; Rh matching preferred

Key uses of whole blood
- Hemorrhage
- Trauma
- Major burns

Key uses of packed RBCs
- Restoring or maintaining oxygen-carrying capacity of blood in patients with anemic conditions
- Correcting blood losses during or after surgery

Key uses of fresh frozen plasma
- Hemorrhage
- Plasma volume expander
- Correcting undetermined coagulation factor deficiencies
- Replacing specific clotting factors
- Correcting factor deficiencies resulting from liver disease

Key uses of platelets
- Platelet dysfunctions or thrombocytopenia
- Multiple transfusions of stored blood
- Acute leukemia or bone marrow abnormalities

- Cryoprecipitate
  - Insoluble portion of plasma recovered from fresh frozen plasma; also called *factor VIII*
  - Used to treat various disorders
    - von Willebrand's disease
    - Hypofibrinogenemia
    - Factor VIII deficiency (antihemophilic factor)
    - Hemophilia A
    - Disseminated intravascular coagulation
  - ABO compatibility testing and Rh matching unnecessary
- Albumin
  - Colloidal solution extracted from plasma
  - Contains globulin and other proteins
  - Used for patients with one of several disorders or conditions
    - Acute liver failure
    - Burns
    - Trauma
    - Patients who have had surgery
    - Neonates with hemolytic disease when crystalloids prove ineffective
    - Hypoproteinemia with or without edema
  - Large albumin molecules: increase plasma oncotic pressure, coaxing fluid from the interstitial space across normal capillary membranes and into the intravascular space; may actually do more harm than good in shock patients by leaking through damaged capillary membranes and dragging intravascular fluid along to worsen interstitial edema
  - ABO compatibility and Rh matching unnecessary

- **Uses**
  - Replace blood loss
  - Replace RBC loss
  - Treat anemia
  - Expand blood volume

- **Administration routes**
  - Peripheral or central I.V.

- **Nursing interventions**
  - Make sure the patient or a responsible family member has signed an informed consent form
  - Use standard precautions when handling blood and blood products
  - Use a blood filter when administering blood or blood products
  - Infuse blood products through an I.V. catheter at least 18G or 20G; never use a smaller-gauge catheter or needle
  - Inspect the blood bag's contents for discoloration

- Before administration, check blood identification and compatibility information against patient information with another nurse, following institutional protocol
- Assess blood temperature before administering, and use blood-warming equipment when necessary
- Take and record baseline vital signs before blood administration, including temperature, pulse, blood pressure, and respirations; repeat after 15 minutes and at completion
- Flush with normal saline solution before and after infusing blood products; don't use a dextrose solution (which can cause hemolysis) or lactated Ringer's solution (which contains calcium and can clog the tubing)
- When starting the transfusion, remain with the patient and observe him carefully for the first 15 minutes; most acute adverse reactions occur within that time period, although delayed reactions can occur up to 2 weeks later (continue to assess vital signs per institutional policy)
- Adjust the infusion rate to prevent the risk of bacterial growth and RBC hemolysis from the infusion hanging too long
  - Maximum infusion time: 4 hours
  - Use infusion pump: to regulate flow rate according to institutional protocol
- Assess for signs and symptoms of blood transfusion reaction, such as fever, chills, shortness of breath, headache, and hematuria (see *Guide to blood transfusion reactions,* pages 254 and 255)
  - If reactions occur
    - Stop infusion immediately; use new administration set to infuse normal saline solution to keep vein open
    - Take vital signs
    - Notify physician
    - Take further actions according to institutional policies
- Monitor for signs and symptoms of anaphylactic reaction, including respiratory distress, hypotension, rash, flushing, chills, and pruritus
- Watch for possible complications of massive transfusion, such as hyperkalemia, acidosis, hypothermia, citrate toxicity, and 2,3-diphosphoglycerate deficiency
- Obtain laboratory tests as ordered to determine the effectiveness of the treatment
  - Hemoglobin level of adult patient receiving 1 unit of packed RBCs: should increase by 1 g/dl; hematocrit by 3%
  - Platelets: should increase 5,000 to 10,000/mm³ with each unit transfused platelets
  - Prothrombin time and partial thromboplastin time: should improve after giving clotting factors

Key nursing interventions for a patient receiving blood and blood products

- Have consent form signed.
- Use standard precautions.
- Use a blood filter.
- Check blood identification and compatibility information against patient information with another nurse.
- Assess blood temperature.
- Take and record baseline vital signs after 15 minutes and at completion.
- Flush with normal saline solution before and after infusing blood products.
- Observe the patient for the first 15 minutes.
- Remember that maximum infusion time is 4 hours.
- Assess for signs and symptoms of blood transfusion reaction.
- Obtain laboratory tests to determine the effectiveness of the treatment.

Common causes of blood transfusion reactions

- Allergic reaction
- Bacterial contamination
- Febrile
- Hemolytic
- Plasma protein incompatibility
- Bleeding tendencies
- Circulatory overload
- Hypocalcemia
- Hypothermia
- Potassium intoxication

Guide to blood transfusion reactions

This chart describes endogenous reactions (those caused by antigen-antibody reactions) and exogenous reactions (those caused by external factors in administered blood).

CAUSES	ASSESSMENT FINDINGS	NURSING INTERVENTIONS
Allergic reaction • Allergen in donated blood • Donor blood hypersensitive to certain medication	Anaphylaxis (anxiety, chills, facial swelling, laryngeal edema, pruritus, urticaria, wheezing), fever, nausea, vomiting	• Stop the infusion. • Give antihistamines as ordered. • Monitor vital signs and continue to assess the patient. • Give epinephrine and corticosteroids as ordered.
Bacterial contamination • Organisms that survive the cold, such as Pseudomonas and Staphylococcus	Abdominal cramping, chills, diarrhea, fever, shock, signs of renal failure, vomiting	• Stop the infusion. • Give antibiotics, corticosteroids, and epinephrine as prescribed. • Maintain strict blood-storage control. • Change the administration set and filter every 4 hours or every 2 units. • Infuse each unit of blood over 2 to 4 hours; stop the infusion if it lasts more than 4 hours. • Maintain sterile technique.
Febrile • Bacterial lipopolysaccharides • Antileukocyte recipient antibodies directed against donor white blood cells	Chest tightness, chills, cough, facial flushing, fever up to 104° F (40° C) or an increase in temperature of 1.8° F (1° C), flank pain, headache, increased pulse rate, palpitations	• Stop the infusion. • Administer antipyretics and antihistamines as ordered. • If the patient needs further transfusions, use frozen red blood cells (RBCs) and a leukocyte. filter, and give acetaminophen (Tylenol) as ordered.
Hemolytic • ABO or Rh incompatibility • Intradonor incompatibility • Improper crossmatching • Improperly stored blood	Bloody oozing at infusion site, burning along the vein receiving blood, chest pain, chills, dyspnea, tachycardia, tachypnea, facial flushing, fever, flank pain, nausea, hypotension, hemoglobinuria, oliguria, shock, signs of renal failure	• Stop the infusion. • Monitor vital signs, including pulse oximetry, as well as hourly urine output. • Manage shock with I.V. fluids, oxygen, epinephrine, and vasopressors as ordered. • Obtain a posttransfusion reaction blood sample and urine specimen for analysis. • Observe for signs of hemorrhage from disseminated intravascular coagulation.
Plasma protein incompatibility • Immunoglobulin A incompatibility	Abdominal pain, chills, diarrhea, dyspnea, fever, flushing, hypotension	• Stop the infusion. • Administer oxygen, fluids, epinephrine, and corticosteroids as ordered.

Guide to blood transfusion reactions *(continued)*

CAUSES	ASSESSMENT FINDINGS	NURSING INTERVENTIONS
Bleeding tendencies ● Low platelet count in stored blood, causing thrombocytopenia	Abnormal bleeding and oozing from cuts or breaks in the skin or the gums, abnormal bruising and petechiae	● Give platelets, fresh frozen plasma, or cryoprecipitate as ordered. ● Monitor platelet count.
Circulatory overload ● Possibly from infusing whole blood too rapidly	Back pain, chest pain or tightness, chills, distended jugular veins, dyspnea, cough, fever, flushed feeling, headache, tachycardia, hypertension, increased central venous pressure, increased plasma volume	● Slow or stop the infusion. ● Monitor vital signs. ● Use packed RBCs instead of whole blood. ● Give diuretics as ordered.
Hypocalcemia ● Citrate toxicity, which occurs when citrate-treated blood is infused too rapidly and binds with calcium, causing a calcium deficiency	Arrhythmias, hypotension, muscle cramps, muscle tremors, nausea, seizures, tingling in fingers, vomiting	● Slow or stop the transfusion if ordered; expect a more severe reaction in hypothermic patients or patients with elevated potassium levels. ● Give calcium gluconate I.V. slowly if ordered.
Hypothermia ● Rapid infusion of large amounts of cold blood, which decreases body temperature	Arrhythmias (especially bradycardia), cardiac arrest if core temperature falls below 86° F (30° C), chills, hypotension, shaking	● Stop the transfusion. ● Warm the patient. ● Obtain an ECG. ● Warm the blood if the transfusion is resumed.
Potassium intoxication ● An abnormally high level of potassium in stored plasma caused by hemolysis of RBCs	Bradycardia, cardiac arrest, diarrhea, electrocardiogram (ECG) changes (such as tall, peaked T waves), flaccidity, nausea, intestinal colic, muscle twitching, oliguria, signs of renal failure	● Stop the infusion. ● Obtain an ECG and serum electrolyte levels, such as potassium and glucose. ● Give sodium polystyrene sulfonate (Kayexalate) as ordered. ● Give glucose 50% and insulin, bicarbonate, or calcium, as ordered, to force potassium into cells. ● Give mannitol (Osmitrol) and maintain vigorous hydration to force diuresis and prevent renal damage.

TOP 10

Items to study for your next test on fluid and electrolyte replacement therapy

1. Specific examples of isotonic, hypotonic, and hypertonic solutions
2. Methods and techniques of fluid and electrolyte replacement—oral, gastric, parenteral
3. Differences among crystalloids, colloids, electrolytes, nutrition, and blood products
4. Advantages of each method of delivery for replacement therapy
5. Limitations or complications of each method of delivery for replacement therapy
6. Diagnostics used to support the effectiveness of replacement therapy
7. Nursing assessments for each method and technique of replacement therapy
8. Drugs that are impacted by or need modification with each delivery method of replacement therapy
9. Key facts concerning blood replacement therapy, including diagnostics, signs and symptoms of incompatibility, flow rate, universal donors and recipients, and administration guidelines
10. Contents of and management during TPN replacement

NCLEX CHECKS

It's never too soon to begin your NCLEX preparation. Now that you've reviewed this chapter, carefully read each of the following questions and choose the best answer. Then compare your responses to the correct answers.

1. When administering 5% albumin to a client with normal capillaries, which effect on intravascular fluid volume can be expected?
- [ ] **1.** Fluid will be drawn into blood vessels.
- [ ] **2.** Extra fluid will be excreted from the body.
- [ ] **3.** There will be no effect on intravascular fluid volume.
- [ ] **4.** Fluid will leak into the interstitial space.

2. A client is receiving I.V. fluid, and has reported feeling pain at the insertion site. Upon inspection, the nurse notes that the site is red and edematous. What should the nurse's next actions be? Select all that apply.
- [ ] **1.** Slow the infusion to a rate to keep the vein open, and notify the physician.
- [ ] **2.** Stop the infusion.
- [ ] **3.** Check the I.V. line for blood return.
- [ ] **4.** Elevate the extremity.
- [ ] **5.** Place the extremity below the level of the heart.
- [ ] **6.** Apply warm compresses.

3. Which solution should be selected to flush an I.V. line immediately following a blood transfusion?
- [ ] **1.** D_5W
- [ ] **2.** $D_{10}W$
- [ ] **3.** Normal saline solution
- [ ] **4.** Lactated Ringer's solution

4. Clients with which blood type are known as "universal recipients?"
- [ ] **1.** A
- [ ] **2.** B
- [ ] **3.** AB
- [ ] **4.** O

5. Which is the only blood type suitable for administration in an emergency situation when there's no time to perform crossmatching?
- [ ] **1.** A positive
- [ ] **2.** O positive
- [ ] **3.** B negative
- [ ] **4.** O negative

6. Some blood products require ABO compatibility testing before administration, whereas others don't. Which group of blood products requires ABO compatibility testing before administration?
- [ ] **1.** Whole blood and platelets
- [ ] **2.** Fresh frozen plasma and albumin
- [ ] **3.** Whole blood and packed RBCs
- [ ] **4.** Packed RBCs and albumin

7. Administration of a colloid solution places the client at risk for which complication?

☐ **1.** Hyperkalemia
☐ **2.** Hypervolemia
☐ **3.** Hypernatremia
☐ **4.** Hypovolemia

8. Which key step must be performed before administration of an enteral feeding through an NG tube?

☐ **1.** Flush the tube with normal saline solution.
☐ **2.** Check the pH of a small amount of gastric aspirate.
☐ **3.** Leave the NG tube cap off to allow for air ventilation.
☐ **4.** Withdraw and discard any remaining gastric contents from the previous feeding.

9. A client receiving NG tube feedings has developed diarrhea. What's the most appropriate intervention?

☐ **1.** Slow the flow rate of the feedings.
☐ **2.** Provide the patient with additional fluids.
☐ **3.** Increase the client's fruit and vegetable intake.
☐ **4.** Flush the tube with water after each feeding.

10. Which blood product would be appropriate to administer to treat a client with anemia?

☐ **1.** Packed RBCs
☐ **2.** Whole blood
☐ **3.** Platelets
☐ **4.** Fresh frozen plasma

ANSWERS AND RATIONALES

1. CORRECT ANSWER: 1
Albumin's large molecules increase plasma oncotic pressure, coaxing fluid from the interstitial space across normal capillary membranes and into the intravascular space. Therefore, the intravascular volume can be expected to increase.

2. CORRECT ANSWER: 2, 4, 6
Pain, redness, and edema are all signs that the I.V. has infiltrated into surrounding tissues. The most appropriate actions include stopping the infusion, elevating the extremity, and applying warm compresses to promote venous return and absorption of the extra fluid. Slowing the infusion would allow fluid to continue to infiltrate. Checking the I.V. for blood return wouldn't be helpful because the line must come out due to signs and symptoms. Placing the extremity below the level of the heart would worsen signs and symptoms.

3. CORRECT ANSWER: 3

Normal saline solution should be used to flush the I.V. line before and after infusing blood products. Dextrose solutions can cause hemolysis, and lactated Ringer's solution, which contains calcium, can clog the tubing.

4. CORRECT ANSWER: 3

Clients with type AB blood have no antibodies and, therefore, can receive blood types O, A, B, or AB without having an ABO reaction. For this reason, they're known as *universal recipients*.

5. CORRECT ANSWER: 4

Type O, Rh-negative blood is the only blood type suitable to administer without crossmatching during a crisis situation. This blood is from a universal donor, meaning that it's suitable to administer to clients with any blood type. A positive, O positive, and B negative blood types all contain antigens that can cause hemolytic reactions.

6. CORRECT ANSWER: 3

ABO compatibility testing is required before administration of whole blood and packed RBCs to prevent an ABO incompatibility reaction. ABO compatibility testing isn't necessary for fresh frozen plasma, albumin, or platelets, although some of these products require Rh matching.

7. CORRECT ANSWER: 2

Because colloids pull fluid into the bloodstream, clients receiving them are at risk for hypervolemia, and should be monitored closely for increased blood pressure, dyspnea, and bounding pulse during a colloid infusion.

8. CORRECT ANSWER: 2

Proper placement of the NG tube must be verified each time before using the tube (to prevent aspiration). A gastric pH of less than 4 confirms NG tube placement in the stomach.

9. CORRECT ANSWER: 1

To reduce or prevent diarrhea, the nurse may slow the flow rate of the feeding. Providing additional fluids and increasing fruit and vegetable intake can help to prevent or relieve constipation. Flushing the tube with water after feedings helps to prevent tube clogging.

10. CORRECT ANSWER: 1

Packed RBCs can help restore or maintain the oxygen-carrying capacity of the blood in clients with anemic conditions. Whole blood, rarely used, is indicated to treat hemorrhage, trauma, or major burns. Fresh frozen plasma is used to treat hemorrhage and expand plasma volume. Platelets are used for clients with platelet dysfunctions or thrombocytopenia.

Glossary
Selected references
Index

Glossary

absorption: taking up of a substance by cells or tissues

acid: substance that donates hydrogen ions

acid-base balance: mechanism by which the body's acids and bases are kept in balance

acidosis: condition resulting from acid accumulation or base loss

active transport: movement of solutes from an area of lower concentration to one of higher concentration (the solutes are said to move against the concentration gradient)

adenosine triphosphate (ATP): vital phosphorus-containing compound that represents stored energy in the cells; needed to carry out the body's functions

albumin: protein that can't pass through capillary walls and that draws water into the capillaries by osmosis during reabsorption

aldosterone: hormone secreted by the adrenal cortex that regulates sodium reabsorption by the kidneys (the renin-angiotensin system responds to decreased blood flow and decreased blood pressure to stimulate aldosterone secretion)

alkalosis: condition resulting from base accumulation or acid loss

anaphylactic reaction (anaphylaxis): severe allergic reaction that may include flushing, chills, anxiety, agitation, generalized itching, palpitations, paresthesia, throbbing in the ears, wheezing, coughing, seizures, and cardiac arrest

anion: negatively charged ion, of which proteins, chloride, bicarbonate, and phosphorus are among the body's most plentiful

anion gap: measurement of the difference between the amount of sodium and the amount of bicarbonate and chloride in the blood

antidiuretic hormone (ADH): hormone made by the hypothalamus and released by the pituitary gland that decreases urine production by increasing the reabsorption of water by the renal tubules

anuria: absence of urine formation or output of less than 100 ml of urine in 24 hours

base: substance that accepts hydrogen ions

2,3-biphosphoglycerate (2,3-BPG): compound in red blood cells that contains phosphorus and facilitates the transfer of oxygen from hemoglobin to the tissues

blood type: usually, one of the four blood types in the ABO system, including A, B, AB, and O, which is named for the antigen—A, B, both of these, or neither—that's carried on a person's red blood cells

buffer: substance that, when combined with acids or bases, minimizes changes in pH

calcification: deposit of calcium phosphate in soft tissues that can occur with prolonged high serum phosphorus levels; can lead to organ dysfunction

calcium: positively charged ion involved in the structure and function of bones, impulse transmission, the blood-clotting process, and the normal function of heart and skeletal muscles

carboxyhemoglobin: molecule of carbon monoxide and hemoglobin that prevents the normal transfer of oxygen and carbon dioxide; can result in asphyxiation or death

cation: positively charged ion, of which sodium, potassium, calcium, magnesium, and hydrogen are the body's most plentiful

cation-exchange resin: medication used to lower serum potassium levels by exchanging sodium ions for potassium ions in the GI tract

central venous (CV) therapy: treatment in which drugs or fluids are infused directly into a major vein; used in emergencies, when a patient's peripheral veins are inaccessible, or when a patient needs infusion of a large volume of fluid, multiple infusion therapies, or long-term venous access (in CV therapy, a catheter is inserted with its tip in the superior vena cava, inferior vena cava, or right atrium of the heart)

chloride: most abundant anion in extracellular fluid; maintains serum osmolality and fluid, electrolyte, and acid-base balance

Chvostek's sign: abnormal spasm of facial muscles that may indicate hypocalcemia or tetany; tested by lightly tapping the facial nerve (upper cheek, below the zygomatic bone)

colloid: large molecule, such as albumin, that normally doesn't cross the capillary membrane

colloid osmotic pressure: osmotic, or pulling, force of albumin in the intravascular space that draws water into the capillaries during reabsorption

compensation: process by which one system (renal or respiratory) attempts to correct an acid-base disturbance in the other system

crystalloid: solute, such as sodium or glucose, that crosses the capillary membrane in solution

diffusion: movement of solutes from an area of higher concentration to one of lower concentration by passive transport (a fluid movement process that requires no energy)

diuretics: class of medications acting at various points along the nephron to increase urine output, resulting in the loss of water and electrolytes

electrolyte: solute that separates in a solvent into electrically charged particles called *ions*

extracellular fluid (ECF): any fluid in the body that isn't contained inside the cells, including interstitial fluid, plasma, and transcellular fluid

factor VIII (cryoprecipitate): antihemophilic factor recovered from fresh frozen plasma; instrumental in blood clotting

fluid balance: constant and approximately equal distribution of fluids between the intracellular and extracellular fluid compartments

glomerular filtration rate (GFR): rate at which the glomeruli in the kidneys filter blood; normally occurs at a rate of 125 ml/minute

granulocytopenia: fewer than normal number of granular leukocytes in the blood

hemolytic reaction: life-threatening reaction to transfusions that occurs as a result of incompatible ABO or Rh blood or improper blood storage

hydrostatic pressure: pressure exerted by fluid in the blood vessels

hypercapnia: partial pressure of arterial carbon dioxide that's greater than 45 mm Hg

hyperchloremic metabolic acidosis: condition resulting from a deficit in bicarbonate ions and an increase in chloride ions, which causes a decrease in pH

hyperglycemia: high blood glucose level; a possible complication of parenteral nutrition; commonly an early warning sign of sepsis

hypertonic solution: a solution with higher osmolarity (concentration) than the normal range of serum (275 to 295 mOsm/L), such as dextrose 5% in half-normal saline solution, dextrose 5% in normal saline solution, and dextrose 5% in lactated Ringer's solution

hypervolemia: excess fluid and solutes in extracellular fluid; can be caused by increased fluid intake, fluid shifts in the body, or renal failure

hypocalcemia: calcium deficiency; signs and symptoms include tingling in the fingers, muscle cramps, nausea, vomiting, hypotension, cardiac arrhythmias, and seizures

hypocapnia: partial pressure of arterial carbon dioxide that's less than 35 mm Hg

hypochloremic metabolic alkalosis: condition caused by a deficit in chloride and a subsequent increase in bicarbonate that ultimately causes an increase in pH

hypoglycemia: low blood glucose level; a possible complication of parenteral nutrition; signs and symptoms include sweating, shaking, and irritability

hypokalemia: low blood potassium level; a possible complication of parenteral nutrition; signs and symptoms include muscle weakness, paralysis, paresthesia, and arrhythmias

hypomagnesemia: low blood magnesium level; a possible complication of parenteral nutrition; patient may complain of tingling around the mouth or paresthesia in the fingers and may show signs of mental changes, hyperreflexia, tetany, and arrhythmias

hypophosphatemia: low blood phosphate level; a possible complication of parenteral nutrition; patient may be irritable or weak and may have paresthesia; in extreme cases, coma and cardiac arrest can occur

hypotonic: solution that has fewer solutes than another solution

hypotonic solution: a solution with lower osmolarity (concentration) than the normal range of serum (275 to 295 mOsm/L)—such as half-normal saline solution, 0.33% saline solution, or dextrose 2.5% in water—which hydrates cells while reducing fluid in the circulatory system

hypovolemia: condition marked by the loss of fluid and solutes from extracellular fluid that, if left untreated, can progress to hypovolemic shock

hypovolemic shock: potentially life-threatening condition in which decreased blood volume leads to low cardiac output and poor tissue perfusion

hypoxemia: oxygen deficit in arterial blood (lower than 80 mm Hg)

hypoxia: oxygen deficit in the tissues

interstitial fluid: fluid surrounding cells that, with plasma, makes up extracellular fluid

isotonic solution: solution that has the same concentration as normal serum range (275 to 295 mOsm/L), such as dextrose 5% in water or normal saline solution

magnesium: cation located primarily in intracellular fluid that promotes efficient energy use, aids protein synthesis, regulates nerve and muscle impulses, and promotes cardiovascular function

metabolic acidosis: condition in which excess acid or reduced bicarbonate in the blood lowers the arterial blood pH below 7.35

metabolic alkalosis: condition in which excess bicarbonate or reduced acid in the blood increases the arterial blood pH above 7.45

oliguria: low urine output; less than 400 ml/24 hours

osmolality: concentration of a solution; expressed in milliosmols per kilogram of solution

osmolarity: concentration of a solution; expressed in milliosmols per liter of solution

osmoreceptors: special sensing cells in the hypothalamus that respond to changes in the osmolality of blood

osmosis: passive transport of fluid across a membrane from an area of lower concentration to one of higher concentration that stops when the solute concentrations are equal

osmotic pressure: pressure exerted by a solute in solution on a semipermeable membrane

osteomalacia: softening of bone tissues due to demineralization; commonly accompanies chronic hypocalcemia

parenteral: any route other than the GI tract by which drugs, nutrients, or other solutions may enter the body (for example, I.V., I.M., or subcutaneously)

parenteral nutrition: I.V. therapy that provides calories from dextrose and one or more nutrients that keep the body functioning; ordered when a nutritional assessment reveals a nonfunctional GI tract, increased metabolic need, or a combination of both

pH: measurement of the percentage of hydrogen ions in a solution; normal pH of body fluids is 7.35 to 7.45, arterial blood gas analysis is used to evaluate acid-base balance

phosphorus: anion located primarily in intracellular fluid; involved in maintaining bone and cell structure, maintaining storage of energy in cells, and aiding oxygen delivery to tissue

potassium: major intracellular cation involved in skeletal muscle contraction, fluid distribution, osmotic pressure, and acid-base balance as well as heartbeat regulation

pulmonary edema: abnormal fluid accumulation in the lungs; life-threatening condition

reabsorption: taking in, or absorbing, a substance again

renin: enzyme that's released by the kidneys into the blood; it triggers a series of reactions that produce angiotensin II, a potent vasoconstrictor

resorption: loss of a substance through physiologic or pathologic means such as loss of calcium from bone

respiratory acidosis: acid-base disturbance caused by failure of the lungs to eliminate sufficient carbon dioxide; partial pressure of arterial carbon dioxide above 45 mm Hg and pH below 7.35

respiratory alkalosis: acid-base imbalance that occurs when the lungs eliminate more carbon dioxide than normal; partial pressure of arterial carbon dioxide below 35 mm Hg and pH above 7.45

sodium: major cation of extracellular fluid involved in regulating extracellular fluid volume, transmitting nerve impulses, and maintaining acid-base balance

solvent: fluid in which a solute is dissolved

tetany: condition caused by abnormal calcium metabolism; characterized by painful muscle spasms, cramps, and sharp flexion of the wrist and ankle joints

third-space fluid shift: movement of fluid out of the intravascular space into another body space such as the abdominal cavity

Trousseau's sign: carpal (wrist) spasm elicited by applying a blood pressure cuff to the upper arm and inflating it to a pressure 20 mm Hg above the patient's systolic blood pressure; indicates the presence of hypocalcemia

uremia: excess of urea and other nitrogenous waste in the blood

uremic frost: powdery deposits of urea and uric acid salts on the skin, especially the face; caused by the excretion of nitrogenous compounds in sweat

water intoxication: condition in which excess water in the cells results in cellular swelling

Selected references

Bickley, L.S., and Szilagyi, P.G. *Bates' Guide to Physical Examination and History Taking,* 9th ed. Philadelphia: Lippincott Williams & Wilkins, 2007.

Burger, C.M. "Hypokalemia: Averting Crisis with Early Recognition and Intervention," *AJN* 104(11):61-65, November 2004.

Despins, L.A., et al. "Acute Pancreatitis: Diagnosis and Treatment of a Potentially Fatal Complication," *AJN* 105(11):54-57, November 2005.

Diseases: A Nursing Process Approach to Excellent Care, 4th ed. Philadelphia: Lippincott Williams & Wilkins, 2006.

Fluids & Electrolytes Made Incredibly Easy, 3rd ed. Philadelphia: Lippincott Williams & Wilkins, 2005.

Ignatavicius, D.D., and Workman, M.L. *Medical-Surgical Nursing: Critical Thinking for Collaborative Care,* 5th ed. Philadelphia: W.B. Saunders Co., 2006.

Infusion Nurses Society. "Infusion Nursing Standards of Practice," *Journal of Infusion Nursing* 29(1S), Supplement to January-February 2006.

Kasper, D.L., et al., eds. *Harrison's Principles of Internal Medicine,* 16th ed. New York: McGraw-Hill Book Co., 2005.

McCarley, P.B., and Salai, P.B. "Cardiovascular Disease in Chronic Kidney Disease: Recognizing and Reducing the Risk of a Common CKD Comorbidity," *AJN* 105(4):40-52, April 2005.

Monahan, F.D., et al. *Phipp's Medical-Surgical Nursing: Health and Illness Perspectives,* 8th ed. St. Louis: Mosby–Year Book, Inc., 2007.

Nurse's Quick Check: Signs & Symptoms. Philadelphia: Lippincott Williams & Wilkins, 2006.

Porth, C.M. *Pathophysiology: Concepts of Altered Health States,* 7th ed. Philadelphia: Lippincott Williams & Wilkins, 2005.

Potter, P.A., and Perry, A.G. *Fundamentals of Nursing,* 6th ed. St. Louis: Mosby–Year Book, Inc., 2005.

Smeltzer, S.C., and Bare, B.G. *Brunner & Suddarth's Textbook of Medical-Surgical Nursing,* 10th ed. Philadelphia: Lippincott Williams & Wilkins, 2004.

Thibodeau, G.A., and Patton, K.T. *The Human Body in Health and Disease,* 4th ed. St. Louis: Mosby–Year Book, Inc., 2005.

Index

A
ABO blood group, 249
Acid-base balance, 55-64
  blood pH and, 56, 56i
  buffer regulation of, 58
  definition of, 56
  developmental considerations and, 64
  hydrogen ion concentration and, 56
  measurement of, 60-64, 63i
  potassium's role in, 43i
  renal system regulation of, 59-60
  respiratory system regulation of, 59
Acid-base imbalances, 136-161
  patients at risk for, 161
  renal system compensation for, 60, 137
  respiratory system compensation for, 59, 137
  types of, 57, 57i, 137, 140-161
Acidosis. *See also* Metabolic acidosis *and* Respiratory acidosis.
  pH in, 57, 57i
  potassium and, 43i
Acids, 56
Acquired immunodeficiency syndrome, 166-170
  assessment findings in, 168
  causes of, 166
  diagnostic findings in, 168-169
  nursing interventions for, 169-170
  pathophysiologic changes in, 166-167
  potential imbalances in, 167-168
  treatment of, 169
Active transport mechanisms, 7, 8i

Acute renal failure, 170-177
  assessment findings in, 174-175
  causes of, 170-171, 172i
  complications of, 170
  diagnostic findings in, 175-176
  nursing interventions for, 176-177
  pathophysiologic changes in, 171-173
  potential imbalances in, 173-174
  treatment of, 176
Additives in total parenteral nutrition, 247
Adrenal glands, electrolyte balance and, 35
Adult blood volume, 248
AIDS. *See* Acquired immunodeficiency syndrome.
Air embolism as I.V. therapy complication, 239t
Albumin
  composition of, 250-251
  level of, in relation to calcium level, 46
  transfusion of, 252
  uses of, 252
Alcohol solutions, parenteral nutritional supplementation and, 246
Aldosterone
  chloride regulation and, 45
  fluid regulation and, 22, 23i
  production of, 22i
  sodium regulation and, 40-41
Alkalosis. *See also* Metabolic alkalosis *and* Respiratory alkalosis.
  pH in, 57, 57i
  potassium and, 43i

Allergic reaction as I.V. therapy complication, 240t
Allergic transfusion reaction, 254t
Alveolar hypoventilation, respiratory failure and, 217i
Anion gap
  calculating, 63i
  identification of, 63
  interpretation of, 63-64
  metabolic acidosis and, 130i
  result of, 62
Anions, 4, 5i
Antidiuretic hormone
  fluid regulation and, 20-21, 21i
  sodium regulation and, 40-41
Arterial blood gas analysis, 61-62
  avoiding inaccurate results of, 62
  interpreting results of, 62
  metabolic acid-base imbalances and, 139i, 150i, 154, 156i, 159
  parameters measured in, 61-62
  purpose of, 61, 137
  respiratory acid-base imbalances and, 138i, 140i, 143, 145i, 148
  sources of samples for, 61
Arterial blood pH, 10
Arterial catheter, blood pressure measurement with, 26
Aspiration of gastric secretions as tube feeding complication, 232t
Atrial natriuretic peptide, fluid regulation and, 22
Automated blood pressure unit, 25

B
Bacteremia as I.V. therapy complication, 239t
Bacterial contamination as transfusion reaction, 254t

---
i refers to an illustration; t refers to a table.

i refers to an illustration; t refers to a table.

i refers to an illustration; t refers to a table.

i refers to an illustration; t refers to a table.

i refers to an illustration; t refers to a table.

i refers to an illustration; t refers to a table.

i refers to an illustration; t refers to a table.

The enclosed CD-ROM is just one more reason why the *Straight A's* series is at the head of its class. The more than 250 additional NCLEX-style questions contained on the CD provide you with another opportunity to review the material and gauge your knowledge. The program allows you to:

- take tests of varying lengths on subject areas of your choice
- learn the rationales for correct and incorrect answers
- print the results of your tests to measure progress over time.

Minimum system requirements

To operate the *Straight A's* CD-ROM, we recommend that you have the following minimum computer equipment:

- Windows XP-Home
- Pentium 4
- 256 MB RAM
- 10 MB of free hard-disk space
- SVGA monitor with High Color (16-bit)
- CD-ROM drive
- mouse.

Installation

Before installing the CD-ROM, make sure that your monitor is set to High Color (16-bit) and your display area is set to 800 × 600. If it isn't, consult your monitor's user's manual for instructions about changing the display settings. (The display settings are typically found in Start/Settings/Control Panel/Display/Settings tab.)

To run this program, you must install it onto the hard drive of your computer, following these three steps:

1. Start Windows XP-Home (minimum).
2. Place the CD in your CD-ROM drive. After a few moments, the install process will automatically begin. *Note:* If the install process doesn't automatically begin, click the Start menu and select Run. Type *D:\setup.exe* (where *D:* is the letter of your CD-ROM drive) and then click OK.
3. Follow the on-screen instructions for installation.

Technical support

For technical support, call toll-free 1-800-638-3030, Monday through Friday, 8:30 a.m. to 5 p.m. Eastern Time. You may also write to Lippincott Williams & Wilkins Technical Support, 351 W. Camden Street, Baltimore, MD 21201-2436, or e-mail us at *technicalsupport3@wolterskluwer.com.*